Portal Hypertension

Editor

SAMMY SAAB

CLINICS IN LIVER DISEASE

www.liver.theclinics.com

Consulting Editor
NORMAN GITLIN

November 2019 • Volume 23 • Number 4

ELSEVIER

1600 John F. Kennedy Boulevard ● Suite 1800 ● Philadelphia, Pennsylvania, 19103-2899

http://www.theclinics.com

CLINICS IN LIVER DISEASE Volume 23, Number 4
November 2019 ISSN 1089-3261, ISBN-13: 978-0-323-71034-3

Editor: Kerry Holland
Developmental Editor: Donald Mumford

Clinics in Liver Disease (ISSN 1089-3261) is published quarterly by Elsevier Inc., 360 Park Avenue South, New York, NY 10010-1710. Months of issue are February, May, August, and November. Business and Editorial Offices: 1600 John F. Kennedy Blvd., Ste. 1800, Philadelphia, PA 19103-2899. Customer Service Office: 3251 Riverport Lane, Maryland Heights, MO 63043. Periodicals postage paid at New York, NY and additional mailing offices. Subscription prices are $304.00 per year (U.S. individuals), $100.00 per year (U.S. student/resident), $542.00 per year (U.S. institutions), $409.00 per year (international individuals), $200.00 per year (international student/resident), $672.00 per year (international instituitions), $343.00 per year (Canadian individuals), $200.00 per year (Canadian student/resident), and $672.00 per year (Canadian institutions). Foreign air speed delivery is included in all *Clinics* subscription prices. All prices are subject to change without notice. **POSTMASTER:** Send address changes to *Clinics in Liver Disease*, Elsevier Health Sciences Division, Subscription Customer Service, 3251 Riverport Lane, Maryland Heights, MO 63043. **Customer Service: Telephone: 1-800-654-2452 (U.S. and Canada); 314-447-8871 (outside U.S. and Canada). Fax: 314-447-8029. E-mail: journalscustomer service-usa@elsevier.com (for print support); journalsonlinesupport-usa@elsevier.com (for online support).**

Reprints. For copies of 100 or more of articles in this publication, please contact the Commercial Reprints Department, Elsevier Inc., 360 Park Avenue South, New York, NY 10010-1710. Tel.: 212-633-3874; Fax: 212-633-3820; E-mail: reprints@elsevier.com.

Clinics in Liver Disease is covered in *MEDLINE/PubMed (Index Medicus)*, Science Citation Index Expanded, Journal Citation Reports/Science Edition, and Current Contents/Clinical Medicine.

Contributors

CONSULTING EDITOR

NORMAN GITLIN, MD, FRCP (LONDON), FRCPE (EDINBURGH), FAASLD, FACP, FACG
Head of Hepatology, Southern California Liver Centers, San Clemente, California, USA

EDITOR

SAMMY SAAB, MD, MPH, AGAF, FAASLD, FACG
Professor of Medicine and Surgery, Head, Outcomes Research in Hepatology, David Geffen School of Medicine at UCLA, Adjunct Professor of Nursing, UCLA School of Nursing, Los Angeles, California, USA

AUTHORS

ELIZABETH S. ABY, MD
Department of Medicine, University of California, Los Angeles, UCLA Medical Center, Los Angeles, California, USA

DANIELLE ADEBAYO, BSc (Hons), MBBS, MRCP
Division of Gastroenterology, Department of Medicine, Toronto General Hospital, University of Toronto, Toronto, Ontario, Canada

SANDRA BOUTROS
Department of Surgery, University of California, Los Angeles, Los Angeles, California, USA

CHALERMRAT BUNCHORNTAVAKUL, MD
Division of Gastroenterology and Hepatology, Associate Professor, Department of Medicine, Rajavithi Hospital, College of Medicine, Rangsit University, Bangkok, Thailand; Division of Gastroenterology and Hepatology, Department of Medicine, University of Pennsylvania, Philadelphia, Pennsylvania, USA

RONALD W. BUSUTTIL, MD, PhD
Professor, Chief, Division of Liver and Pancreas Transplantation, Chair, Department of Surgery, David Geffen School of Medicine at UCLA, University of California, Los Angeles, The Dumont-UCLA Transplant Center, Los Angeles, California, USA

RODRIGO CARTIN-CEBA, MD, MSc
Associate Professor of Medicine, Division of Pulmonary and Critical Care Medicine, Mayo Clinic, Scottsdale, Arizona, USA

GUADALUPE GARCIA-TSAO, MD
Section of Digestive Diseases, Yale School of Medicine, New Haven, Connecticut, USA; Professor of Medicine (Digestive Diseases), Chief, Section of Digestive Diseases, VA Connecticut Healthcare System, West Haven, Connecticut, USA

MATTHEW L. HUNG, MD
Division of Interventional Radiology, Department of Radiology, UCLA Medical Center, David Geffen School of Medicine at UCLA, Ronald Reagan UCLA Medical Center, Los Angeles, California, USA

DENNIS M. JENSEN, MD
Staff Physician, Medicine-GI, VA Greater Los Angeles Healthcare System, Professor of Medicine, David Geffen School of Medicine at UCLA, Ronald Reagan UCLA Medical Center, Key Investigator and Director, Human Studies Core and GI Hemostasis Research Unit, VA/CURE Digestive Disease Research Center, Los Angeles, California, USA

RAJEEV KHANNA, MD, PDCC
Associate Professor, Department of Pediatric Hepatology, Institute of Liver & Biliary Sciences (ILBS), New Delhi, India

THOMAS O.G. KOVACS, MD
Division of Digestive Diseases, Professor of Medicine, David Geffen School of Medicine at UCLA, Ronald Reagan UCLA Medical Center, Olive View-UCLA Medical Center, Sylmar, California, USA

MICHAEL J. KROWKA, MD
Professor of Medicine, Division of Pulmonary and Critical Care Medicine, Mayo Clinic, Rochester, USA

EDWARD WOLFGANG LEE, MD, PhD
Associate Professor, Division of Interventional Radiology, Department of Radiology, UCLA Medical Center, David Geffen School of Medicine at UCLA, Department of Surgery, Division of Liver and Pancreas Transplant Surgery, Ronald Reagan UCLA Medical Center, Los Angeles, California, USA

SHUET FONG NEONG, MBBS, MRCP
Division of Gastroenterology, Department of Medicine, Toronto General Hospital, University of Toronto, Toronto, Ontario, Canada

K. RAJENDER REDDY, MD
Ruimy Family President's Distinguished Professor of Medicine, Division of Gastroenterology and Hepatology, Department of Medicine, University of Pennsylvania, Philadelphia, Pennsylvania, USA

DON C. ROCKEY, MD
Chairman, Department of Medicine, Medical University of South Carolina, Charleston, South Carolina, USA

SAMMY SAAB, MD, MPH, AGAF, FAASLD, FACG
Professor of Medicine and Surgery, Head, Outcomes Research in Hepatology, David Geffen School of Medicine at UCLA, Adjunct Professor of Nursing, UCLA School of Nursing, Los Angeles, California, USA

SHIV KUMAR SARIN, MD, DM, DSc, FNASc, FAASLD
Senior Professor, Department of Hepatology, Institute of Liver & Biliary Sciences (ILBS), New Delhi, India

LAURA TURCO, MD
Division of Gastroenterology, Azienda Ospedaliero-Universitaria di Modena, PhD Program in Clinical and Experimental Medicine, University of Modena and Reggio Emilia, Modena, Italy

ADAM WINTERS, MD
Department of Medicine, University of California, Los Angeles, Los Angeles, California, USA

FLORENCE WONG, MBBS, MD, FRACP, FRCPC
Division of Gastroenterology, Department of Medicine, Toronto General Hospital, University of Toronto, Toronto, Ontario, Canada

MELISSA WONG, MD
Assistant Professor, Division of Transplant Surgery, Department of Surgery, Medical College of Wisconsin, Transplant Center, Milwaukee, Wisconsin, USA

BESHOY YANNY, MD
Department of Medicine, University of California, Los Angeles, Los Angeles, California, USA

Contents

Preface: Portal Hypertension xiii

Sammy Saab

Portal Hypertension: Pathogenesis and Diagnosis 573

Laura Turco and Guadalupe Garcia-Tsao

Portal hypertension (PH) is an increase in the pressure gradient between portal vein and inferior vena cava. Increased resistance occurs at different levels within the portal venous system, followed by increased portal venous inflow. PH is the main driver of cirrhosis decompensation. Varices on endoscopy or portosystemic collaterals on imaging indicate PH. Although its cause is determined mostly via noninvasive tests, the gold standard to measure portal pressure in cirrhosis and determine its severity is hepatic vein catheterization with determination of the hepatic venous pressure gradient. Measuring portal pressure is essential in proof-of-concept studies of portal pressure-lowering drugs.

Frailty, Sarcopenia, and Malnutrition in Cirrhotic Patients 589

Elizabeth S. Aby and Sammy Saab

Sarcopenia, frailty, and malnutrition are prevalent complications in patients with end-stage liver disease (ESLD) and are associated with increased risk of morbidity and mortality. It is valuable to measure nutritional status, sarcopenia, and frailty over time in order to create interventions tailored to individuals with ESLD. Evaluating sarcopenia and frailty in patients with ESLD is challenging. Further work is needed to perfect these assessments so that clinicians can incorporate these assessments into their decision-making and management plans for cirrhotic patients.

Hepatic Encephalopathy Challenges, Burden, and Diagnostic and Therapeutic Approach 607

Beshoy Yanny, Adam Winters, Sandra Boutros, and Sammy Saab

Hepatic encephalopathy (HE) is an important cause of morbidity and mortality in patients with cirrhosis. The impact of HE on the health care system is similarly profound. The number of hospital admissions for HE has increased in the last 10-year period. HE is a huge burden to the patients, care givers, and the health care system. HE represents a "revolving door" with readmission, severely affects care givers, and has effects on cognition that can persists after liver transplant. This article reviews the current literature to discuss the challenges and diagnostic and therapeutic approaches to HE.

Varices: Esophageal, Gastric, and Rectal 625

Thomas O.G. Kovacs and Dennis M. Jensen

Gastrointestinal varices are associated with cirrhosis and portal hypertension. Variceal hemorrhage is a substantial cause of morbidity and mortality, with esophageal and gastric varices the most common source and rectal varices a much less common cause of severe gastrointestinal bleeding. The goals of managing variceal hemorrhage are control of active bleeding and prevention of rebleeding. This article focuses on reviewing the current management strategies, including optimal medical, endoscopic, and angiographic interventions and their clinical outcomes to achieve these goals. Evidence based discussion is used with current references as much as possible.

An Update: Portal Hypertensive Gastropathy and Colopathy   643

Don C. Rockey

Complications of portal hypertension include portal hypertensive gastropathy and colopathy. These disorders may cause chronic or acute gastrointestinal bleeding. The diagnosis is made endoscopically; therefore, there is great variability in their assessment. Portal hypertensive gastropathy can range from a mosaic-like pattern resembling snakeskin mucosa to frankly bleeding petechial lesions. Portal hypertensive colopathy has been less well-described and is variably characterized (erythema, vascular lesions, petechiae). Treatment is challenging and results are inconsistent. Currently, available evidence does not support the use of beta-blockers for primary prevention. Further investigation of the pathogenesis, natural history, and treatment of these disorders is needed.

Ascites and Hepatorenal Syndrome   659

Danielle Adebayo, Shuet Fong Neong, and Florence Wong

Ascites occurs in up to 70% of patients during the natural history of cirrhosis. Management of uncomplicated ascites includes sodium restriction and diuretic therapy, whereas that for refractory ascites (RA) is regular large-volume paracentesis with transjugular intrahepatic portosystemic shunt being offered in appropriate patients. Renal impairment occurs in up to 50% of patients with RA with type 1 hepatorenal syndrome (HRS) being most severe. Liver transplant remains the definitive treatment of eligible candidates with HRS, whereas combined liver and kidney transplant should be considered in patients requiring dialysis for more than 4 to 6 weeks or those with underlying chronic kidney disease.

Pulmonary Complications of Portal Hypertension   683

Rodrigo Cartin-Ceba and Michael J. Krowka

The most common pulmonary complications of chronic liver disease are hepatic hydrothorax, hepatopulmonary syndrome, and portopulmonary hypertension. Hepatic hydrothorax is a transudative pleural effusion in a patient with cirrhosis and no evidence of underlying cardiopulmonary disease. Hepatic hydrothorax develops owing to the movement of ascitic fluid into the pleural space. Hepatopulmonary syndrome and portopulmonary hypertension are pathologically linked by the presence of portal hypertension; however, their pathophysiologic mechanisms are significantly different. Hepatopulmonary syndrome is characterized by low pulmonary vascular resistance secondary to intrapulmonary vascular dilatations and hypoxemia; portopulmonary hypertension features elevated pulmonary vascular resistance and constriction/obstruction within the pulmonary vasculature.

Pharmacologic Management of Portal Hypertension   713

Chalermrat Bunchorntavakul and K. Rajender Reddy

Terlipressin, somatostatin, or octeotide are recommended as pharmacologic treatment of acute variceal hemorrhage. Nonselective β-blockers decrease the risk of variceal hemorrhage and hepatic decompensation, particularly in those 30% to 40% of patients with good hemodynamic response. Carvedilol, statins, and anticoagulants are promising agents in the management of portal hypertension. Recent advances in the pharmacologic treatment of portal hypertension have mainly focused on modifying an increased intrahepatic resistance through nitric oxide and/or modulation of vasoactive substances. Several novel pharmacologic agents for portal hypertension are being evaluated in humans.

Role of Transjugular Intrahepatic Portosystemic Shunt in the Management of Portal Hypertension: Review and Update of the Literature   737

Matthew L. Hung and Edward Wolfgang Lee

Transjugular intrahepatic portosystemic shunt (TIPS) is a well-established procedure used in the management of complications of portal hypertension. Although the most robust evidence supports the use of TIPS as salvage therapy in variceal hemorrhage, secondary prophylaxis of variceal bleeding, and treatment of refractory ascites, there is also data to suggest its efficacy in other indications such as hepatic hydrothorax, hepatorenal syndrome, and Budd-Chiari syndrome. Recent literature also suggests that TIPS may improve survival for certain subpopulations if placed early after variceal bleeding. This article provides an updated evidence-based review of the indications for TIPS. Outcomes, complications, and adequate patient selection are also discussed.

Surgery in Patients with Portal Hypertension   755

Melissa Wong and Ronald W. Busuttil

Patients with portal hypertension will increasingly present for nontransplant surgery because of the increasing incidence of, and improving long-term survival for, chronic liver disease. Such patients have increased perioperative morbidity and mortality caused by the systemic pathophysiology of liver disease. Preoperative assessment should identify modifiable causes of liver injury and distinguish between compensated and decompensated cirrhosis. Risk stratification, which is crucial to preparing patients and their families for surgery, relies on scores such as Child-Turcotte-Pugh and Model for End-stage Liver Disease to translate disease severity into quantified outcomes predictions. Risk factors for postoperative complications should also be recognized.

Noncirrhotic Portal Hypertension: Current and Emerging Perspectives   781

Rajeev Khanna and Shiv Kumar Sarin

Idiopathic portal hypertension (IPH) and extrahepatic portal venous obstruction (EHPVO) are prototype noncirrhotic causes of portal hypertension (PHT), characterized by normal hepatic venous pressure gradient, variceal bleeds, and moderate to massive splenomegaly with preserved liver synthetic functions. Infections, toxins, and immunologic, prothrombotic and genetic disorders are possible causes in IPH, whereas prothrombotic and local factors around the portal vein lead to EHPVO. Growth failure, portal biliopathy, and minimal hepatic encephalopathy are long-term concerns in EHPVO. Surgical shunts and transjugular intra-hepatic portosystemic shunt resolve the complications secondary to PHT. Meso-Rex shunt is now the standard-of-care surgery in children with EHPVO.

CLINICS IN LIVER DISEASE

FORTHCOMING ISSUES

February 2020
Drug Hepatotoxicity
Pierre Gholam, *Editor*

May 2020
Hepatic Encephalopathy
Vinod K. Rustgi, *Editor*

August 2020
Consultations in Liver Disease
Steven Flamm, *Editor*

RECENT ISSUES

August 2019
Hepatitis B Virus Update
Tarek I. Hassanein, *Editor*

May 2019
Liver in Systemic Diseases
Jorge L. Herrera, *Editor*

February 2019
Alcoholic Liver Disease
Norman L. Sussman and
Michael R. Lucey, *Editors*

THE CLINICS ARE AVAILABLE ONLINE!
Access your subscription at:
www.theclinics.com

Preface

Portal Hypertension

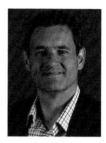

Sammy Saab, MD, MPH, AGAF, FAASLD, FACG
Editor

Portal hypertension is defined as increased blood pressure in the portal venous system, most often seen in the setting of advanced liver disease, such as cirrhosis. The development of portal hypertension is one of the major complications with advanced liver disease. Patients can be asymptomatic for years and considered compensated. However, the overt clinical manifestation of portal hypertension defines hepatic decompensation. The onset of hepatic decompensation represents a major turning point in patients with advanced liver disease, with a substantially negative impact on patients' life expectancy and quality.

In this issue of *Clinics in Liver Disease*, experts discuss the major signs of hepatic decompensation. The first article lays the foundation for the issue with an in-depth review of the pathogenesis and diagnosis of portal hypertension by Drs Turco and Garcia-Tsao. Drs Aby and Saab review the diagnosis and clinical implications of frailty and sarcopenia in patients with cirrhosis. Indeed, this decompensation manifestation unfortunately negatively contributes to posttransplant outcomes. Another important sign of decompensation is the development of hepatic encephalopathy. We learn from Dr Yanny and his colleagues how hepatic encephalopathy is a contributor to increased caregiver burden and health care utilization. Equally important, the authors highlight treatment approaches to hepatic encephalopathy, including those who are refractory to common therapy. Drs Kovacs and Jensen address one of the most dreaded and feared manifestations of decompensated liver disease: variceal bleed. The authors provide a rational approach to diagnosis and treatment. Dr Rockey discusses portal hypertensive gastropathy and colopathy, another cause of gastrointestinal bleeding, which is an often overlooked but serious complication of portal hypertension. The development of ascites is the most common initial presentation of hepatic decompensation. Dr Wong and her colleagues not only provide insight into the pathogenesis of ascites and but also review downstream complications, such as refractoriness and hepatorenal syndrome. Drs Cartin-Ceba and Krowka address the

Clin Liver Dis 23 (2019) xiii–xiv
https://doi.org/10.1016/j.cld.2019.08.001
1089-3261/19/© 2019 Published by Elsevier Inc.

pulmonary complications of cirrhosis. These complications can be clinically subtle but can be associated with a significant impact on life expectancy. The treatment of portal hypertension is addressed in 2 separate but equally essential articles: pharmacologic therapy by Drs Bunchorntavakul and Reddy and radiologic intervention by Drs Hung and Lee. Drs Bunchorntavakul and Reddy critically assess current therapy and offer insight into upcoming therapies. Drs Hung and Lee examine the specific role of transjugular intrahepatic portosystemic shunt in directly alleviating portal hypertension. Because patients with cirrhosis are living longer, it is very likely that many will require surgery. Drs Wong and Busuttil highlight predictive models of outcomes related to surgery and describe the evaluation process to mitigate surgical-related risks. The issue ends with a discussion of noncirrhotic causes of portal hypertension by Drs Khanna and Sarin.

We hope you will enjoy the story of portal hypertension in this issue of *Clinics in Liver Disease*.

Sammy Saab, MD, MPH, AGAF, FAASLD, FACG
Pfleger Liver Institute
UCLA Medical Center
200 Medical Plaza, Suite 214
Los Angeles, CA 90095, USA

E-mail address:
SSaab@mednet.ucla.edu

Portal Hypertension
Pathogenesis and Diagnosis

Laura Turco, MD[a,b], Guadalupe Garcia-Tsao, MD[c,d],*

KEYWORDS

- Cirrhosis • Gastroesophageal varices • Bleeding • Ascites
- Hepatic venous pressure gradient • Liver stiffness

KEY POINTS

- Portal hypertension is defined as an increase in portal pressure at any level in the portal venous system. The site of increased resistance or obstruction is the basis of its classification.
- The most common cause of portal hypertension is cirrhosis in which the site of increased resistance is intrahepatic, leading to an increase in portal pressure that, in turn, leads to splanchnic vasodilation, increase in portal blood inflow, and a hyperdynamic circulation that further aggravates portal hypertension.
- The presence of varices (on endoscopy) and/or other abdominal portosystemic collaterals (on imaging) establish the diagnosis of portal hypertension.
- The cause of portal hypertension can be established by a combination of noninvasive and imaging tests and, when uncertainty remains regarding its cause or severity (in cirrhosis), measurement of sinusoidal pressure via catheterization of the hepatic vein and determination of the hepatic venous pressure gradient will be essential.

INTRODUCTION

Portal hypertension (PH) is a clinical syndrome characterized by an increase in the portal pressure gradient (PPG), defined as the gradient between the portal vein at the site downstream of the site of obstruction (proximal to the thrombus in the case of portal

Grants or Financial Support: L. Turco is a recipient of a grant from the University of Modena and Reggio Emilia (PI Prof Filippo Schepis and Prof Erica Villa). This review was partially supported by the Yale Liver Center NIH P30 DK34989.
Conflicts of Interest: The authors disclose no conflicts.
[a] Division of Gastroenterology, Azienda Ospedaliero-Universitaria di Modena, University of Modena and Reggio Emilia, Via del Pozzo 71, Modena 41125, Italy; [b] PhD Program in Clinical and Experimental Medicine, University of Modena and Reggio Emilia, Via del Pozzo n 71, Modena 41125, Italy; [c] Section of Digestive Diseases, Yale School of Medicine, Yale University School of Medicine, PO Box 208056, 333 Cedar Street -1080 LMP, New Haven, CT 06520-8056, USA; [d] Section of Digestive Diseases, VA Connecticut Healthcare System, 950 Campbell Avenue, West Haven, CT 06516, USA
* Corresponding author. Yale University School of Medicine, PO Box 208056, 333 Cedar Street -1080 LMP, New Haven, CT 06520-8056.
E-mail address: guadalupe.garcia-tsao@yale.edu

Clin Liver Dis 23 (2019) 573–587
https://doi.org/10.1016/j.cld.2019.07.007
1089-3261/19/© 2019 Elsevier Inc. All rights reserved.

liver.theclinics.com

vein thrombosis and at the hepatic sinusoids in the case of cirrhosis) and the inferior vena cava.

The most common cause of PH is cirrhosis. Normal PPG values range between 1 to 5 mm Hg and values greater than 5 mm Hg indicate the presence of PH. In cirrhosis, values greater than 5 but less than 10 mm Hg are considered mild or nonclinically significant, whereas values greater than or equal to 10 mm Hg are considered clinically significant because they are associated with the development of gastroesophageal varices (GEVs) and clinical events that define decompensation (ascites, variceal hemorrhage, encephalopathy).[1] As proof-of-concept, reductions in portal pressure induced by pharmacologic therapy in patients with both compensated and decompensated cirrhosis,[2] or by placement of the transjugular intrahepatic portosystemic shunt (TIPS) in patients with decompensated cirrhosis,[3,4] have resulted in a reduction in the development of decompensating events and/or in an improvement in survival.

PATHOGENESIS

As in any vascular system, pressure in the portal venous system follows dynamic Ohm's law in which pressure gradient (ΔP) is the result of the amount of blood flow circulating through system (Q) and the resistance opposing this flow (R) ($\Delta P = Q \times R$). In all causes of PH, the primum movens is an increase in resistance to portal blood flow followed by an increase in portal venous inflow.[5] The site of increased resistance is the basis of the classification of PH (see later discussion). In the case of portal vein thrombosis (the second most common cause of PH), an obstruction in the main portal vein (thrombus) is the initiating event and pathogenesis is therefore clearer. Because cirrhosis is the main cause of PH and its pathogenesis is more complex (**Fig. 1**), this article refers to the pathogenesis of PH in cirrhosis.

Increased Intrahepatic Resistance

In cirrhosis, increased intrahepatic resistance results from a combination of structural (fixed) alterations in the hepatic sinusoids (sinusoidal fibrosis, regenerative nodules)

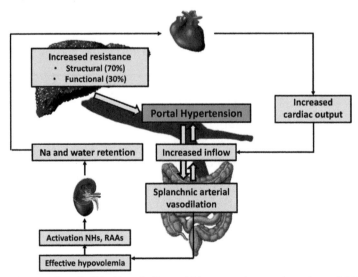

Fig. 1. Pathogenesis of PH. Na, Sodium; NHs, neurohumoral system; RAAs, renin-angiotensin-aldosterone system.

and functional (dynamic) vasoconstriction of the intrahepatic circulation resulting from a decreased production of vasodilators from sinusoidal cells.

Architectural disruption

Progression of chronic liver disease of any cause contributes to protean changes in the hepatic sinusoids,[5] mostly due to phenotypic and functional alterations in hepatic stellate cells (HSCs) and sinusoidal endothelial cells (SECs). HSCs respond to liver injury[6] with an activation that consists of a switch in activity from vitamin A production or storage to matrix deposition in the hepatic sinusoids. Additionally. SECs, which normally contain fenestrae, also respond to injury by losing fenestrae, leading to capillarization of the sinusoids by deposition of basement membrane. Capillarization may act as a very early player both in increasing intrahepatic resistance and in promoting fibrosis formation.[6] Changes also occur at the level of the plasma membrane of hepatocytes adjacent to the sinusoid that can lose their microvilli as a response to liver injury.

The role of angiogenesis consists of the growth and proliferation of endothelial cells that contribute to increased intrahepatic resistance and fibrosis.[7] Angiogenic endothelial cells may stimulate HSC activation through the vascular endothelial growth factor (VEGF), a potent angiogenic molecule.[7]

These changes and cross-talk between HSCs and the SECs, with resultant matrix deposition and narrowing of the sinusoids, account for the fixed increase in intrahepatic resistance.

Endothelial dysfunction (vasoconstriction)

In addition to the fixed component, there is a dynamic component that contributes to intrahepatic resistance that arises from contraction of myofibroblasts within the space of Disse.[8] Inflammation and cytokines released from injured hepatocytes stimulate the recruitment of HSCs and lead to their transformation into contractile myofibroblasts. In response to liver injury, SECs can also increase the contractility of perisinusoidal cells. Endothelial dysfunction further contributes to contractility through decreased production of potent vasodilators, such as nitric oxide (NO), and increased release of vasoconstrictors, such as endothelins.[9] This potentially reversible component of PH represents up one-third of the increased hepatic resistance.

Intrahepatic microthrombi

The traditional view of cirrhosis as a prohemorrhagic condition has recently changed, recognizing that cirrhosis is both a prohemorrhagic and prothrombotic entity in a very precarious equilibrium.[10] Several data indicate a close relationship between prothrombotic status and worsening of hepatic fibrosis and PH, both in experimental and clinical models.[11] In patients with cirrhosis, the thrombotic occlusion of intrahepatic veins and sinusoids causes intimal fibrosis and vein obstruction, leading to parenchymal extinction defined as the loss of contiguous hepatocytes and their replacement by fibrous tissue.[11] Moreover, the development of thrombi in the hepatic sinusoids can activate HSCs by protease-activated receptors, responsible for extracellular matrix deposition.[11] These theories are supported by studies showing that anticoagulation leads to a reduction in hepatic fibrosis and PH.[12,13]

Splanchnic Vasodilation

The increased intrahepatic vascular resistance leads to an increased pressure in the portal vein system that induces shear stress in the splanchnic vessels and the release of vasodilators such as NO.[14] Consequent splanchnic arterial vasodilation[15] is the core factor in the progression and worsening of PH, leading to the development of clinically significant PH (CSPH). Splanchnic vasodilatation also affects the systemic circulation, leading to a decrease in mean arterial pressure and a decrease in effective arterial blood volume that, in turn, leads to activation of neurohumoral systems, sodium and water retention, and an increase in cardiac output, a hyperdynamic circulatory state that further increases portal pressure.[16]

Role of Systemic Inflammation or Bacterial Translocation

Translocation of bacterial or bacterial products from the intestinal lumen into the system circulation is more prominent in decompensated cirrhosis but may also occur at the compensated stage.[17] It is currently considered that bacterial translocation is a consequence and an aggravating factor for PH.[18] Gut-derived bacterial products stimulate HSCs and Kupffer cells (KCs), leading to changes in HSCs into a fibrogenic and contractile phenotype, as well as the KCs activation stimulating fibrogenesis.[18] Activated HSCs produce local mediators (VEGF, angiopoietin-1), which stimulate angiogenesis in the SECs, aggravating PH.[19] Additionally, bacterial-induced inflammation contributes to a deterioration of the systemic hyperdynamic circulation and to a dysfunction of extraintestinal organs (ie, heart, kidney, brain).[20] Markers of inflammation have been shown to predict decompensation in patients with compensated cirrhosis and death in patients with decompensated cirrhosis.[16]

CLASSIFICATION OF PORTAL HYPERTENSION

PH is caused by an obstruction of portal blood flow that can occur in different portions of the portal venous system. The pressure proximal to the obstructed portion will be hypertensive, whereas, distal to the obstruction, pressure will be normal. Based on the site of obstruction, PH is classified in prehepatic (if the obstruction occurs in the splenic vein, portal vein before the liver, or mesenteric vein; ie, before reaching the liver), intrahepatic (if the obstruction is at the liver), or posthepatic (if the obstruction involves the hepatic venous outflow; ie, after the liver). Intrahepatic PH is subclassified according to the site of the obstruction within the hepatic sinusoid as presinusoidal (portal-based illnesses; eg, schistosomiasis), sinusoidal (cirrhosis), or postsinusoidal (illnesses affecting the central vein).

As shown in **Table 1**, different types of PH are caused by different etiological factors and have different clinical presentations. In adults, cirrhosis accounts for more than 90% of cases of PH, whereas the second most common cause is portal vein thrombosis.

Because liver function and sinusoidal pressure are normal in patients with prehepatic or presinusoidal types of PH, ascites is not a main clinical feature of these entities and they are, in general, associated with a better prognosis than sinusoidal and postsinusoidal or posthepatic causes of PH.

In the remaining types of PH (sinusoidal, postsinusoidal, posthepatic), patients may develop GEVs and variceal bleeding; however, ascites development is a sine qua non and may be accompanied by liver insufficiency.

DIAGNOSIS OF PORTAL HYPERTENSION

The diagnosis of PH is established when the presence of abdominal portosystemic collaterals can be visualized by upper endoscopy (GEVs) or on imaging studies. PH also forms a part of the differential diagnosis of splenomegaly and/or thrombocytopenia.

Because the portal venous system is located between 2 capillary beds, the hepatic sinusoids and the splanchnic capillaries, direct access to the portal vein is complicated and different invasive approaches have been established to measure portal

Table 1
Portal hypertension classification

Type	Most Common Causes	Clinical Presentation	Hemodynamic Characteristics
Prehepatic	Portal vein occlusion (thrombosis or neoplasm) Splenic vein occlusion (thrombosis or neoplasm) Portal vein stenosis	Splenomegaly GEVs Collaterals Variceal bleeding	Normal HVPG Normal WHVP Normal FHVP
Intrahepatic			
Presinusoidal	Schistosomiasis Primary biliary cholangitis (early stages) Primary sclerosing cholangitis Focal nodular hyperplasia Idiopathic PH Sarcoidosis	Splenomegaly GEVs Collaterals Variceal bleeding	Normal HVPG Normal or slightly elevated WHVP Normal FHVP
Sinusoidal	Cirrhosis (viral, alcoholic, NASH-related) Alcoholic hepatitis Primary biliary cholangitis (advanced stages)	Splenomegaly GEVs Collaterals Variceal bleeding Ascites Hepatic encephalopathy	Elevated HVPG Elevated WHVP Normal FHVP
Postsinusoidal	Venoocclusive disease	Splenomegaly Collaterals Ascites	Normal HVPG Elevated WHVP Elevated FHVP
Posthepatic			
Vascular obstruction	Hepatic vein thrombosis (Budd-Chiari syndrome)	Ascites Intrahepatic collaterals	Not possible to catheterize hepatic veins
Liver congestion	Chronic right heart failure Chronic constrictive pericarditis Restrictive cardiomyopathy Tricuspid insufficiency	Ascites	Normal HVPG Elevated WHVP Elevated FHVP

Abbreviations: FHVP, free hepatic venous pressure; HVPG, hepatic venous pressure gradient; NASH, nonalcoholic steatohepatitis; WHVP, wedged hepatic venous pressure.

pressure to confirm the presence PH and/or to determine its severity in cirrhosis. Noninvasive methods that correlate with invasive measurements of portal pressure in cirrhosis have been investigated more recently (see later discussion). Therefore, tests to diagnose PH and to stratify risk in cirrhosis are based on invasive and noninvasive tests (NITs).

Invasive Tests

Esophagogastroduodenoscopy
The incidental finding of GEVs on esophagogastroduodenoscopy (EGD) establishes the diagnosis of PH and leads to investigative tests to determine its cause (mainly

investigations to diagnose cirrhosis and, if negative, imaging studies to rule out portal vein thrombosis). Varices due to PH are larger in the lower esophagus and are of progressively smaller size as the endoscope is withdrawn. Varices that are larger in the upper esophagus and smaller at the level of the lower esophageal sphincter (downhill varices) are not due to PH but may be due to superior vena cava obstruction, which is most commonly caused by tumors or thrombosis from vascular catheterization.

In patients with cirrhosis, finding GEVs establishes the presence of CSPH because it has been shown that patients with GEVs have an hepatic venous pressure gradient (HVPG) of at least 10 to 12 mm Hg.[21]

Patients with compensated cirrhosis who require prophylaxis to prevent bleeding are those with high-risk varices (HRVs), defined as medium or large GEVs or any size varices with red wale marks. In patients with decompensated cirrhosis, GEVs of any size require prophylaxis.[21]

Compensated patients without GEVs at screening EGD should have it repeated every 2 to 3 years according to the presence or not of ongoing liver injury (abstinence in alcoholics, viral elimination in viral cirrhosis, absence of cofactors such as obesity). In compensated patients with small varices at screening endoscopy, EGD should be repeated every 1 to 2 years according to the presence or not of ongoing liver injury. Decompensated patients without GEVs should have an EGD repeated every year.

In the last decade, a growing number of studies have suggested that endoscopic ultrasound (EUS) may be useful in the evaluation of PH. Paraesophageal varices and the left gastric vein can be better visualized by EUS, which not only correlates with variceal size[22] but seems to predict variceal recurrence after ligation or sclerotherapy.[23] Moreover, it has been recently shown in animal models[24] and in humans[25] that PPG can be measured directly by placing a needle through the gastric or duodenal wall into the portal vein and then into the right hepatic vein. This method seems to be safe and correlates well with pressure values obtained by the transjugular approach. Although it has the potential of screening for varices and measuring portal pressure (useful in those without varices) during the same procedure, it requires further evaluation.

Portal pressure measurements

Portal pressure measurement applies to measurements in patients with cirrhosis. However, the absence of sinusoidal PH in a patient with GEVs or collaterals establishs the presence of prehepatic or presinusoidal PH.

The first measurement of PH was performed in 1937, inserting a needle catheter directly into a branch of portal vein during abdominal surgery.[26] Other direct approaches to the portal vein have been proposed over time, including catheterization of the umbilical vein[27] and transcutaneous transhepatic catheterization of portal vein branches (percutaneous or via jugular vein).[28] The measurement of PH directly into the portal vein or one of its branches provides an uncorrected measure of portal pressure that can be affected by the positioning of the pressure transducer and increases in intraabdominal pressure (eg, ascites). Additionally, these techniques are invasive, technically challenging, potentially risky, and, if executed under general anesthesia, could affect portal pressure owing to the effect of deep sedation on splanchnic hemodynamics. Currently, direct measures of portal vein pressure are routinely performed at the time of TIPS placement; however, in these instances, it should always be corrected by subtracting the inferior vena cava pressure, thereby correctly reflecting a pressure gradient. However, TIPS placement has very specific indications and a transjugular approach to measure only pressure seems too invasive.

Hepatic venous pressure gradient The HVPG is the most commonly used indirect method to assess portal pressure and is considered the gold standard. HVPG is calculated by subtracting the free hepatic venous pressure (FHVP), a measure of systemic pressure, from the wedged hepatic venous pressure (WHVP), a measure of hepatic sinusoidal pressure. It was first described in 1951,[29] when a small catheter was advanced into the hepatic vein until it could not be advanced further; that is, the catheter was wedged into the most distal portion of the hepatic vein branch. The catheter thus wedged measures the pressure in the hepatic sinusoid, which in cirrhosis is a measure of main portal vein pressure. In fact, it has been shown that WHVP correlates very closely ($r = 0.95$) with the pressure measured by direct catheterization of the main portal vein in alcoholic and viral cirrhosis.[30] The advantage is that measures of the pressure when the catheter is free in the hepatic vein allows a systemic pressure that acts as an internal zero and corrects for extravenous factors such as ascites.

In 1979, Groszmann and colleagues[31] described a method that involved the use of a balloon catheter instead of a straight catheter that would occlude rather than wedge the hepatic vein and, by inflating the balloon, repeated measures of free and occluded pressure could be obtained without the need to move the catheter.

Normal HVPG values are between 3 and 5 mm Hg. Values above 5 mm Hg indicate PH. In a patient with chronic liver disease, the presence of PH should be diagnostic of cirrhosis. However, there is a percentage of patients ($\sim 10\%$)[32] with histologic cirrhosis with a normal HVPG. The reason for this is unclear and may be related to venovenous shunts or to a poor HVPG technique. As previously mentioned, an HVPG equal or greater than 10 mm Hg in patients with compensated cirrhosis without GEVs predicts development of GEVs, clinical decompensation, and hepatocellular carcinoma.[1] In compensated patients with CSPH (with or without varices), an HVPG greater than 16 mm Hg predicts clinical decompensation,[16] whereas in patients with acute variceal hemorrhage, an HVPG greater than 20 mm Hg[33,34] predicts variceal rebleeding, treatment failure, and higher mortality.

As mentioned previously, in patients with prehepatic or presinusoidal PH, in which pressure in the sinusoids is normal, the HVPG will be normal or only slightly elevated (see **Table 1**). In patients with posthepatic PH, mainly in those with heart failure, HVPG will also be normal because the hepatic sinusoidal pressure is high as a reflection of high systemic pressure (see **Table 1**).

Other than for diagnostic purposes, HVPG is not widely used and is not recommended in the clinical evaluation of patients with cirrhosis.[21] However, its use is essential in proof-of-concept studies investigating drugs with a potential portal pressure lowering effect.[14]

Noninvasive Tests

Determining the presence of GEVs is essential in patients with cirrhosis and determining the severity of PH is useful in their management and in discussions regarding prognosis. However, EGD is not free of risk and performance of HVPG is generally limited to specialized centers (and specialized providers) because it is a nuanced procedure that can lead to erroneous values in inexperienced hands. Therefore, many studies have looked for NITs to determine the presence of varices or PH.

Liver stiffness measurements

The progressive accumulation of liver fibrosis that leads to cirrhosis is associated with progressive increases in liver stiffness. This stiffness can be measured by vibration-controlled transient elastography (TE), which is the most used and validated NIT and has been very useful in staging liver fibrosis in patients with chronic liver disease.[35]

It has also been used to assess the presence of varices or degree of PH in patients with cirrhosis.

Correlation with hepatic venous pressure gradient Overall, a good correlation has been reported between HVPG and liver stiffness measurement (LSM) in patients with advanced liver fibrosis or cirrhosis ($r = 0.55$–0.86).[35]

The best correlation between HVPG and LSM occurs with HVPG values between 5 and 10 to 12 mm Hg ($r = 0.91$), which is the range described for mild PH, the stage driven by increase in intrahepatic resistance.[36] The correlation persists but decreases markedly with levels above 12 mm Hg ($r = 0.17$) when increased hepatic blood flow is an additional factor contributing to PH (CSPH).[36]

Ability to identify the presence of clinically significant portal hypertension Importantly, LSM can discriminate between patients with and without CSPH with an area under the receiver operating characteristic (AUROC) curve ranging from 0.82 to 0.94.[35] Cut off values of LSM greater than 13.6 kPa[36] or LSM greater than 21 Kpa[35] have been found to have a 90% sensitivity and a 90% specificity in the diagnosis of CSPH. Considering all studies, which were mostly performed in subjects with hepatitis C virus (HCV)-related cirrhosis, the most recent Baveno VI Consensus Conference recommended that an LSM greater than or equal to 21 kPa be used rule in CSPH in these subjects.[37]

Ability to identify the presence high-risk varices Many studies have aimed at identifying patients with HRVs. A multicenter large cohort study provided the most validated criteria[38] that led to the Baveno VI consensus recommendation to consider patients with an LSM less than 20 kPa and a platelet count greater than 150.000/mm³ as being very unlikely to have HRV.[37] With these criteria, 21% EGDs could be avoided and only less than 5% patients with HRV would be missed. Other criteria have been proposed in studies that have included subjects with all causes of cirrhosis and in studies including subjects with specific causes of cirrhosis (**Table 2**). Notably, these studies included mostly subjects with HCV-related cirrhosis and were carried out before the availability of effective antiviral therapy. Because viral elimination has been shown to decrease LSM and increase platelet count,[46] concerns have been raised regarding the applicability of these criteria in the setting of patients with HCV-related cirrhosis who have attained sustained virological response (SVR). However, a recent study performed in 94 subjects with HCV-related cirrhosis who achieved SVR and in 98 treated subjects with hepatitis B virus (HBV)-related cirrhosis, demonstrated that Baveno VI criteria can also be applied to these subjects, showing that 25% of EGDs could have been avoided and only 1% subjects with HRV would have been missed.[45]

Spleen stiffness measurements
With the development of PH, there is a progressive increase in spleen size due not only to backflow into the spleen but also due to hyperplasia, increased angiogenesis, and fibrogenesis of the spleen that increases its stiffness.[35] Spleen stiffness measurement (SSM) can be detected by TE and has been used to assess the presence of varices or degree of PH in patients with cirrhosis. Importantly, SSM seem to be useful in prehepatic and presinusoidal causes of PH.[35]

Correlation with hepatic venous pressure gradient In a cohort of subjects with HCV-related cirrhosis, spleen stiffness was found to correlate significantly with HVPG (multivariate coefficient [r^2] = 0.78).[47]

Table 2
Noninvasive criteria to rule out high-risk varices in compensated cirrhosis

Study	Number of Subjects	Cause	Prevalence of HRV	Noninvasive Criteria to Rule Out High-Risk Varices	Number of Spared EGDs	Missing HRV
Abraldes et al,[38] 2016	499	Any; 70% viral	14%	LSM <20 kPa and PLT >150.000/mm^3	21%	<5%
Jangouk et al,[39] 2017	161 (US cohort) 101 (Italian cohort)	Any; >65% viral	9% (US cohort) 17% (Italian cohort)	MELD = 6/PLT >150.000/mm^3	54% (US cohort) 30% (Italian cohort)	0% (US cohort) 1% (Italian cohort)
Augustin et al,[40] 2017	925	Any; 60% viral	10%	LSM <25 kPa and PLT >110.000/mm^3	40%	2%
Colecchia et al,[42] 2018	498	Any; 90% viral	20%	LSM <20 kPa and PLT >150.000/mm^3 SSM ≤46 kPa	44%	<5%
Lee et al,[41] 2019	1218	Any; 50% viral	20%	LSM <20 kPa and PLT >110.000/mm^3 Or LSM <25 kPa and PLT >120.000/mm^3	39%	<5%
Petta et al,[43] 2018	790	NASH	11%	LSM <30 kPa and PLT >110.000/mm^3 (using M probe) LSM <25 kPa and PLT >110.000/mm^3 (using XL probe)	>50%	<5%
Moctezuma-Velazquez et al,[44] 2019	227	PBC and PSC	13%	LSM <20 kPa and PLT >150.000/mm^3	30%–40%	0%
Thabut et al,[45] 2019	200	HCV and HBV after SVR	8%	LSM <20 kPa and PLT >150.000/mm^3	25%	1%

Abbreviations: EGDs, esophagogastroduodenoscopies; HBV, hepatitis B virus; M, medium; MELD, model for end-stage liver disease; PBC, primary biliary cholangitis; PLT, platelet (count); PSC, primary sclerosing cholangitis; SSM, spleen stiffness measurement; SVR, sustained viral response; XL, extra large; US, United States.

Ability to identify the presence of clinically significant portal hypertension SSM seems to perform better than LSM in the identification of CSPH. A cutoff SSM value of less than 40 kPa rules out CSPH with a sensitivity of 98%, whereas a cutoff of greater than or equal to 53 kPa rules in CSPH with a specificity of 97%.[47] SSM also seems to be useful in distinguishing patients with and without GEVs. A cutoff SSM value of less than 41.3 kPa rules out the presence of GEVs with a sensitivity of 98% and a cutoff value of greater than or equal to 55 kPa, and rules in varices at 96%.[47] Moreover, SSM together with the model for end-stage liver disease (MELD) have been found to be independent predictors of clinical decompensation in a cohort of subjects with HCV-related cirrhosis,[48] with an SSM cutoff less than 54 kPa able to identify patients with a lower risk of decompensation (negative predictive value of 98%).

Ability to identify the presence high-risk varices SSM less than our equal to 46 kPa rules out HRV with a high sensitivity (98%).[42] As shown in **Table 2**, a stepwise approach of Baveno VI and SSM criteria increases the number of subjects (up to 44%) in whom EGD can be safely avoided while missing only less than 5% of the subjects with HRV.

One of the main limitations of SSM by TE is the high rate of unsuccessful examinations (15%–20%), which can be avoided by using ultrasound guidance, which is the case with point shear wave elastography when using acoustic radiation force impulse (ARFI). SSM by ARFI has been shown to correlate with various markers of PH, such as GEVs,[35] HVPG,[35] and HVPG changes pre-TIPS and post-TIPS.[35] It has also been shown to predict decompensation (cutoff 3.25 m/s) and death (cutoff 3.43 m/s).[35] However, the number of subjects studied is not large and it has not been used to identify HRVs.

Combination of tests

Combinations of NITs have been proposed to detect the presence and severity of PH in patients with cirrhosis. A combination of LSM by TE, platelet count and spleen diameter (calculated as LSM × spleen size or platelet count [LSPS]) at cutoffs of 1.72 and of 3.21 correctly identifies patients with CSPH and GEVs, respectively, with good sensitivity and specificity (both >80%).[49] In the ANTICIPATE study,[38] LSPS showed an excellent ability in identifying HRV (AUROC = 0.79) with a cutoff of 1.33 avoiding 26% of EGDs. Platelet count or spleen ratio was found having good power in predicting the presence of HRV (cutoff of 1.64 with AUROC = 0.74),[38] with the advantage of not requiring TE, technology that is not widely available. Other criteria that have been proposed in the absence of TE is the combination of MELD and platelet count that was able to avoid up to 54% endoscopies while missing only 1% of patients with HRV[38] (see **Table 2**).

Indocyanine green test

Indocyanine green (ICG) is a water-soluble organic dye secreted unchanged into bile and removed exclusively by the liver. Its clearance from blood depends on hepatic blood flow and is used to evaluate liver function before partial hepatic resection for malignancy.[50] A study including subjects with compensated cirrhosis of various causes, demonstrated that, when using an ICG-retention test, after 15 minutes its intravenous injection (ICG-r15) correlated fairly well with HVPG ($r^2 = 0.571$).[51]

ICG retention also performs very well in detecting CSPH: a cutoff value of ICG-r15 less than 6.7% can rule-out CSPH with a 96% sensitivity and 2 cutoffs of ICG-r15 less than 10% and ICG-r15 greater than 23% can rule-out (98% sensitivity) and rule-in (90% specificity) GEV, respectively. ICG-r15 cutoffs of less than 13.3% could rule out (100% sensitivity) and rule in (73% specificity) the presence large varices.[51] The number of subjects included in these studies is not large and the technique is not well established or standardized in most centers.

ICG-r15 together with HVPG measurement and GEVs have been shown to be independent predictors of decompensation in patients with compensated cirrhosis.[52] However, in Child B and C patients, in which the ICG clearance could be influenced by the progressive deterioration of liver function, ICG-r15 shows less accuracy in predicting CSPH than in Child A patients.[53]

MRI

Liver architecture, perfusion of the liver and spleen, and blood flow in the splenic artery determined by MRI have been shown to correlate with portal pressure assessed by HVPG.

In a study performed in subjects with advanced fibrosis and cirrhosis (60%), liver longitudinal relaxation time and splenic artery velocity were found to correlate significantly with HVPG ($r = 0.90$) and with CSPH ($r = 0.85$).[54] MRI could be integrated with MR elastography of both the liver and the spleen. SSM by MRI can identify patients with cirrhosis and an HVPG greater than 12 mm Hg (AUROC = 0.81) and with HRV (AUROC = 0.93).[55]

These exploratory studies need to be confirmed in a larger number of subjects and issues of cost and feasibility (TE being a point-of-care test) require evaluation.

SUMMARY

Patients with PH are identified by the presence of varices or variceal hemorrhage and/ or by the presence of portosystemic collaterals on imaging (**Fig. 2**). Because the main cause of PH is cirrhosis, clinical tests, imaging studies, and LSMs should be first used to rule out or rule in cirrhosis. If negative, imaging studies to rule out portal vein thrombosis should be performed and, if these are negative, HVPG measurements should be

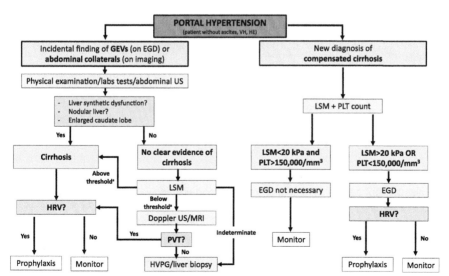

Fig. 2. PH: diagnostic algorithm.[a] LSM thresholds vary depending on cause of chronic liver disease.[35] HE, hepatic encephalopathy; PLT, platelets (count); PVT, portal vein thrombosis; US, ultrasound; VH, variceal hemorrhage.

performed with simultaneous liver biopsy. In cirrhosis, NITs can safely rule out the presence of HRVs and avoid endoscopy; however, in general, EGD is still necessary to screen for varices. The presence of varices or collaterals establishes the presence of CSPH. In the absence of varices, only HVPG can accurately determine the presence of CSPH.

REFERENCES

1. Ripoll C, Groszmann R, Garcia-Tsao G, et al. Hepatic venous pressure gradient predicts clinical decompensation in patients with compensated cirrhosis. Gastroenterology 2007;133:481–8.
2. Turco L, Villanueva C, La Mura V, et al. Lowering portal pressure improves outcomes of patients with cirrhosis, with or without ascites: a meta-analysis. Clin Gastroenterol Hepatol 2019 [pii:S1542-3565(19)30601-9].
3. García-Pagán JC, Caca K, Bureau C, et al. Early use of TIPS in patients with cirrhosis and variceal bleeding. N Engl J Med 2010;362(25):2370–9.
4. Bureau C, Thabut D, Oberti F, et al. Transjugular intrahepatic portosystemic shunts with covered stents increase transplant-free survival of patients with cirrhosis and recurrent ascites. Gastroenterology 2017;152(1):157–63.
5. Iwakiri Y, Shah V, Rockey DC. Vascular pathobiology in chronic liver disease and cirrhosis – current status and future directions. J Hepatol 2014;61:912–24.
6. DeLeve LD. Liver sinusoidal endothelial cells in hepatic fibrosis. Hepatology 2015;61(5):1740–6.
7. Fernandez M, Semela D, Bruix J, et al. Angiogenesis in liver disease. J Hepatol 2009;50:604–20.
8. Reynaert H, Thompson MG, Thomas T, et al. Hepatic stellate cells: role in microcirculation and pathophysiology of portal hypertension. Gut 2002;50:571–81.
9. Gupta TK, Toruner M, Chung MK, et al. Endothelial dysfunction and Decreased Production of Nitric Oxide in the intrahepatic microcirculation of cirrhotic rats. Hepatology 1998;28:926–31.
10. Tripodi A, Mannucci PM. The coagulopathy of chronic liver disease. N Engl J Med 2011;365(2):147–56.
11. Turco L, Schepis F, Villa E. The role of anticoagulation in treating portal hypertension. Curr Hepatol Rep 2018;17(3):200–8.
12. Cerini F, Vilaseca M, Lafoz EE, et al. Enoxaparin reduces hepatic vascular resistance and portal pressure in cirrhotic rats. J Hepatol 2016;64(4):834–42.
13. Vilaseca M, García-Calderó H, Lafoz E, et al. The anticoagulant rivaroxaban lowers portal hypertension in cirrhotic rats mainly by deactivating hepatic stellate cells. Hepatology 2017;65:2031–44.
14. Abraldes JG, Trebicka J, Chalasani N, et al. Prioritization of therapeutic targets and trial design in cirrhotic portal hypertension. Hepatology 2019;69(3):1287–99.
15. Schrier RW, Arroyo V, Bernardi M, et al. Peripheral Arterial vasodilation hypothesis: a proposal for the initiation of renal sodium and water retention in cirrhosis. Hepatology 1988;8:1151–7.
16. Turco L, Garcia-Tsao G, Magnani I, et al. Cardiopulmonary hemodynamics and C-reactive protein as prognostic indicators in compensated and decompensated cirrhosis. J Hepatol 2018;68(5):949–58.
17. Wiest R, Garcia-Tsao G. Bacterial translocation (BT) in cirrhosis. Hepatology 2005;41:422–33.
18. Mehta G, Gustot T, Mookerjee RP, et al. Inflammation and portal hypertension - the undiscovered country. J Hepatol 2014;61(1):155–63.

19. Taura K, De Minicis S, Seki E, et al. Hepatic stellate cells secrete angiopoietin 1 that induces angiogenesis in liver fibrosis. Gastroenterology 2008;135:1729–38.
20. Albillos A, de la Hera A, González M, et al. Increased lipopolysaccharide binding protein in cirrhotic patients with marked immune and hemodynamic derangement. Hepatology 2003;37:208–17.
21. Garcia-Tsao G, Abraldes JG, Berzigotti A, et al. Portal hypertensive bleeding in cirrhosis: risk stratification, diagnosis, and management: 2016 practice guidance by the American Association for the study of liver diseases. Hepatology 2017; 65(1):310–35.
22. Hino S, Kakutani H, Ikeda K, et al. Hemodynamic assessment of the left gastric vein in patients with esophageal varices with color Doppler EUS: factors affecting development of esophageal varices. Gastrointest Endosc 2002;55(04):512–7.
23. Kuramochi A, Imazu H, Kakutani H, et al. Color Doppler endoscopic ultrasonography in identifying groups at a high-risk of recurrence of esophageal varices after endoscopic treatment. J Gastroenterol 2007;42(03):219–24.
24. Huang JY, Samarasena JB, Tsujino T, et al. EUS-guided portal pressure gradient measurement with a novel 25-gauge needle device versus standard transjugular approach: a comparison animal study. Gastrointest Endosc 2016;84(02):358–62.
25. Huang JY, Samarasena JB, Tsujino T, et al. EUS-guided portal pressure gradient measurement with a simple novel device: a human pilot study. Gastrointest Endosc 2017;85(05):996–1001.
26. Thompson WP, Caughey JL, Whipple AO, et al. Splenic vein pressure in congestive splenomegaly. J Clin Invest 1937;16:571–2.
27. Gonzalez CO. Portography: a preliminary report of a new technique via the umbilical vein. Clin Proc Child Hosp Dist Columbia 1959;15:120–2.
28. Boyer TD, Triger DR, Horisawa M, et al. Direct transhepatic measurement of portal vein pressure using a thin needle. Comparison with wedged hepatic vein pressure. Gastroenterology 1977;72:584–9.
29. Myers JD, Taylor WJ. An estimation of portal venous pressure by occlusive catheterization of a hepatic venule. J Clin Invest 1951;30:662–3.
30. Perelló A, Escorsell A, Bru C, et al. Wedged hepatic venous pressure adequately reflects portal pressure in hepatitis C virus-related cirrhosis. Hepatology 1999; 30(6):1393–7.
31. Groszmann RJ, Glickman M, Blei AT, et al. Wedged and free hepatic venous pressure measured with a balloon catheter. Gastroenterology 1979;76:253–8.
32. Calvaruso V, Burroughs AK, Standish R, et al. Computer-assisted image analysis of liver collagen: relationship to Ishak scoring and hepatic venous pressure gradient. Hepatology 2009;49(4):1236–44.
33. Monescillo A, Martínez-Lagares F, Ruiz-del-Arbol L, et al. Influence of portal hypertension and its early decompression by TIPS placement on the outcome of variceal bleeding. Hepatology 2004;40(4):793–801.
34. Abraldes JG, Villanueva C, Banares R, et al. Hepatic venous pressure gradient and prognosis in patients with acute variceal bleeding treated with pharmacologic and endoscopic therapy. J Hepatol 2008;48:229–36.
35. Ferraioli G, Wong VW, Castera L, et al. Liver ultrasound elastography: an update to the World Federation for Ultrasound in Medicine and Biology guidelines and recommendations. Ultrasound Med Biol 2018;44(12):2419–40.
36. Vizzutti F, Arena U, Romanelli RG, et al. Liver stiffness measurement predicts severe portal hypertension in patients with HCV-related cirrhosis. Hepatology 2007; 45:1290–7.

37. de Franchis R, Baveno VI Faculty. Expanding consensus in portal hypertension: report of the Baveno VI Consensus Workshop: stratifying risk and individualizing care for portal hypertension. J Hepatol 2015;63(3):743–52.

38. Abraldes JG, Bureau C, Stefanescu H, et al. Noninvasive tools and risk of clinically significant portal hypertension and varices in compensated cirrhosis: the "Anticipate" study. Hepatology 2016;64(6):2173–84.

39. Jangouk P, Turco L, De Oliveira A, et al. Validating, deconstructing and refining Baveno criteria for ruling out high-risk varices in patients with compensated cirrhosis. Liver Int 2017;37(8):1177–83.

40. Augustin S, Pons M, Maurice JB, et al. Expanding the Baveno VI criteria for the screening of varices in patients with compensated advanced chronic liver disease. Hepatology 2017;66(6):1980–8.

41. Lee HA, Kim SU, Seo YS, et al. Prediction of the varices needing treatment with noninvasive tests in patients with compensated advanced chronic liver disease. Liver Int 2019;39(6):1071–9.

42. Colecchia A, Ravaioli F, Marasco G, et al. A combined model based on spleen stiffness measurement and Baveno VI criteria to rule out high-risk varices in advanced chronic liver disease. J Hepatol 2018;69(2):308–17.

43. Petta S, Sebastiani G, Bugianesi E, et al. Non-invasive prediction of esophageal varices by stiffness and platelet in non-alcoholic fatty liver disease cirrhosis. J Hepatol 2018;69(4):878–85.

44. Moctezuma-Velazquez C, Saffioti F, Tasayco-Huaman S, et al. Non-invasive prediction of high-risk varices in patients with primary biliary cholangitis and primary sclerosing cholangitis. Am J Gastroenterol 2019;114(3):446–52.

45. Thabut D, Bureau C, Layese R, et al. Validation of Baveno VI criteria for screening and surveillance of esophageal varices in patients with compensated cirrhosis and a sustained response to antiviral therapy. Gastroenterology 2019;156(4): 997–1009.

46. Mauro E, Crespo G, Montironi C, et al. Portal pressure and liver stiffness measurements in the prediction of fibrosis regression after sustained virological response in recurrent hepatitis C. Hepatology 2018;67(5):1683–94.

47. Colecchia A, Montrone L, Scaioli E, et al. Measurement of spleen stiffness to evaluate portal hypertension and the presence of esophageal varices in patients with HCV-related cirrhosis. Gastroenterology 2012;143(3):646–54.

48. Colecchia A, Colli A, Casazza G, et al. Spleen stiffness measurement can predict clinical complications in compensated HCV-related cirrhosis: a prospective study. J Hepatol 2014;60(6):1158–64.

49. Berzigotti A, Seijo S, Arena U, et al. Elastography, spleen size, and platelet count identify portal hypertension in patients with compensated cirrhosis. Gastroenterology 2013;144(1):102–11.

50. Burczynski FJ, Pushka KL, Sitar DS, et al. Hepatic plasma flow: accuracy of estimation from bolus injections of indocyanine green. Am J Physiol 1987;252: H953–62.

51. Lisotti A, Azzaroli F, Buonfiglioli F, et al. Indocyanine green retention test as a noninvasive marker of portal hypertension and esophageal varices in compensated liver cirrhosis. Hepatology 2014;59:643–50.

52. Lisotti A, Azzaroli F, Cucchetti A, et al. Relationship between indocyanine green retention test, decompensation and survival in patients with Child-Pugh A cirrhosis and portal hypertension. Liver Int 2016;36(9):1313–21.

53. Pind ML, Bendtsen F, Kallemose T, et al. Indocyanine green retention test (ICG-r15) as a noninvasive predictor of portal hypertension in patients with different severity of cirrhosis. Eur J Gastroenterol Hepatol 2016;28(8):948–54.
54. Palaniyappan N, Cox E, Bradley C, et al. Non-invasive assessment of portal hypertension using quantitative magnetic resonance imaging. J Hepatol 2016; 65(6):1131–9.
55. Ronot M, Lambert S, Elkrief L, et al. Assessment of portal hypertension and high-risk oesophageal varices with liver and spleen three-dimensional multifrequency MR elastography in liver cirrhosis. Eur Radiol 2014;24(6):1394–402.

Frailty, Sarcopenia, and Malnutrition in Cirrhotic Patients

Elizabeth S. Aby, MD[a], Sammy Saab, MD, MPH[a,b],*

KEYWORDS

- Sarcopenia • Frailty • Malnutrition • Liver transplantation/hepatology
- Rehabilitation

KEY POINTS

- Frailty, sarcopenia, and malnutrition are frequent complications in end-stage liver disease (ESLD) that adversely affect morbidity and mortality.
- Several tools can be used to evaluate and quantify frailty and sarcopenia, including the liver frailty index. The liver frailty index is a disease-specific model that predicts mortality in patients with ESLD.
- Assessment of muscle mass, muscle function, and nutritional status is valuable, because they are modifiable risk factors.
- Interventions such as nutritional supplementation and physical training show promise in improving muscle mass and exercise capacity.

INTRODUCTION

Cirrhosis of the liver is a major global health burden associated with high rates of morbidity and mortality.[1] Cirrhotic patients often have manifestations of portal hypertension, including ascites, hepatic encephalopathy, and esophageal varices; however, cirrhosis takes a toll on patients in other ways. Cirrhotic patients often suffer from undernutrition, cachexia, and chronic protein synthetic dysfunction, which make them susceptible to developing frailty. Frailty is defined as a clinical state of decreased reserve and decreased ability to endure stressors such as cumulative declines across multiple systems.[2] Frailty, a concept originally described in the geriatric literature, has

Disclosure Statement: The authors have nothing to disclose.
a Department of Medicine, University of California at Los Angeles, UCLA Medical Center, 757 Westwood Plaza, Suite 7501, Los Angeles, CA 90095, USA; b Department of Surgery, University of California at Los Angeles, Los Angeles, CA, USA
* Corresponding author. Pfleger Liver Institute, UCLA Medical Center, 200 Medical Plaza, Suite 214, Los Angeles, CA 90095.
E-mail address: SSaab@mednet.ucla.edu
; @lizabmn47 (E.S.A.)

Clin Liver Dis 23 (2019) 589–605
https://doi.org/10.1016/j.cld.2019.06.001
1089-3261/19/© 2019 Elsevier Inc. All rights reserved.

liver.theclinics.com

since been validated in cohorts of patients with chronic diseases, such as end-stage liver disease (ESLD), and is associated with adverse health outcomes.[3,4] Frailty is common in patients with chronic liver disease; 17% of patients awaiting liver transplantation were categorized as frail based on the Fried Frailty Index (FFI).[3]

Sarcopenia, defined as the progressive and generalized loss of skeletal muscle mass, strength, and function, is a component of frailty.[5–7] Sarcopenia is characterized by loss of muscle mass alone or in combination with increased fat mass.[7] Sarcopenia is often associated with aging; however, sarcopenia may also be present in the setting of chronic diseases such as ESLD.[8] Sarcopenia is a common complication of cirrhosis; it is estimated to occur in 30% to 70% of patients with ESLD, and has been shown to be an independent predictor of mortality in cirrhotic patients.[9–13] Based on anatomic assessments in patients with ESLD, sarcopenia is more frequently found in men compared with women, patients with low body mass index (BMI), and in patients with alcoholic liver disease.[10,13–17] Not only is sarcopenia associated with increased mortality in patients cirrhosis, it is also independently associated with increased health-related costs for patients on the waiting list for liver transplantation.[18] Furthermore, given the increasing prevalence of obesity in cirrhosis, patients can develop low muscle mass and increased fat mass, often called sarcopenic obesity.[19,20] The prevalence of sarcopenia obesity is estimated to be between 20% and 35% and associated with increased mortality.[21,22] The awareness that sarcopenia can exist in the presence of obesity is valuable given clinicians often rely on the eyeball test to assess muscle mass, which can be challenging in the presence of obesity.

Malnutrition also plays a role in the complex development of sarcopenia and frailty in patients with ESLD. The prevalence of malnutrition in cirrhosis is high, estimated to be 65% to 90%.[23,24] Malnutrition and sarcopenia often present simultaneously given they have similar physiologic mechanisms. Malnutrition differs from sarcopenia in that malnutrition is defined by an imbalance of energy, protein, and other nutrients, whereas sarcopenia is based on muscle mass, strength, and performance. Malnutrition has been shown to negatively impact patient outcomes. For instance, preoperative malnutrition has been shown to negatively impact liver transplant outcomes after surgery.[25,26]

The assessments of frailty, sarcopenia, and malnutrition have become a growing field of interest given the association between these clinical states and adverse outcomes in ESLD and liver transplantation (**Fig. 1**). Frailty is not only linked to increases in falls, fractures, but also with increased waitlist mortality and decreased quality of life in patients awaiting liver transplantation.[3,27–29] In cirrhotic patients on the liver transplant list, frailty is predictive of hospitalization and total hospitalized days per year, independent of liver disease severity; this suggests that frailty also leads to increased health care utilization in cirrhotic patients.[28] Frailty is an important concept in patients with ESLD given that frailty often progresses over time. There is an increasing understanding that objective assessments of nutrition and frailty are needed to improve prognostication in cirrhotic patients and create appropriate interventions. Conventionally, the Child Turcotte Pugh (CTP) classification and the model for end-stage liver disease (MELD) score are used to predict prognosis and mortality in cirrhotic patients; however, one of the drawbacks of these scores is that nutritional status and functional status are not incorporated.[30–34] A recent study found that the MELD score and CTP class were useful prognostic tools for survival in patients with ESLD without sarcopenia, but not in patients with severe sarcopenia.[35] Research is ongoing to develop tools to evaluate muscle mass and function with the goal of better informing patients of their prognosis and to create interventions to improve patient outcomes.

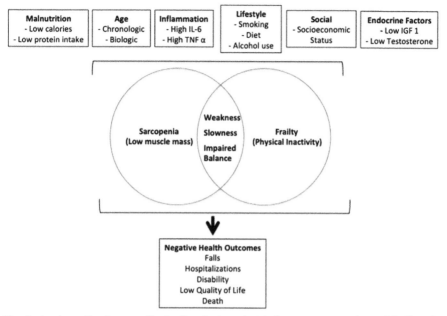

Fig. 1. A schematic diagram illustrating factors that influence sarcopenia and frailty, the intersection between frailty and sarcopenia, and the health outcomes that result.

SARCOPENIA ASSESSMENTS

Sarcopenia is characterized by the loss of skeletal muscle mass, strength, and function. Given the challenge of creating a single assessment that captures muscle mass, strength, and function, several different measurements have been created to characterize components of sarcopenia.

One technique for measuring anatomic sarcopenia uses cross-sectional imaging with either computed tomography (CT) scan or MRI to determine skeletal muscle mass.[36] Given that cirrhotic patients may have salt and water retention and an elevated BMI, cross-sectional imaging offers advantages for evaluating muscle mass; it is objective, not influenced by fluid retention, and effort-independent. Several methods of muscle measurement and sarcopenia have been used, including cross-sectional muscle area with corresponding skeletal muscle index (SMI), psoas muscle area, and the dorsal muscle group area.[10,13,15,16,37–50] Single-slice imaging above the level of the fourth and fifth lumbar vertebra was found to correlate with whole-body skeletal muscle; thus, the technique of characterizing muscle mass using single-slice imaging has been used to more broadly characterize total body muscle composition.[51] SMI has been found to be a suitable indicator of total body muscle mass and predictor of mortality in cirrhotic patients.[13,51,52] A recent study carried out by the Fitness, Life Enhancement, and Exercise in Liver Transplantation (FLEXIT) consortium looked at the association of psoas muscle index (PMI) with SMI and the capability of PMI to predict mortality in patients with ESLD awaiting liver transplantation.[53] Their data showed that PMI has a poor ability to identify patients with higher waitlist mortality for cirrhosis and that SMI is a stronger measurement for predicting waitlist mortality.[53]

A systematic review and meta-analysis looking at the impact of skeletal muscle mass, assessed by cross-sectional imaging in patients awaiting or undergoing liver transplantation found that low muscle mass was independently associated with post-transplantation and waiting list mortality.[54] An advantage of cross-section imaging for sarcopenia assessments is that it minimizes confounding factors, such as volume status and hepatic encephalopathy; however, these assessments are limited by their inability to assess muscle function. In addition, there is no established method for skeletal muscle measurement in cirrhotic patients and no consensus regarding cutoffs to classify patients as sarcopenic or nonsarcopenic. If anatomic sarcopenia is to be used as a tool for patient assessment, more work is needed to determine definitions and cutoffs for sarcopenia, especially given that definitions may vary based on age, gender, or etiology of cirrhosis.

In addition to cross-sectional imaging, dual x-ray absorptiometry (DEXA) and bioelectrical impedance analysis (BIA) are used to measure body composition in cirrhosis. DEXA quantifies sarcopenia by measuring body fat, fat-free mass, and bone mineral content; however, fluid overload may impact the reliability of this assessment.[55,56] Bioelectrical impedance analysis evaluates muscle mass and sarcopenia by measuring the body's resistance to flow of electrical current. It is easy to perform and noninvasive, has high interobserver reliability, and is correlated with DEXA.[57]

Despite the lack of a gold standard tool for evaluating body composition in patients with cirrhosis, there is consistent evidence that lower skeletal muscle mass is associated with impaired survival independent of other factors, such as MELD score.[54]

FRAILTY ASSESSMENTS

Whereas sarcopenia assessments more commonly evaluate body composition, frailty assessments test physical strength and function (**Table 1**).

One of the original and most frequently used instruments for frailty assessment is the FFI, which combines 5 domains of physical frailty: weakness, exhaustion, weight loss, low activity, and slowness, into a 5-point score.[2] Frailty, defined by an FFI of at least 3, has been shown to be independently associated with mortality in patients with ESLD.[3] It is valuable, given that it can be easily performed in the outpatient setting in a short amount of time. One downside of this tool is that it incorporates subjective, patient-reported domains.

The Short Physical Performance Battery (SPPB), another frailty assessment tool, is an objective instrument to evaluate lower-extremity physical performance status.[58] The test evaluates performance on 3 timed tasks: walking speed, standing balance, and chair stand tests. The SPPB is convenient tool that can be used in the outpatient setting to measure several motor domains, including strength, coordination, and balance. Results from a systemic review and meta-analysis suggest that poor performance on the SPPB in the general population is associated with an increased risk of all-cause mortality.[59]

The Liver Frailty Index (LFI), designed specifically for patients with liver disease, consists of 3 performance-based tests of physical frailty, including grip strength, chair stands, and balance testing. Weak grip strength is a marker of nutritional status; slow chair stands are a marker of lower extremity strength, and impaired balance is a marker of neuromotor function. Given its simple nature, it can be feasibly carried out in the outpatient setting at baseline and be followed over time. Moreover, the LFI is advantageous given it is performance based and measures multiple aspects of frailty, including muscle wasting, neuromotor coordination, and malnutrition. The LFI has been shown to have construct validity for frailty and improves risk prediction of 3-month waitlist mortality for liver transplantation over MELD-Na alone.[60] One disadvantage of the LFI and the SPPB, however, is that these tests may measure other systems involved with movement, such as cardiovascular fitness and pulmonary

Table 1
Measures of frailty

Disease Measure	Type	Special Devices/ Training	Components	Scoring
Fried Frailty Instrument[2]	Performance-based + self-report	Yes	Slowness, low levels of physical activity, weight loss, exhaustion, weakness	Scored from 0 to 1 in 5 sections Minimum score: 0 Maximum score: 5 (most frail)
Short Physical Performance Battery[50]	Performance-based	Yes	Chair stands, gait speed, balance test	Scored from 0 to 4 in 3 sections Minimum score: 0 (most frail) Maximum score: 12
Activities of daily living[107]	Self-report	No	Ability to perform basic activities of self-care without assistance (feeding, transferring, continence, bathing, dressing, and toileting)	Scored from 0 to 1 in 6 activities Minimum score: 0 (most frail) Maximum score: 6
Instrumental activities of daily living[108]	Self-report	No	Ability to perform activities to live within society without assistance (using the telephone, shopping, laundry, preparing food, housekeeping, using transportation, managing medications, and managing finances)	Scored from 0 to 1 in 8 activities Minimum score: 0 (most frail) Maximum score: 8
Liver Frailty Index[52]	Performance-based	Yes	Grip strength, chair stands, balance	(-0.330*gender-adjusted grip strength) + (−2.529*number of chair stands per second) + (−0.040*balance time) + 6

* Multiplication.

function. Hepatic encephalopathy can also interfere with the executive functioning needed to carry out these tasks.

Adding LFI to clinician assessments of frailty can improve predictions of waitlist mortality. Traditionally, clinicians often rely on the eyeball test to assess muscle mass and physical ability. However, this appraisal is subjective, varies between clinicians, and may miss subtle signs of muscle wasting or incoordination valuable for prognostication. LFI testing and subjective clinician assessment of the patient's health were compared in over 500 cirrhotic patients; although clinician assessment can predict liver transplant mortality, it was found to be subjective and variable between hepatologists.[61] When the LFI was added to the clinician assessment, the predictions of waitlist mortality significantly improved, suggesting that the addition of the LFI to the eyeball test would enhance decision making and management.[61]

The LFI has also been used to examine how pretransplant frailty impacts post-transplant frailty.[62] Lai and colleagues[62] studied over 200 adult patients who underwent liver transplantation. They found that frailty worsens at 3 months after liver transplantation, but improves modestly 1 year after transplantation, with patients maintaining or slightly improving their pretransplantation frailty score. Patients defined as robust prior to transplantation were likely to be robust after transplant.[62] Those who were frail prior to transplantation were likely to remain nearly frail or frail, with only 14% of patients achieving a robust status.[62] Overall, pretransplant LFI was found to be a predictor of post-transplant robust status. This work suggests that pretransplant assessment and interventions are needed to optimize frailty prior to transplantation to ensure the best possible outcome after transplantation.

EXERCISE CAPACITY IN PATIENTS WITH CIRRHOSIS

Patients with chronic conditions, such as ESLD, experience a decline in exercise capacity because of physiologic changes and physical inactivity associated with their underlying disease.[63] Several studies have looked at the relationship between severity of liver disease and exercise capacity. One standard for assessing exercise capacity is measurement of maximal oxygen consumption (Vo_2). Studies have shown negative correlations between CTP score and the absolute Vo_2 peak value, Vo_2 peak value as a percentage of the predicted value, and Vo_2 at anaerobic threshold as a percentage of the predicted peak value.[64–67] There are several possible explanations for the reduction in peak Vo_2 during maximal exercise in cirrhotic patients, such as cirrhotic cardiomyopathy, cardiac chronotropic incompetence, decreased peripheral oxygen utilization in the setting of muscle wasting and decondition, and oxygen delivery abnormalities in the setting of hepatopulmonary syndrome.[68,69] Additionally, cirrhotic patients with ascites tend to have lower exercise capacities compared with cirrhotic patients without ascites, with Vo_2 peak values of 46% versus 86%, respectively, compared with control subjects.[70]

Reduced exercise capacity prior to liver transplantation, measured by Vo_2 peak, has been shown to be independently associated with short-term mortality in multivariate analysis.[71] Work by Dharancy and colleagues[72] suggests that severely impaired pretransplant exercise capacity, defined as peak Vo_2 values less than 60% predicted, in patients with ESLD was independently associated with 1-year mortality after transplant. A recent study looking at the 6-minute walk test found that for every 100 m increase in the walk distance at baseline, there was a significant increase in survival in patients awaiting transplantation.[4]

Not only do patients with cirrhosis have decreased exercise capacity, they also have decreased muscle strength. Muscle strength was assessed in upper and lower extremities in patients with alcoholic cirrhosis; in all areas tested, cirrhotic patients were noted to be significantly weaker compared with healthy controls.[73]

NUTRITIONAL ASSESSMENTS

Malnutrition is estimated to affect between 50% and 90% of patients with ESLD, and can lead to decreased skeletal muscle mass.[74] Malnutrition is caused by a combination of decreased caloric intake, increased protein requirements, increased muscle protein catabolism, decreased muscle protein synthesis, and poor absorption of nutrients.[75–78]

In addition, those with ascites have an increased resting energy expenditure, yet their food intake is often decreased because of early satiety in the setting of raised abdominal pressure, which can prevent gastric food accomodation.[79] Furthermore, inflammation in the setting of cirrhosis can promote catabolism, which promotes disease-related malnutrition.[80–82]

Malnutrition negatively impacts survival and increases complications related to cirrhosis. For instance, malnutrition is associated with a higher risk of postoperative mortality in patients with ESLD undergoing liver transplantation.[68–70] Not only does malnutrition affect post-transplant outcomes, it also affects quality of life. Malnourished cirrhotic patients experience a lower quality of life compared with those who are not malnourished.[83]

Unfortunately, ESLD confounds the common markers of nutritional status, such as prealbumin, albumin, and prothrombin time. For example, albumin and prealbumin depend on hepatocyte synthetic function, which is impaired in ESLD. Furthermore, assessments of weight are challenging given common complications of cirrhosis, including peripheral edema and ascites, which can mask the development of cachexia. Given this, common assessments of nutritional status, such as BMI and weight, do not provide an adequate assessment of nutritional status in patients with cirrhosis with fluid retention. In patients with fluid retention, dry body weight should be determined after paracentesis, or it can be determined by subtracting a percentage of weight based upon the severity of ascites (mild 5%, moderate 10%, severe 15%), with an additional 5% subtracted if bilateral lower extremity edema is present.[10,52]

Because of the challenges of these nutritional assessments, the subjective global assessment (SGA) was developed in 1987.[84] The SGA incorporates physical examination findings and history, including symptoms, weight changes, and nutrient intake. The SGA is simple, can be performed quickly at bedside, and is noninvasive. One weakness is that some components of the SGA are subjective. In a prospective study by Stephenson and colleagues,[85] postoperative length of stay was significantly longer in those with severe malnutrition, as measured by the SGA, compared with patients with mild or moderate malnutrition. There were also more deaths in patients who were severely malnourished, but the difference in mortality was not statistically significant because of lack of power.[85] A recent study found a weak concordance between malnutrition defined based on SGA and sarcopenia defined based on cross-sectional imaging.[86] They also found that sarcopenia, but not malnutrition defined by SGA, was associated with mortality.[86] These results imply that despite the advantages of the SGA, it may have a more limited role given it is not associated with mortality in patients with ELSD.

Nutritional status can also be evaluated using anthropometric techniques, such as midarm muscle circumference (MAMC). MAMC has been shown to be an independent predictor of mortality in patients with cirrhosis in some studies, but not others.[87,88] Despite some of the benefits of anthropometric methods, it can be affected by edema and has a high interobserver variability, which makes it challenging to monitor changes over time.

Malnutrition assessments are crucial in patients with ESLD to identify and treat those who are nutritionally deficient.

INTERVENTIONS FOR SARCOPENIA, FRAILTY, AND MALNUTRITION

Early diagnosis of loss of muscle function and strength as well as malnutrition is necessary to allow for appropriate intervention, given these factors are predictive of complications of liver disease and mortality. Hepatic and extrahepatic factors that contribute to sarcopenia and frailty need to be assessed in the outpatient setting to provide an accurate prognosis and support care planning.

Nutrition

Protein energy malnutrition is common in patients with ESLD and is associated with risk for morbidity and mortality after liver transplantation; thus, it is important to provide adequate protein and calorie supplementation prior to liver transplant to optimize nutritional status.[25,89–91]

Evidence has demonstrated that the recommend intake for cirrhosis is 25 to 40 kcal/kg/d and 1.20 to 1.5 g/kg/d of protein, with adjustment based on comorbid conditions such as encephalopathy.[92–94] It is recommended that patients with recurrent or persistent hepatic encephalopathy consume a diet low in animal protein and rich in vegetable protein.[95] Patients with cirrhosis should also be counseled to avoid consumption of raw seafood given the risk of Vibrio vulnificus infection.[96]

If patients are unable to obtain the recommended intake with dietary adjustments, the European Society of Clinical Nutrition and Metabolism guidelines recommend the addition of oral supplements or overnight enteral feeds to optimize nutritional status. Total parenteral nutrition (TPN) should only be used in cirrhotic patients with contraindications to oral or enteral nutrition who are unable to maintain adequate oral or enteral caloric intake despite their best efforts. TPN increases infection risk and when used for prolonged periods of time can cause worsening liver function; thus it should only be used when enteral optimization fails. Cirrhotic patients are often deficient in fat-soluble vitamin supplementation as well as zinc and selenium, so diet supplementation is recommended.[93,97] In those with ongoing or a history of alcohol abuse, thiamine and folic acid supplementation should be considered.[93,97]

Recent evidence suggests beneficial effects of nutritional interventions in patients with cirrhosis. A randomized controlled trial from India showed that 6 months of nutritional support (30–35 kcal/kg/d, 1.0–1.5 g/kg/d of vegetable protein) led to an significant increase in health-related quality of life ,and fewer patients progressed to overt hepatic encephalopathy, compared with the control group.[98] This study did not, however, examine the impact of nutritional therapy on muscle mass.

Cirrhotic patients have increased protein requirements given they exhibit gluconeogenesis after short-term fasting. Increased fatty acid oxidation and enhanced gluconeogenesis are thought to occur during overnight fasting in cirrhotic patients, which can lead to poor nutritional status. Consequently, Plank and colleagues[99] compared nutritional supplementation of 710 kcal per day in the late evening compared in the daytime. They found that total body protein, measured by neutron activation analysis, increased significantly in the late evening group compared with the day group when examined over a 12-month period.[99] Despite the encouraging results of increased total body protein with late evening nutritional supplementation, the study was limited by poor adherence to appropriate timing of the supplement and a high dropout rate. Further studies have supported the implementation of late evening snack as an intervention to reverse anabolic resistance and sarcopenia of cirrhosis.[100] In addition, cirrhotic patients are recommend to have several small meals per day to reduce the possibility of nausea, vomiting, or protein overload.[101]

In addition to nutritional support and altering the timing of nutritional intake, branched chain amino acid (BCAA) supplementation has showed promise in improving muscle mass in cirrhotic patients. BCAAs are necessary for regulation of energy, protein synthesis, and protein turnover.[102] In patients with ESLD, there is an imbalance in BCAA and aromatic amino acids (AAAs) because of AAA accumulation secondary to impaired hepatocyte function and decreased BCAA levels because of uptake into skeletal muscles in the process of ammonia degradation.[102] Fixing the imbalance in the BCAA to AAA ratio may have the potential to improve nutritional status in patients with ESLD. A randomized, multicenter trial looked at the effect of BCAA supplementation in cirrhotic patients and found that BCAA supplementation led to increased muscle mass, as measured by midarm muscle circumference (MAMC).[103] Hanai and colleagues[14] evaluated cirrhotic patients retrospectively to determine the impact of BCAA supplementation on patients with sarcopenia. They found that BCAA supplementation improved survival of sarcopenia patients in a subgroup analysis. Despite the potential benefits with the use of oral BCAA supplementation, it is expensive and not palatable, making it poorly tolerated by patients.

A multitude of factors contribute to malnutrition in patients with cirrhosis. It is essential to identify, prevent, and treat malnutrition to improve muscle mass, survival, and quality of life.

Exercise

Reduced exercise tolerance in cirrhotic patients is an independent prognostic factor of morbidity and mortality before and after transplantation.[104,105] Therefore, optimizing muscle mass and function through exercise is imperative in the management of patients with ESLD.

There is scant literature on the effect of physical training on exercise capacity and muscle mass in patients with ESLD. One study evaluated the impact of a 12-week moderate exercise regimen in cirrhotic patients. Patients who underwent the 12-week exercise program experienced an increase in exercise capacity (measured by a 6-minute walk test and 2-minute step test), an increase in muscle mass (measured by lower thigh circumference), and an enhanced health-related quality of life.[106] A randomized control trial looked at the effect of 12 weeks of moderate exercise in patients with cirrhosis and found that a moderate exercise program improves functional capacity, increases muscle mass, and decreases body fat.[107] Another group assessed the impact of an 8-week supervised exercise program on peak Vo_2, muscle mass, and quality of life in patients with CTP class A or B cirrhosis.[108] They found that patients who participated in the exercise program had increased peak Vo_2, increased muscle mass, and reduced fatigued compared with usual care.[108] Another study looked at the effect of an exercise program on Vo_2 max in patients with compensated cirrhosis; they found that after 4 to 6 weeks and 10 to 12 weeks of training, there was a statically significant increase in Vo_2 max at both time points.[109] Debette-Gratien and colleagues[110] evaluated the impact of a 12-week personalized exercise program in cirrhotic patients before liver transplantation. They found an improvement in physical fitness and muscular strength with the personalized exercise program based on increased peak Vo_2, 6-minute walk test, and muscle strength.

A systematic review and meta-analysis were done to assess the impact of adapted physical activity on hospital stay and 1-year mortality and morbidity after liver transplantation.[111] Four randomized control trials with 81 patients total were included.[106–108,112] Given the lack of available evidence, no conclusions were derived regarding the effect of physical activity prior to liver transplantation on outcomes; however, the evidence suggests that physical activity is safe in cirrhotic patients.[111]

These studies suggest that muscle mass and exercise capacity can be improved with exercise training. These modifiable factors can be adapted to improve the outcomes of patients with ESLD. Patients with cirrhosis would benefit from baseline physical capacity assessments, customized exercise programming, and subsequent monitoring of progress. Duarte-Rojo and colleagues[113] recommend 30- to 60-minute sessions combining both aerobic and resistance training to achieve at least 150 minutes per week for patients with ESLD. For those with severe sarcopenia and frailty, balance training and strength training are advised prior to aerobic and resistance training.[113] However, it is necessary that exercise programs be tailored thoughtfully for cirrhotic patients.[114]

Transjugular Intrahepatic Portosystemic Stent

A recent study by Tsien and colleagues[115] looked at the impact of transjugular intrahepatic portosystemic stent (TIPS) on sarcopenia in cirrhotic patients. Psoas muscle mass increased significantly in those who underwent TIPS compared with cirrhotic patients who did not.[115] It is important to note that TIPS was not performed for malnutrition or sarcopenia, but for indications such as refractory variceal bleeding or refractory ascites; the unintended benefit was improvement in muscle mass. The increase in the total skeletal muscle area was independently associated with a reduction in mortality.[115] Two other studies have showed similar results, noting an increase in muscle mass measured by bioelectrical impedance after TIPS placement.[116,117] The mechanisms of sarcopenia reversal following TIPS are unknown, but possible explanations include reduction in portal pressure, reduction in ascites, and increased appetite.[115] Despite these encouraging results, this study was retrospective in nature; therefore, a well-designed randomized controlled trial would be helpful to validate these findings. At this time, TIPS is not recommended as an intervention to improve muscle mass.

Based on the current literature regarding sarcopenia and frailty assessments and potential interventions, the authors have devised an approach to frailty in the outpatient setting in cirrhotic patients. It is described in **Fig. 2.**

Assessment
1. Evaluate objective data
   a. Vital signs
   b. Laboratory data (INR, serum creatinine, albumin, total bilirubin, and sodium)
   c. Imaging and procedural data (such as esophagogastroduodenoscopy, transthoracic echocardiogram, and abdominal ultrasound)
2. History and physical examination
   a. Evaluation for signs of complications (such as hepatic encephalopathy, ascites, variceal bleeding, or hepatopulmonary syndrome)
3. Perform functional assessment
   a. Liver Frailty Index
4. Discussion with patient regarding lifestyle and social factors (including diet, exercise, alcohol, tobacco, and finances).
5. Assessment of co-morbid conditions and social situation

Interventions
1. Discuss caloric intake recommendations (25–40 kcal/kg/day and 1.20–1.5 g/kg/day of protein), sodium restriction, and late evening snacks
   a. Consider referral to a nutritionist
   b. Consider branch chain amino acid supplementation
2. Discuss moderate exercise regimen
   a. Create personalized exercise regimens
   b. Consider referral to specialized physical therapy
3. If moderate to severe frailty or fall history, consider home safety evaluation
4. Trend weights and liver frailty index scores to monitor progress

Fig. 2. Approach to frailty in the clinical setting in patients with cirrhosis.

SUMMARY

Sarcopenia, frailty, and malnutrition are prevalent in cirrhotic patients and are determinants of morbidity and mortality in this patient population. Frailty, sarcopenia, and malnutrition may modifiable risk factors; therefore, gaining a better understanding of a patient's muscle mass, muscle function, and nutritional status is essential to individualizing nutritional and exercise interventions with the aim of improving patient outcomes. Research is ongoing to develop and refine frailty and nutritional assessments to allow clinicians to incorporate these metrics into their decision making and management plans for patients with cirrhosis.

The tools established to assess that risk (eg, MELD) incompletely capture its magnitude, while investigational tools (eg, acute physiology and chronic health evaluation [APACHE]) require expertise and are unfamiliar to most clinicians.

REFERENCES

1. Mokdad AA, Lopez AD, Shahraz S, et al. Liver cirrhosis mortality in 187 countries between 1980 and 2010: a systematic analysis. BMC Med 2014;12(1). https://doi.org/10.1186/s12916-014-0145-y.
2. Fried LP, Tangen CM, Walston J, et al. Frailty in older adults: evidence for a phenotype. J Gerontol A Biol Sci Med Sci 2001;56(3):M146–57.
3. Lai JC, Feng S, Terrault NA, et al. Frailty predicts waitlist mortality in liver transplant candidates. Am J Transplant 2014;14(8):1870–9.
4. Carey EJ, Steidley DE, Aqel BA, et al. Six-minute walk distance predicts mortality in liver transplant candidates. Liver Transpl 2010;16(12):1373–8.
5. Morley JE, Vellas B, Abellan van Kan G, et al. Frailty consensus: a call to action. J Am Med Dir Assoc 2013;14(6):392–7.
6. Cruz-Jentoft AJ, Baeyens JP, Bauer JM, et al. Sarcopenia: European consensus on definition and diagnosis: report of the European Working Group on sarcopenia in older people. Age Ageing 2010;39(4):412–23.
7. Fielding RA, Vellas B, Evans WJ, et al. Sarcopenia: an undiagnosed condition in older adults. Current consensus definition: prevalence, etiology, and consequences. International Working Group on Sarcopenia. J Am Med Dir Assoc 2011;12(4):249–56.
8. Lang T, Streeper T, Cawthon P, et al. Sarcopenia: etiology, clinical consequences, intervention, and assessment. Osteoporos Int 2010;21(4):543–59.
9. Bhanji RA, Carey EJ, Yang L, et al. The long winding road to transplant: how sarcopenia and debility impact morbidity and mortality on the waitlist. Clin Gastroenterol Hepatol 2017;15(10):1492–7.
10. Tandon P, Ney M, Irwin I, et al. Severe muscle depletion in patients on the liver transplant wait list: its prevalence and independent prognostic value. Liver Transpl 2012;18(10):1209–16.
11. Campillo B, Paillaud E, Uzan I, et al. Value of body mass index in the detection of severe malnutrition: influence of the pathology and changes in anthropometric parameters. Clin Nutr 2004;23(4):551–9.
12. Merli M, Giusto M, Gentili F, et al. Nutritional status: its influence on the outcome of patients undergoing liver transplantation. Liver Int 2010;30(2):208–14.
13. Montano-Loza AJ, Meza-Junco J, Prado CMM, et al. Muscle wasting is associated with mortality in patients with cirrhosis. Clin Gastroenterol Hepatol 2012;10(2):166–73.e1.
14. Hanai T, Shiraki M, Nishimura K, et al. Sarcopenia impairs prognosis of patients with liver cirrhosis. Nutrition 2015;31(1):193–9.

15. Andrea DiMartini M. Muscle mass predicts outcomes following liver transplantation. Liver Transpl 2013;73(4):389–400.

16. Montano-Loza AJ, Meza-Junco J, Baracos VE, et al. Severe muscle depletion predicts postoperative length of stay but is not associated with survival after liver transplantation. Liver Transpl 2014;20(6):640–8.

17. Riggio O, Andreoli A, Diana F, et al. Whole body and regional body composition analysis by dual-energy x-ray absorptiometry in cirrhotic patients. Eur J Clin Nutr 1997;51(12):810–4.

18. van Vugt JLA, Buettner S, Alferink LJM, et al. Low skeletal muscle mass is associated with increased hospital costs in patients with cirrhosis listed for liver transplantation–a retrospective study. Transpl Int 2018;31(2):165–74.

19. Choi KM. Sarcopenia and sarcopenic obesity. Korean J Intern Med 2016;31(6):1054–60.

20. Zamboni M, Rubele S, Rossi AP. Sarcopenia and obesity. Curr Opin Clin Nutr Metab Care 2019;22(1):13–9.

21. Kaibori M, Ishizaki M, Iida H, et al. Effect of intramuscular adipose tissue content on prognosis in patients undergoing hepatocellular carcinoma resection. J Gastrointest Surg 2015;19(7):1315–23.

22. Montano-Loza AJ, Angulo P, Meza-Junco J, et al. Sarcopenic obesity and myosteatosis are associated with higher mortality in patients with cirrhosis. J Cachexia Sarcopenia Muscle 2015;126–35. https://doi.org/10.1002/jcsm.12039.

23. Caregaro L, Alberino F, Amodio P, et al. Malnutrition. Am J Clin Nutr 1996;63:602–9.

24. Campillo B, Richardet J, Scherman E, et al. Evaluation of nutritional practice in hospitalized cirrhotic patients : results of a prospective study. Nutrition 2003;19:515–21.

25. Pikul J, Sharpe MD, Lowndes R, et al. Degree of preoperative malnutrition is predictive of postoperative morbidity and mortality in liver transplant recipients. Transplantation 1994;57(3):469–72.

26. Müller MJ, Lautz HU, Plogmann B, et al. Energy expenditure and substrate oxidation in patients with cirrhosis: the impact of cause, clinical staging and nutritional state. Hepatology 1992;15(5):782–94.

27. Derck JE, Thelen AE, Cron DC, et al. Quality of life in liver transplant candidates: frailty is a better indicator than severity of liver disease. Transplantation 2015;99(2):340–4.

28. Sinclair M, Poltavskiy E, Dodge JL, et al. Frailty is independently associated with increased hospitalisation days in patients on the liver transplant waitlist. World J Gastroenterol 2017;23(5):899–905.

29. Trivedi HD, Tapper EB. Interventions to improve physical function and prevent adverse events in cirrhosis. Gastroenterol Rep (Oxf) 2018;6(1):13–20.

30. Pugh RNH, Murray-Lyon IM, Dawson JL, et al. Transection of the oesophagus for bleeding oesophageal varices. Br J Surg 1973;60(8):646–9.

31. Christensen E. Prognostic models including the Child-Pugh, MELD and Mayo risk scores - where are we and where should we go? J Hepatol 2004;41(2):344–50.

32. Malinchoc M, Kamath PS, Gordon FD, et al. A model to predict poor survival in patients undergoing transjugular intrahepatic portosystemic shunts. Hepatology 2000;31(4):864–71.

33. Kamath PS, Wiesner RH, Malinchoc M, et al. A model to predict survival in patients with end-stage liver disease. Hepatology 2001;33(2):464–70.

34. Botta F, Giannini E, Romagnoli P, et al. MELD scoring system is useful for predicting prognosis in patients with liver cirrhosis and is correlated with residual liver function: a European study. Gut 2003;52(1):134–9.
35. Kang SH, Jeong WK, Baik SK, et al. Impact of sarcopenia on prognostic value of cirrhosis: going beyond the hepatic venous pressure gradient and MELD score. J Cachexia Sarcopenia Muscle 2018;9(5):860–70.
36. Heymsfield SB. Development of imaging methods to assess adiposity and metabolism. Int J Obes 2008;32:S76–82.
37. Bergerson JT, Lee JG, Furlan A, et al. Liver transplantation arrests and reverses muscle wasting. Clin Transpl 2015;29(3):216–21.
38. Cruz RJ, Dew MA, Myaskovsky L, et al. Objective radiologic assessment of body composition in patients with end-stage liver disease: going beyond the BMI. Transplantation 2013;95(4):617–22.
39. Durand F, Buyse S, Francoz C, et al. Prognostic value of muscle atrophy in cirrhosis using psoas muscle thickness on computed tomography. J Hepatol 2014;60(6):1151–7.
40. Englesbe MJ, Patel SP, He K, et al. Sarcopenia and mortality after liver transplantation. J Am Coll Surg 2010;211(2):271–8.
41. Giusto M, Lattanzi B, Albanese C, et al. Sarcopenia in liver cirrhosis. Eur J Gastroenterol Hepatol 2015;27(3):328–34.
42. Hamaguchi Y, Kaido T, Okumura S, et al. Impact of quality as well as quantity of skeletal muscle on outcomes after liver transplantation. Liver Transpl 2014;20:1413–9.
43. Krell RW, Kaul DR, Martin AR, et al. Association between sarcopenia and the risk of serious infection among adults undergoing liver transplantation. Liver Transpl 2013;19(12):1396–402.
44. Masuda T, Shirabe K, Ikegami T, et al. Sarcopenia is a prognostic factor in living donor liver transplantation. Liver Transpl 2014;20(4):401–7.
45. Meza-Junco J, Montano-Loza AJ, Baracos VE, et al. Sarcopenia as a prognostic index of nutritional status in concurrent cirrhosis and hepatocellular carcinoma. J Clin Gastroenterol 2013;47(10):861–70.
46. Toshima T, Shirabe K, Kurihara T, et al. Profile of plasma amino acids values as a predictor of sepsis in patients following living donor liver transplantation: special reference to sarcopenia and postoperative early nutrition. Hepatol Res 2015;45(12):1170–7.
47. Tsien C, Garber A, Narayanan A, et al. Post-liver transplantation sarcopenia in cirrhosis: a prospective evaluation. J Gastroenterol Hepatol 2014;29(6):1250–7.
48. Valero V, Amini N, Spolverato G, et al. Sarcopenia adversely impacts postoperative complications following resection or transplantation in patients with primary liver tumors. J Gastrointest Surg 2015;19(2):272–81.
49. Waits SA, Kim EK, Terjimanian MN, et al. Morphometric age and mortality after liver transplant. JAMA Surg 2014;149(4):335.
50. Yadav A, Chang Y-H, Carpenter S, et al. Relationship between sarcopenia, six-minute walk distance and health-related quality of life in liver transplant candidates. Clin Transpl 2015;29(2):134–41.
51. Shen W. Total body skeletal muscle and adipose tissue volumes: estimation from a single abdominal cross-sectional image. J Appl Physiol (1985) 2004;97(6):2333–8.
52. Tandon P, Low G, Mourtzakis M, et al. A model to identify sarcopenia in patients with cirrhosis. Clin Gastroenterol Hepatol 2016;14(10):1473–80.e3.

53. Ebadi M, Wang CW, Lai JC, et al. Poor performance of psoas muscle index for identification of patients with higher waitlist mortality risk in cirrhosis. J Cachexia Sarcopenia Muscle 2018;9(6):1053–62.

54. van Vugt JLA, Levolger S, de Bruin RWF, et al. Systematic review and meta-analysis of the impact of computed tomography-assessed skeletal muscle mass on outcome in patients awaiting or undergoing liver transplantation. Am J Transplant 2016;16(8):2277–92.

55. Newman AB, Kupelian V, Visser M, et al. Sarcopenia: alternative definitions and associations with lower extremity function. J Am Geriatr Soc 2003;51(11): 1602–9.

56. Shaw KA, Srikanth VK, Fryer JL, et al. Dual energy X-ray absorptiometry body composition and aging in a population-based older cohort. Int J Obes 2007; 31(2):279–84.

57. Kaido T, Ogawa K, Fujimoto Y, et al. Impact of sarcopenia on survival in patients undergoing living donor liver transplantation. Am J Transplant 2013;13(6): 1549–56.

58. Guralnik JM, Simonsick EM, Ferrucci L, et al. A short physical performance Battery assessing lower extremity function: association with self-reported disability and prediction of mortality and nursing home admission. J Gerontol 1994;49(2): M85–94.

59. Pavasini R, Guralnik J, Brown JC, et al. Short physical performance Battery and all-cause mortality: systematic review and meta-analysis. BMC Med 2016;14(1). https://doi.org/10.1186/s12916-016-0763-7.

60. Lai JC, Covinsky KE, Dodge JL, et al. Development of a novel frailty index to predict mortality in patients with end-stage liver disease. Hepatology 2017; 66(2):564–74.

61. Lai JC, Covinsky KE, McCulloch CE, et al. The liver frailty index improves mortality prediction of the subjective clinician assessment in patients with cirrhosis. Am J Gastroenterol 2017;113(2):235–42.

62. Lai JC, Segev DL, McCulloch CE, et al. Physical frailty after liver transplantation. Am J Transplant 2018. https://doi.org/10.1111/ajt.14675.

63. Jones JC, Coombes JS, MacDonald GA. Exercise capacity and muscle strength in patients with cirrhosis. Liver Transpl 2012;18(2):146–51.

64. Wiesinger GF, Quittan M, Zimmermann K, et al. Physical performance and health-related quality of life in men on a liver transplantation waiting list. J Rehabil Med 2001;33(6):260–5.

65. Terziyski K, Andonov V, Marinov B, et al. Exercise performance and ventilatory efficiency in patients with mild and moderate liver cirrhosis. Clin Exp Pharmacol Physiol 2008;35(2):135–40.

66. Campillo B, Fouet P, Bonnet JC, et al. Submaximal oxygen consumption in liver cirrhosis. Evidence of severe functional aerobic impairment. J Hepatol 1990; 10(2):163–7.

67. Epstein SK, Ciubotaru RL, Zilberberg MD, et al. Analysis of impaired exercise capacity in patients with cirrhosis. Dig Dis Sci 1998;43(8):1701–7.

68. Epstein SK, Zilberberg MD, Jacoby C, et al. Response to symptom-limited exercise in patients with the hepatopulmonary syndrome. Chest 1998;114(3): 736–41.

69. Ma Z, Lee SS. Cirrhotic cardiomyopathy: getting to the heart of the matter. Hepatology 1996;24(2):451–9.

70. Wong F, Girgrah N, Graba J, et al. The cardiac response to exercise in cirrhosis. Gut 2001;49(2):268–75.

71. Epstein SK, Freeman RB, Khayat A, et al. Aerobic capacity is associated with 100-day outcome after hepatic transplantation. Liver Transpl 2004;10(3): 418–24.

72. Dharancy S, Lemyze M, Boleslawski E, et al. Impact of impaired aerobic capacity on liver transplant candidates. Transplantation 2008;86(8):1077–83.

73. Andersen H, Borre M, Jakobsen J, et al. Decreased muscle strength in patients with alcoholic liver cirrhosis in relation to nutritional status, alcohol abstinence, liver function, and neuropathy. Hepatology 1998;27(5):1200–6.

74. Montano-Loza AJ. Clinical relevance of sarcopenia in patients with cirrhosis. World J Gastroenterol 2014;20(25):8061–71.

75. Zoli M, Marchesini G, Dondi C, et al. Myofibrillar protein catabolic rates in cirrhotic patients with and without muscle wasting. Clin Sci 1982;62(6):683–6.

76. Kohno M, Fujii T, Hirayama C. [15N]glycine metabolism in normal and cirrhotic subjects. Biochem Med Metab Biol 1990;43(3):201–13.

77. Morrison WL, Bouchier IA, Gibson JN, et al. Skeletal muscle and whole-body protein turnover in cirrhosis. Clin Sci (Lond) 1990;78:613–9.

78. Kallwitz ER. Sarcopenia and liver transplant: the relevance of too little muscle mass. World J Gastroenterol 2015;21(39):10982–93.

79. Dolz C, Raurich JM, Ibanez J, et al. Ascites increases the resting energy expenditure in liver cirrhosis. Gastroenterology 1991;100(3):738–44.

80. Tandon P, Raman M, Mourtzakis M, et al. A practical approach to nutritional screening and assessment in cirrhosis. Hepatology 2017;65(3):1044–57.

81. Akerman PA, Jenkins RL, Bistrian BR. Preoperative nutrition assessment in liver transplantation. Nutrition 1993;9(4):350–6.

82. Porayko MK, DiCecco S, O'Keefe SJD. Impact of malnutrition and its therapy on liver transplantation. Semin Liver Dis 1991;11(4):305–14.

83. Norman K, Kirchner H, Lochs H, et al. Malnutrition affects quality of life in gastroenterology patients. World J Gastroenterol 2006;12(21):3380–5.

84. Detsky a S, McLaughlin JR, Baker JP, et al. What is subjective global assessment of nutritional status? JPEN J Parenter Enteral Nutr 1987;11(1):8–13.

85. Stephenson GR, Moretti EW, El-Moalem H, et al. Malnutrition in liver transplant patients: preoperative subjective global assessment is predictive of outcome after liver transplantation. Transplantation 2001;72(4):666–70.

86. Moctezuma-Velazquez C, Ebadi M, Bhanji RA, et al. Limited performance of subjective global assessment compared to computed tomography-determined sarcopenia in predicting adverse clinical outcomes in patients with cirrhosis. Clin Nutr 2018. https://doi.org/10.1016/j.clnu.2018.11.024.

87. Alberino F, Gatta A, Amodio P, et al. Nutrition and survival in patients with liver cirrhosis. Nutrition 2001;17(6):445–50.

88. Bakshi N, Singh K. Nutrition assessment and its effect on various clinical variables among patients undergoing liver transplant. Hepatobiliary Surg Nutr 2016;5(4):358–71.

89. Sanchez AJ, Aranda-Michel J. Nutrition for the liver transplant patient. Liver Transpl 2006;12(9):1310–6.

90. Selberg O, Böttcher J, Tusch G, et al. Identification of high- and low-risk patients before liver transplantation: a prospective cohort study of nutritional and metabolic parameters in 150 patients. Hepatology 1997;25(3):652–7.

91. Helton WS. Nutritional issues in hepatobiliary surgery. Semin Liver Dis 1994; 14(2):140–57.

92. Nompleggi DJ, Bonkovsky HL. Nutritional supplementation in chronic liver disease: an analytical review. Hepatology 1994;19(2):518–33.

93. Gottschlich M, Mattox T, Mueller C. The A.S.P.E.N. NUTRITION SUPPORT CORE CURRICULUM. ASPEN Nutr Support core Curric a case-based approach - adult patient. 2007:495–500.

94. Vilstrup H, Amodio P, Bajaj J, et al. Hepatic encephalopathy in chronic liver disease: 2014 practice guideline by the European association for the study of the liver and the American Association for the Study of Liver Diseases. J Hepatol 2014;61(3):642–59.

95. Amodio P, Bemeur C, Butterworth R, et al. The nutritional management of hepatic encephalopathy in patients with cirrhosis: International Society for Hepatic Encephalopathy and Nitrogen Metabolism Consensus. Hepatology 2013; 58(1):325–36.

96. Haq SM, Dayal HH. Chronic liver disease and consumption of raw oysters: a potentially lethal combination - a review of Vibrio vulnificus septicemia. Am J Gastroenterol 2005;100(5):1195–9.

97. Cheung K, Lee SS, Raman M. Prevalence and mechanisms of malnutrition in patients with advanced liver disease, and nutrition management strategies. Clin Gastroenterol Hepatol 2012;10(2):117–25.

98. Maharshi S, Sharma BC, Sachdeva S, et al. Efficacy of nutritional therapy for patients with cirrhosis and minimal hepatic encephalopathy in a randomized trial. Clin Gastroenterol Hepatol 2016;14(3):454–60.e3.

99. Plank LD, Gane EJ, Peng S, et al. Nocturnal nutritional supplementation improves total body protein status of patients with liver cirrhosis: a randomized 12-month trial. Hepatology 2008;48(2):557–66.

100. Tsien CD, Mccullough AJ, Dasarathy S. Late evening snack: exploiting a period of anabolic opportunity in cirrhosis. J Gastroenterol Hepatol 2012;27(3):430–41.

101. Rivera Irigoin R, Abilés J. [Nutritional support in patients with liver cirrhosis]. Gastroenterol Hepatol 2012;35(8):594–601.

102. Tsiaousi ET, Hatzitolios AI, Trygonis SK, et al. Malnutrition in end stage liver disease: recommendations and nutritional support. J Gastroenterol Hepatol 2008; 23(4):527–33.

103. Les I, Doval E, García-Martínez R, et al. Effects of branched-chain amino acids supplementation in patients with cirrhosis and a previous episode of hepatic encephalopathy: a randomized study. Am J Gastroenterol 2011;106(6):1081–8.

104. Neviere R, Edme JL, Montaigne D, et al. Prognostic implications of preoperative aerobic capacity and exercise oscillatory ventilation after liver transplantation. Am J Transplant 2014;14(1):88–95.

105. Bernal W, Martin-Mateos R, Lipcsey M, et al. Aerobic capacity during cardiopulmonary exercise testing and survival with and without liver transplantation for patients with chronic liver disease. Liver Transpl 2014;20(1):54–62.

106. Román E, Torrades MT, Nadal MJ, et al. Randomized pilot study: effects of an exercise programme and leucine supplementation in patients with cirrhosis. Dig Dis Sci 2014;59(8):1966–75.

107. Roman E, Garcia-Galceran C, Torrades T, et al. Effects of an exercise programme on functional capacity, body composition and risk of falls in patients with cirrhosis: a randomized clinical trial. PLoS One 2016;11(3):1–15.

108. Zenith L, Meena N, Ramadi A, et al. Eight weeks of exercise training increases aerobic capacity and muscle mass and reduces fatigue in patients with cirrhosis. Clin Gastroenterol Hepatol 2014;12(11):1920–6.e2.

109. Ritland S, Petlund CF, Knudsen T, et al. Improvement of physical capacity after long-term training in patients with chronic active hepatitis. Scand J Gastroenterol 1983;18(8):1083–7.

110. Debette-Gratien M, Tabouret T, Antonini MT, et al. Personalized adapted physical activity before liver transplantation: acceptability and results. Transplantation 2015;99(1):145–50.
111. Brustia R, Savier E, Scatton O. Physical exercise in cirrhotic patients: towards prehabilitation on waiting list for liver transplantation. A systematic review and meta-analysis. Clin Res Hepatol Gastroentero 2018;42(3):205–15.
112. Macías-Rodríguez RU, Ilarraza-Lomelí H, Ruiz-Margáin A, et al. Changes in hepatic venous pressure gradient Induced by physical exercise in cirrhosis: results of a pilot randomized open clinical trial. Clin Transl Gastroenterol 2016; 7(7):e180.
113. Duarte-Rojo A, Ruiz-Margáin A, Montaño-Loza AJ, et al. Exercise and physical activity for patients with end-stage liver disease: improving functional status and sarcopenia while on the transplant waiting list. Liver Transpl 2018;24(1):122–39.
114. García-Pagàn JC, Santos C, Barberá JA, et al. Physical exercise increases portal pressure in patients with cirrhosis and portal hypertension. Gastroenterology 1996;111(5):1300–6.
115. Tsien C, Shah SN, Mccullough AJ, et al. Reversal of sarcopenia predicts survival after a transjugular intrahepatic portosystemic stent. Eur J Gastroenterol Hepatol 2013;25(1):85–93.
116. Plauth M, Schütz T, Buckendahl DP, et al. Weight gain after transjugular intrahepatic portosystemic shunt is associated with improvement in body composition in malnourished patients with cirrhosis and hypermetabolism. J Hepatol 2004; 40(2):228–33.
117. Montomoli J, Holland-Fischer P, Bianchi G, et al. Body composition changes after transjugular intrahepatic portosystemic shunt in patients with cirrhosis. World J Gastroenterol 2010;16(3):348–53.

Hepatic Encephalopathy Challenges, Burden, and Diagnostic and Therapeutic Approach

Beshoy Yanny, MD[a],*, Adam Winters, MD[a], Sandra Boutros[b], Sammy Saab, MD, MPH[a,b,c]

KEYWORDS

- Hepatic encephalopathy • Liver cirrhosis • Portal hypertension
- Refractory hepatic encephalopathy

KEY POINTS

- Hepatic encephalopathy (HE) is an important cause of morbidity and mortality in patients with cirrhosis.
- The impact of HE on the health care system is similarly profound.
- The number of hospital admissions for HE has increased in the last 10-year period.
- Patients with HE are also at high risk of hospital readmission.
- HE is a huge burden to the patients, care givers, and the health care system.

INTRODUCTION

Hepatic encephalopathy (HE) is one of the most common and debilitating complications of liver disease. It is a reversible neurologic condition caused by the failure of the liver to detoxify blood in the portal circulation, either because of an insufficiency of the liver or shunting between the portal and systemic vasculature. Along with variceal hemorrhage, ascites, and jaundice, HE is a manifestation of hepatic

Role in the study: Study concept and design (B. Yanny, S. Saab); acquisition of data (B. Yanny, A. Winters); analysis and interpretation of data (B. Yanny, A. Winters); drafting of the article (B. Yanny, A. Winters, S. Boutros); critical revision of the article for important intellectual content (B. Yanny, A. Winters, S. Saab); administrative, technical, or material support; study supervision (B. Yanny, S. Saab).
Authors have no disclosures to declare.
[a] Department of Medicine, University of California at Los Angeles, 1223 16th street, suite 3100, Santa Monica, CA 90404, USA; [b] Department of Surgery, University of California at Los Angeles, 200 medical plaza, 3rd floor, Los Angeles, CA 90095, USA; [c] Department of Nursing, University of California at Los Angeles, 200 medical plaza, 3rd floor, Los Angeles, CA 90095, USA
* Corresponding author.
E-mail address: byanny@mednet.ucla.edu

decompensation in cirrhotic patients. In addition to its broad impact on the health of cirrhotic patients, HE presents a significant, increasing burden to the health care system, highlighting the need for better strategies designed to improve the diagnosis of subclinical disease and subsequent treatment.

Symptoms of HE are wide-ranging, although often subtle, and typically reflect the severity of underlying disease. The most recent joint guidelines from the American Association for the Study of Liver Disease (AASLD) and European Association for the Study of the Liver (EASL) suggest a universal definition of HE: "a brain dysfunction caused by liver insufficiency and/or [portosystemic shunting]; it manifests as a wide spectrum of neurological or psychiatric abnormalities ranging from subclinical alterations to coma."[1] Given the spectrum of clinical manifestations, these guidelines have introduced the terms covert HE (CHE) and overt HE (OHE) to encompass the continuum of disease. OHE represents disease that is readily obvious to providers and family members, comprising symptoms such as confusion and behavioral changes, whereas CHE is subtle and typically requires office-based screening to reliably detect.

EPIDEMIOLOGY AND BURDEN OF DISEASE

HE is a common disorder of cirrhosis and has wide-ranging effects on patients, their caregivers, and the health care system. Because of its often overlapping clinical presentation, the reported epidemiology of HE varies greatly. In 2 studies of patients with alcohol-related disease, the prevalence of OHE at the diagnosis of cirrhosis was between 6% and 13%.[2,3] In decompensated cirrhosis, OHE is estimated to occur in 16% to 21% of patients at the time of diagnosis.[4,5] CHE has been detected in 20% to 53% of cirrhotic patients using various office-based diagnostic tests.[6–10] With regard to patients undergoing transjugular intrahepatic portosystemic shunting, 1-year incidence of OHE is between 27% and 53%.[11,12] Overall, patients' risk of recurrence of OHE increases with each subsequent episode.[13]

HE is an important contributor to mortality in cirrhotic patients. In a study of 111 cirrhotic patients, survival rates at 1 and 3 years for patients who developed HE were 42% and 23%, respectively, in patients who developed grade 3 and 4 HE[14] Patients on the waitlist for liver transplant with more advanced HE (grades 3 and 4) have significantly higher mortalities (66% greater risk of death) than those without HE or with more mild disease.[15] In a study of more than 10,000 patients waitlisted for liver transplant, patients with severe HE (defined as West Haven criteria [WHC] grade 3 to 4) and a Model for End-stage Liver Disease score (MELD) greater than or equal to 30 had a 58% higher 90-day waitlist mortality than those with a MELD greater than or equal to 30 without severe HE.[16] Further, they found that patients with a MELD of 30 to 34 and severe HE (defined as WHC grade 3 to 4) had a similar 90-day mortality (71.1%) to patients with MELD greater than or equal to 35 without severe HE, implicating HE as an important, independent driver of mortality in patients awaiting liver transplant.

The effects of HE encompass not only the patients' physical health but permeates into the psychological, financial, and personal facets of their lives.[17] For example, the presence of prior HE has been shown to drastically lower rates of employment (87.5% vs 19%).[17] Further, HE imposes a greater burden on caregivers compared with cirrhotic patients without a history of HE. Caregivers of patients with a prior diagnosis of HE have significantly higher scores on both the Perceived Caregiver Burden scale and Zarit Burden Interview test than those without.[17] Caregiver scores correlated with the degree of cognitive impairment experienced by the patients.

Despite the importance of the role of the caregiver on the diagnosis and routine care of patients with HE, they may have poor insight into the disease. In a real-world questionnaire-based study of patients with previously diagnosed HE and their caretakers, only 48% of caretakers were aware of a prior diagnosis of HE and, more concerningly, only 6% were aware that their relative was on treatment.[18]

The impact of HE on the health care system is similarly profound. The number of hospital admissions for HE increased in the 10-year period between 2004 and 2014: 95,232 to 156,205.[19] Costs per admission for HE are also increasing. Between the years 2005 and 2009, total inpatient charges increased from $46,663 to $63,108 per case.[20] Total charges during that same period increased from $4.677 billion to more than $7 billion. Average length of stay also increased. Patients with HE are also at high risk of hospital readmission; 38.4% were readmitted within 30 days, and an additional 13.6% reentered the hospital within 31 to 90 days of their last stay.[20] In a study of 1 health care system in Minnesota, HE was the most common reason for readmission of cirrhotic patients to their community centers.[21] In a population-based study of cirrhotic patients with inpatient admissions in 6 states, HE was the complication of liver disease most strongly associated with 30-day and 90-day readmission rates.[22] Another study designed to evaluate readmission rates in cirrhotic patients found HE to be the most common cause of preventable readmissions.[23]

PATHOPHYSIOLOGY

The pathophysiology precipitating HE is complex and incompletely understood. The interplay of increased concentrations of ammonia, alterations in amino acid metabolism, and inflammation are central to the current understanding of the disease.[24] Hyperammonemia in particular forms the primary target of many current therapies.

Most ammonia synthesis occurs in the intestine, with some contribution from muscle and kidney.[25] Amino acids, notably glutamine, from dietary proteins are metabolized to ammonia in the colon. Ammonia-rich blood is directed through the portal circulation, where it is metabolized by the liver and predominantly cleared by the kidneys.[24,26] When the liver experiences injury, hepatic metabolism of ammonia is impaired and the portal hypertension resulting from chronic liver disease causes a shunting of ammonia into the systemic circulation.[27] At high concentrations, ammonia crosses the blood-brain barrier, where it is taken up by astrocytes, the primary driver of neurologic injury in HE.[24] Ammonia is metabolized with glutamate to form glutamine precipitating the formation of reactive oxygen species, which cause inflammation. Second, high concentrations of glutamine cause an osmotic gradient leading to astrocyte swelling and cerebral edema and, thus, neuronal dysfunction.

Other pathogenic mechanisms contributing to HE have been described. In both acute liver failure (ALF) and cirrhosis, alterations are seen in the permeability of the blood-brain barrier, allowing more entry of, in part, glutamate, causing additional formation of toxic glutamine (discussed earlier).[25] Alterations in the production and use of neurotransmitters, specifically γ-aminobutyric acid and serotonin, are also thought to play a role in phenomena such as alterations in the sleep-wake cycle.[28]

CLASSIFICATION AND GRADING

HE is characterized by the cause of underlying disease, severity of each episode, time course of each episode, and whether there is a precipitating cause.[1,29] There are 3 defined types of HE that are based on the cause of disease. Type A encephalopathy occurs in the setting of ALF. Type B refers to encephalopathy in the setting of portal-systemic shunting without organic liver disease. Type C is HE in the presence of cirrhosis.

HE can then be subdivided based on severity using the WHC[16] (**Table 1**). The WHC divides each episode into 4 separate grades. Grade 1 is characterized by a trivial lack of awareness, euphoria or anxiety, shortened attention span, impairment in simple arithmetic, and an altered sleep rhythm. Grade 2 defines episodes featuring lethargy or apathy, disorientation to time, obvious personality changes, inappropriate behavior, dyspraxia, and asterixis. Patients with grade 3 are somnolent or semistuporous, confused, and grossly disoriented, but they are responsive to stimuli. Grade 4 is reserved for comatose patients who do not respond to any stimuli, including pain. A fifth category, minimal HE (MHE), is only detected by psychomotor or neurophysiologic testing without overt clinical symptoms. Together with grade 1, MHE is considered CHE, whereas grades 2 to 4 are consistent with OHE.

HE can further be subdivided based on time course: episodic HE, recurrent HE (episodes occurring within 6 months of each other), or persistent HE (ongoing behavioral alterations that are exacerbated by bouts of OHE). In addition, each HE episode can be nonprecipitated or precipitated (ie, in the setting of concomitant infection or gastrointestinal bleeding).

DIAGNOSIS

The presentation of HE is often nonspecific and shares clinical features with many other disorders. Careful history and physical examination are essential to diagnosis. Care should be taken to assess for the presence of alternative causes as well as other disorders potentiating encephalopathy, such as uremia, hyponatremia, diabetes mellitus, and sepsis.[30–42] Owing to the spectrum of presentations that comprises the continuum of HE, diagnostic testing differs depending on the severity of symptoms.

DIAGNOSIS OF COVERT HEPATIC ENCEPHALOPATHY

CHE (ie, patients with MHE or WHC grade 1 encephalopathy) can be difficult to diagnose given the relative lack of clinically appreciable symptoms. Detecting MHE remains important because of the psychiatric and financial consequences it may incur. For example, patients with cirrhosis and MHE are at higher risk of falls than cirrhotic patients without MHE, leading to increased health care use, including hospitalization.[43] In addition, it serves as an important intervention point for providers to counsel patients and family members or caretakers about HE.[30] One commonly

Table 1			
Hepatic encephalopathy classification and grading according to West Haven criteria			
Grade 1	Grade 2	Grade 3	Grade 4
Mild	Moderate	Severe	Comatose
• Confusion • Short attention span • Irritability	• Disoriented • Fatigue • Personality changes • Obvious disorientation	• Incoordination • Inactive but arousable • Still responsive to vocal stimuli • Muscular rigidity • Hyporeflexia	Complete unresponsiveness

Data from Wong RJ, Gish RG, Ahmed A. Hepatic encephalopathy is associated with significantly increased mortality among patients awaiting liver transplantation. *Liver Transpl.* 2014;20(12):1454-1461.

used tool for diagnosing MHE is the Psychometric Hepatic Encephalopathy Score (PHES). It comprises the sum of 5 subtests designed to detect cognitive impairment: number connection tests A and B, a digit symbol test, serial dotting test, and a line tracing test.[44] Other modalities have been studied for use in CHE, notable the Stroop test, which has been shown to have excellent sensitivity (80%) compared with the PHES.[45] The Stroop test is important in that it is available as a free downloadable smartphone application (EncephalApp Stroop Test), which has shown similarly good sensitivity in detecting MHE.[45,46] This kind of readily available, inexpensive screening test is an important tool in the diagnostic armamentarium, allowing patients and providers to detect HE in the early stages.

DIAGNOSIS OF OVERT HEPATIC ENCEPHALOPATHY

The diagnosis of OHE is clinical and is made based on 3 grades of the WHC (2–4), as discussed earlier.[30] A high index of suspicion for precipitating events, such as infection, kidney injury, or infection, is an essential component of diagnosis and subsequent treatment. Other causes of encephalopathy should be ruled out, such as stroke or electrolyte abnormalities. Clinical presentation varies, although the International Society for Hepatic Encephalopathy and Nitrogen Metabolism (ISHEN) defines the onset of disorientation or asterixis as the characteristics defining OHE.[1,47–55] Asterixis is not specific to HE, because it may occur in other metabolic abnormalities, such as uremia and hypercarbia.[56,57]

THE ROLE OF AMMONIA

Although high levels of serum ammonia contribute to the pathophysiology of HE, there is little diagnostic or prognostic value in measuring ammonia in patients with chronic liver disease.[1] However, patients who show signs of OHE and have normal ammonia concentrations should prompt consideration of alternative diagnoses.

In contrast, in patients with ALF there is evidence that plasma ammonia level does correlate with the severity of HE.[58,59] Increased arterial ammonia levels in ALF are also an independent risk factor for increased intracranial pressure and brain herniation.[31,35,55,59–68] Further, significantly increased ammonia levels on admission may be predictive of mortality in patients presenting with ALF.[69] Increased blood ammonia level alone does not add any diagnostic, staging, or prognostic value for HE in patients with CLD. A normal value calls for diagnostic reevaluation (grade II-3, A, 1).[31] Ammonia level greater than 200 µmol/L is predictive of poor outcome in ALF.[2] Ammonia levels may be altered by inappropriate collection. Appropriate ammonia measurement requires an arterial blood sample that is immediately sent to the laboratory on ice and processed.[31,60] Venous ammonia levels may not correlate well with HE.

REFRACTORY HEPATIC ENCEPHALOPATHY

Refractory HE is often used to describe individuals with severe HE that is not responsive to the widely used and recommended medication regimens.[31,59,60] Studies defining refractory HE are scarce and there is no uniform agreement on treatment duration before diagnosing a patient with refractory HE. Studies have previously coined the diagnosis of refractory HE after 24 to 48 hours of failed lactulose with and without the use of rifaximin therapy in the absence of other precipitating factors.[13,31,32,60,69,70] A proposed diagnostic and therapeutic approach in patients with HE includes identifying any precipitating events in patients with grade 3 to 4 HE, including infection, gastrointestinal bleeding, medications, dehydrations, electrolyte abnormalities, and hypoglycemia, and reversing any precipitating events in addition to lactulose therapy. If there is no improvement in 24 hours, ensure that the patient has an adequate stool output and reevaluate the diagnosis to verify that the patient does have HE.[31,59,60] Strongly consider head imaging with computed tomography or MRI. If work-up is negative and HE is confirmed, add rifaximin if the patient is not already taking rifaximin or neomycin. Rifaximin is preferred to the side effect profile of neomycin (discussed later). If there is no improvement, the diagnosis of refractory HE can be made. If the patient has a MELD of less than 12 to 15, evaluate for a large portosystemic shunt such as a splenorenal shunt; if present, discuss embolization with interventional radiology and embolize if feasible. If there is no improvement, other rescue therapies can be used, including zinc, L-ornithine L-aspartate (LOLA), branched-chain amino acids (BCAAs), and sodium benzoate, and also consider molecular adsorbent recirculating system (MARS) if available. All patients who recover should be on maintenance therapy with lactulose and rifaximin unless otherwise contraindicated.[31,59,60] If the MELD score is high enough based on the United Network for Organ Sharing (UNOS) region, refer for evaluation for for liver transplant and list. On rare occasions, a MELD exception may be obtained with approval of the transplant committee and UNOS. **Fig. 1** outlines the diagnostic approach and management of refractory HE.

TREATMENT
Overt Hepatic Encephalopathy

Most patients require maintenance medications for OHE as secondary prophylaxis on hospital discharge after an episode of HE.[31,60,69] The most widely used regimen during hospital inpatient admission uses the nonabsorbable disaccharide lactulose in addition to rifaximin in some cases.[31,71-79] Treatment modalities, mechanism of action, and side effects are summarized in **Table 2**.

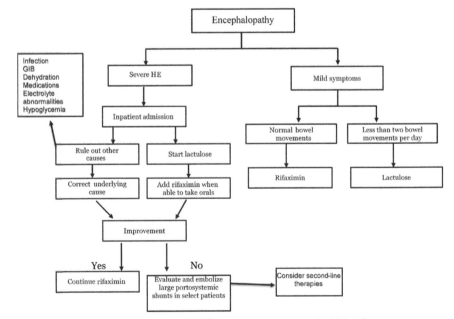

Fig. 1. General approach to patients with HE. GIB, gastrointestinal bleeding.

Table 2
Hepatic encephalopathy treatment modality and efficacy

Treatment Modality	Mechanism of Action	Efficacy Based on Previous Studies	Major Side Effects	References
NADs Lactulose or Lactitol	Lactulose (β-galactosidofructose) and lactitol (β-galactosidosorbitol) reduce ammonia levels by acidification of the colon with resultant conversion of ammonia to ammonium, shifting the colonic flora from urease-producing to non–urease-producing bacterial species, and by its cathartic effect	Considered standard of care Treatment associated with a reduction in mortality in patients with OHE, although not in patients with minimal HE	Use of NADs was associated with nonserious gastrointestinal adverse events	Als-Nielsen et al,[69] 2000; Gluud,[70] 2016
Rifaximin	Poorly absorbed antibiotic that works by altering the gut microbiota and theoretically decreasing the ammonia-producing microorganisms	Treatment with rifaximin maintained remission from HE more than placebo. Reduced the risk of hospitalization involving HE	Infections are of special interest because of known potential side effects of systemic antibiotics	Bass et al,[32] 2010
Neomycin	Neomycin is a poorly absorbed aminoglycoside used to decrease gut bacteria–derived ammonia and is FDA approved for use in acute (episodic), OHE but not chronic HE	FDA approved drug for treatment of acute HE, but not chronic HE. Studies found it not to be as effective as lactulose	May result in nephrotoxicity and ototoxicity	Mcguire & Sibae[80] 2009
Zinc	Ammonia is converted to urea by ornithyl transcarbamylase in the liver and is combined with glutamate by glutamine synthetase in the skeletal muscle to form glutamine	Inversely correlated with blood ammonia. Experimental studies have shown that zinc supplements improve ammonia detoxification	Excessive zinc intake may result in nausea, vomiting, loss of appetite, abdominal cramps, diarrhea, and headaches	Riggio,[81] 2010
LOLA	A compound salt that stimulates ornithine transcarbamoylase and carbamoyl phosphate synthetase, and is a substrate for the formation of urea	In a small trial, the use of LOLA resulted in improvement in mental status and cognitive function in patients with chronic overt and minimal encephalopathy	No major adverse effects reported	Mcguire & Sibae,[80] 2009

(continued on next page)

Table 2
(continued)

Treatment Modality	Mechanism of Action	Efficacy Based on Previous Studies	Major Side Effects	References
SB	SB is thought to be a metabolically active agent in which benzoate is first conjugated by CoA to form benzoyl CoA, which then conjugates with glycine in liver and kidney mitochondria to form hippurate, which, in turn, is rapidly excreted by the kidneys via glomerular filtration and tubular secretion.[12,58,59] One mole of hippurate contains 1 mol of waste nitrogen	SB showed an efficacy similar to lactulose in patients with episodic precipitant-induced HE	The prolonged use of SB can interfere with the management of ascites because it induces a significant sodium load	Riggio,[81] 2010
BCAAs	Theoretically, the plasma amino acid profile in patients with cirrhosis is altered with a decrease in BCAAs and increase in aromatic amino acids	BCAAs increased the number of patients improving from HE compared with control treatments, without any convincing evidence of any effect on survival	No adverse effects. Cannot prevent postoperative HE	Riggio,[81] 2010
MARS	This system was designed to remove protein/albumin-bound toxins such as bilirubin, bile acids, nitrous oxide, and endogenous benzodiazepines and also removes non–protein-bound ammonia that accumulates in liver failure	The FDA approved MARS as a toxin removal device in cases of drug overdose and poisoning; however, it is not approved for HE. The MARS dialysis-treated group had a more significant and rapid improvement in their mental status compared with standard medical therapy	MARS is associated with earlier and more frequent improvement. No adverse effects reported	Leise et al,[31] 2014

Abbreviations: CoA, coenzyme A; FDA, US food and drug administration; NADs, nonabsorbable disaccharides; SB, sodium benzoate.

Nonabsorbable disaccharides

Lactulose (β-galactosidofructose) and lactitol (β-galactosidosorbitol) reduce ammonia levels by acidification of the colon with resultant conversion of ammonia to ammonium, shifting the colonic flora from urease-producing to non–urease-producing bacterial species, and by its cathartic effect. Clinical guidelines recommend lactulose or lactitol as first-line therapy because of their proven efficacy over the years. The results of a large meta-analysis in 2004 showed that nonabsorbable disaccharides were superior to placebo and were associated with beneficial effects on HE, mortality, and serious adverse events.[31,40,60] Nonabsorbable disaccharides are administered orally, by mouth or through a nasogastric tube, or via retention enemas[1,2] initiated at 25 mL every 1 to 2 hours to achieve greater than or equal to 2 soft or loose stools per day.[31]

Rifaximin

Rifaximin a poorly absorbed antibiotic that works by altering the gut microbiota and theoretically decreasing the numbers of ammonia-producing microorganisms. Rifaximin is approved by the US Food and Drug Administration (FDA) for secondary prophylaxis of HE. Secondary prophylaxis is important and appropriate management to reduce the risk of another recurrence in all patients recovering from an episode of OHE. AASLD/EASL recommend secondary prophylaxis with rifaximin to reduce the risk of another OHE recurrence while on lactulose.[34] A 2016 consensus statement on management of HE published in the *European Journal of Gastroenterology & Hepatology* additionally supports the AASLD/EASL guidelines, highlighting that prompt initiation of appropriate management can reduce the duration of admission and reduce the risk of subsequent readmission.[34,69,70] Studies to date are still unable to elucidate the role of rifaximin monotherapy for OHE.[31,42,48–51,82–94] A few clinical trials show that rifaximin is as efficacious as lactulose in the treatment of OHE; however, those clinical trials have not been replicated to date and there is a lack of real-world data.[31,60] The increased use of rifaximin for episodic HE is supported by 1 clinical trial to date that compared lactulose plus placebo with lactulose plus rifaximin in patients hospitalized for HE and showed that 80% of patients had severe HE, grade III or IV, and 70% were Child class C, with the remainder Child class B.[31,33,35,82] Patients in the lactulose and rifaximin group had a higher proportion of complete reversal of HE (76% vs 50.8%; P<.004), shorter hospital stays, and a striking improvement in 10-day mortality (49.1% vs 23.8%; P<.05).[31,82] The very high mortality in the lactulose plus placebo arm raises some concerns about the validity of this study, which should be repeated in a larger number of patients at multiple sites. Clinical guidelines recommend rifaximin as prophylactic therapy for secondary prevention of HE.

Neomycin

Neomycin should be avoided in the routine treatment of HE. However, it may be considered in select patients with refractory HE. Neomycin is a poorly absorbed aminoglycoside used to decrease gut bacteria–derived ammonia. It is FDA approved for use in acute(episodic), OHE but not chronic HE. Real-world studies do not show much efficacy in the use of neomycin. In general, the evidence for neomycin in episodic OHE is weak, and its use is complicated by the risk of ototoxicity and nephrotoxicity. Although FDA approved, the decreased efficacy and high side effect profile compared with other therapies limit its clinical utility.[31,32,60,69,70,80,81] The risk of side effects hinders this agent's use in the armamentarium for HE.[31,32,60,69,70,80,81]

Zinc

Zinc is considered nonstandard therapy for HE, but it may be considered in patients not responsive to initial therapy trials. Ammonia is converted to urea by ornithyl transcarbamylase in the liver and is combined with glutamate by glutamine synthetase in the skeletal muscle to form glutamine.[31] Both ammonia-reduction pathways are impaired by zinc deficiency. Treatment with zinc has been shown to enhance the formation of urea from ammonia and amino acids. Studies show that zinc improved HE in 54% of patients with HE grade I to II that was previously refractory to standard therapy. Overall, there are insufficient data to define the optimal dose of zinc; however, the most frequently used dose was noted to be in zinc sulfate form at 600 mg/d.[31,32,60,69,70,80–82,95,96] Zinc is fairly well tolerated, with the rare side effects of dyspepsia and copper deficiency (with chronic, high-dose use), and it can decrease the effectiveness of ciprofloxacin if taken at the same time, which may pose a problem for patients undergoing spontaneous bacterial peritonitis prophylaxis with ciprofloxacin.[31,96]

L-Ornithine L-aspartate

LOLA is a compound salt that stimulates ornithine transcarbamoylase and carbamoyl phosphate synthetase, and is a substrate for the formation of urea. LOLA also works by stimulating glutamine synthesis in the skeletal muscle and consequently decreasing ammonia levels. The data for the use of this medication are scarce but some small randomized controlled trials show that patients with grade II HE or greater had improvement in HE grade on standard medical therapy (SMT) plus LOLA (79%) versus SMT plus placebo (55%), which was significant ($P = .019$).[31,33]

Sodium benzoate

Small studies show that sodium benzoate may be effective in a select group of patients with HE. Sodium benzoate is thought to be a metabolically active agent in which benzoate is first conjugated by coenzyme A to form benzoyl coenzyme A, which then conjugates with glycine in liver and kidney mitochondria to form hippurate (hippuric acid, N-benzoylglycine), which, in turn, is rapidly excreted by the kidneys via glomerular filtration and tubular secretion.[12,58,59] One mole of hippurate contains 1 mol of waste nitrogen. Thus, 1 mol of nitrogen is removed per mole of benzoate when it is conjugated with glycine (one-half as much nitrogen as is excreted in urea).[31] The data for the use of sodium benzoate are scarce to date. The largest study evaluating the effectiveness of sodium benzoate versus lactulose was a prospective, randomized, double-blind study involving 74 consecutive patients with cirrhosis or surgical portosystemic anastomosis and HE of fewer than 7 days' duration.[70] Recovery was achieved in 80% of patients receiving sodium benzoate after lactulose failure. The limitation of this study is that the number of participants was 74 patients.

Branched-chain amino acids

BCAAs have been previously used as salvage therapy. In theory, the plasma amino acid profile in patients with cirrhosis is altered with a decrease in BCAAs and increase in aromatic amino acids. The BCAAs are a source of glutamate, which helps to metabolize ammonia in skeletal muscle, therefore decreasing systemic ammonia waste. Two randomized controlled trials showed that BCAAs improved important composite end points of death/hospitalization metrics (in 1 study) and hepatic failure, variceal bleeding, HCC, and mortality.[44,45] At present, the European Society for Clinical Nutrition and Metabolism (ESPEN) recommend use of 1.2 g/kg/d of protein for compensated cirrhosis, and 1.5 g/kg/d in decompensated cirrhosis. This recommendation was based on the results of a randomized controlled trial of a normal protein diet (1.2 g/kg/d) versus a restricted diet showing no effect on the outcome of episodic HE, but increased muscle breakdown in the low protein diet group.[56]

Molecular adsorbent recirculating system

MARS is based on the concept of albumin dialysis. This system was designed to remove protein/albumin-bound toxins such as bilirubin, bile acids, nitrous oxide, and endogenous benzodiazepines, and it also removes the non–protein-bound ammonia that accumulates in liver failure.[31] One of the largest trials for the MARS system (RELIEF trial) enrolled 189 patients with acute-on-chronic liver failure and evaluated MARS plus SMT versus SMT alone, on the primary end points of 28-day and 90-day liver transplant–free survival.[31,34] Survival end points were not met, but safety was established. There was a higher proportion of patients with MELD greater than 20 (78.9% vs 69.7%; $P = .16$) and Spontaneous bacterial Peritonitis (14.4% vs 6.7%; $P = .94$) at baseline in the MARS treatment group.[31,34] The proportion of patients with HE grade III to IV HE improvement to HE grade 0 to I was higher in MARS-treated patients (15 out of 24; 62.5%) compared with SMT (13 out of 34; 38.2%) which trended toward statistical significance ($P = .07$).[31]

Shunt embolization

Large portosystemic shunts cause escape of ammonia-rich blood through the shunt to the systemic circulation without liver detoxification, therefore causing HE or worsening existing HE Therefore, embolization of large shunts may be an option for a select group of patients with refractory HE. Two large retrospective series have been published showing the efficacy and safety of embolization of large portosystemic shunts in medically refractory HE. In a European multicenter cohort study (n = 37), 59% of patients were free of HE within 100 days and 48% were HE free over an average of 2 years after embolization.[58] The median MELD in both studies was 13.[31,35] Logistic regression performed in the European study suggested that patients with MELD greater than 11 were at risk of HE recurrence after shunt embolization.[31,35]

There are emerging data on the techniques, safety, and efficacy of this modality, but more data are needed before solidifying the role of this treatment in the management paradigm. Some series have reported an increased risk of portal hypertensive bleeding after embolization of large shunts, whereas others have suggested poor outcomes with mortality within 3 months.[34] In the series with high mortality, it was postulated that these outcomes were related to candidate selection because patients undergoing embolization had Child-Pugh class C cirrhosis. The ideal candidates for shunt embolization are currently not well defined and must be highly selected.[31–35,60,69,70,80–82,95,96]

SUMMARY

HE poses a large burden on the patients and the health care system because of the high costs associated with admissions, work-up needed to reach the diagnosis, and high rate of readmission. Patient and family education is a key component in early recognition, treatment, and prevention of hospital admission. Despite the best efforts of health care professionals, HE remains a devastating complication of liver cirrhosis and portal hypertension. Larger multicenter studies are needed to reach a consensus on the approach to making the diagnosis, defining refractory HE, and management.

REFERENCES

1. Vilstrup H, Amodio P, Bajaj J, et al. Hepatic encephalopathy in chronic liver disease: 2014 practice guideline by the American Association for the Study of Liver Diseases and the European Association for the Study of the Liver. Hepatology 2014;60(2):715–35.

2. Jepsen P, Ott P, Andersen PK, et al. Clinical course of alcoholic liver cirrhosis: a Danish population-based cohort study. Hepatology 2010;51(5):1675–82.

3. Saunders JB, Walters JR, Davies AP, et al. A 20-year prospective study of cirrhosis. Br Med J (Clin Res Ed) 1981;282(6260):263–6.

4. Coltorti M, Del Vecchio-Blanco C, Caporaso N, et al. Liver cirrhosis in Italy. A multicentre study on presenting modalities and the impact on health care resources. National Project on Liver Cirrhosis Group. Ital J Gastroenterol 1991;23(1):42–8.

5. D'Amico G, Morabito A, Pagliaro L, et al. Survival and prognostic indicators in compensated and decompensated cirrhosis. Dig Dis Sci 1986;31(5):468–75.

6. Romero-Gomez M, Cordoba J, Jover R, et al. Value of the critical flicker frequency in patients with minimal hepatic encephalopathy. Hepatology 2007;45(4):879–85.

7. Groeneweg M, Moerland W, Quero JC, et al. Screening of subclinical hepatic encephalopathy. J Hepatol 2000;32(5):748–53.

8. Sharma P, Sharma BC, Puri V, et al. Critical flicker frequency: diagnostic tool for minimal hepatic encephalopathy. J Hepatol 2007;47(1):67–73.

9. Saxena N, Bhatia M, Joshi YK, et al. Auditory P300 event-related potentials and number connection test for evaluation of subclinical hepatic encephalopathy in patients with cirrhosis of the liver: a follow-up study. J Gastroenterol Hepatol 2001;16(3):322–7.

10. Li YY, Nie YQ, Sha WH, et al. Prevalence of subclinical hepatic encephalopathy in cirrhotic patients in China. World J Gastroenterol 2004;10(16):2397–401.

11. Riggio O, Angeloni S, Salvatori FM, et al. Incidence, natural history, and risk factors of hepatic encephalopathy after transjugular intrahepatic portosystemic shunt with polytetrafluoroethylene-covered stent grafts. Am J Gastroenterol 2008;103(11):2738–46.

12. Fonio P, Discalzi A, Calandri M, et al. Incidence of hepatic encephalopathy after transjugular intrahepatic portosystemic shunt (TIPS) according to its severity and temporal grading classification. Radiol Med 2017;122(9):713–21.

13. Bannister CA, Orr JG, Reynolds AV, et al. Natural history of patients taking rifaximin-alpha for recurrent hepatic encephalopathy and risk of future overt episodes and mortality: a post-hoc analysis of clinical trials data. Clin Ther 2016; 38(5):1081–9.e4.

14. Bajaj JS, Wade JB, Gibson DP, et al. The multi-dimensional burden of cirrhosis and hepatic encephalopathy on patients and caregivers. Am J Gastroenterol 2011;106(9):1646–53.

15. Bustamante J, Rimola A, Ventura PJ, et al. Prognostic significance of hepatic encephalopathy in patients with cirrhosis. J Hepatol 1999;30(5):890–5.

16. Wong RJ, Gish RG, Ahmed A. Hepatic encephalopathy is associated with significantly increased mortality among patients awaiting liver transplantation. Liver Transpl 2014;20(12):1454–61.

17. Neff G, Zachry W 3rd. Systematic review of the economic burden of overt hepatic encephalopathy and pharmacoeconomic impact of rifaximin. Pharmacoeconomics 2018;36(7):809–22.

18. Stepanova M, Mishra A, Venkatesan C, et al. In-hospital mortality and economic burden associated with hepatic encephalopathy in the United States from 2005 to 2009. Clin Gastroenterol Hepatol 2012;10(9):1034–41.e1.

19. Chirapongsathorn S, Krittanawong C, Enders FT, et al. Incidence and cost analysis of hospital admission and 30-day readmission among patients with cirrhosis. Hepatol Commun 2018;2(2):188–98.

20. Tapper EB, Halbert B, Mellinger J. Rates of and reasons for hospital readmissions in patients with cirrhosis: a multistate population-based cohort study. Clin Gastroenterol Hepatol 2016;14(8):1181–8.e2.

21. Tapper EB, Jiang ZG, Patwardhan VR. Refining the ammonia hypothesis: a physiology-driven approach to the treatment of hepatic encephalopathy. Mayo Clin Proc 2015;90(5):646–58.

22. Gerber T, Schomerus H. Hepatic encephalopathy in liver cirrhosis: pathogenesis, diagnosis and management. Drugs 2000;60(6):1353–70.

23. Elwir S, Rahimi RS. Hepatic encephalopathy: an update on the pathophysiology and therapeutic options. J Clin Transl Hepatol 2017;5(2):142–51.

24. Wijdicks EF. Hepatic encephalopathy. N Engl J Med 2016;375(17):1660–70.

25. Grippon P, Le Poncin Lafitte M, Boschat M, et al. Evidence for the role of ammonia in the intracerebral transfer and metabolism of tryptophan. Hepatology 1986;6(4): 682–6.

26. Ferenci P, Lockwood A, Mullen K, et al. Hepatic encephalopathy–definition, nomenclature, diagnosis, and quantification: final report of the working party at the 11th World Congresses of Gastroenterology, Vienna, 1998. Hepatology 2002;35(3):716–21.

27. Ferenci P. Hepatic encephalopathy. Gastroenterol Rep (Oxf) 2017;5(2):138–47.

28. Weissenborn K. Diagnosis of minimal hepatic encephalopathy. J Clin Exp Hepatol 2015;5(Suppl 1):S54–9.

29. Allampati S, Duarte-Rojo A, Thacker LR, et al. Diagnosis of minimal hepatic encephalopathy using Stroop EncephalApp: a multicenter US-based, norm-based study. Am J Gastroenterol 2016;111(1):78–86.

30. Bajaj JS, Thacker LR, Heuman DM, et al. The Stroop smartphone application is a short and valid method to screen for minimal hepatic encephalopathy. Hepatology 2013;58(3):1122–32.

31. Leise MD, Poterucha JJ, Kamath PS, et al. Management of hepatic encephalopathy in the hospital. Mayo Clin Proc 2014;89:241–53.

32. Bass MN, Mullen KD, Sanyal A, et al. Rifaximin treatment in hepatic encephalopathy. N Engl J Med 2010;362(12):1071–81.

33. Abid S, Jafri W, Mumtaz K, et al. Efficacy of L-ornithine-L-aspartate as an adjuvant therapy in cirrhotic patients with hepatic encephalopathy. J Coll Physicians Surg Pak 2011;21:666–71.

34. Ruggero MA, Argento AC, Heavner MS, et al. Molecular Adsorbent Recirculating System (MARS((R))) removal of piperacillin/tazobactam in a patient with acetaminophen-induced acute liver failure. Transpl Infect Dis 2013;15:214–8.

35. Laleman W, Simon-Talero M, Maleux G, et al. Embolization of large spontaneous portosystemic shunts for refractory hepatic encephalopathy: a multicenter survey on safety and efficacy. Hepatology 2013;57:2448–57.

36. Suraweera D, Sundaram V, Saab S. Evaluation and management of hepatic encephalopathy: current status and future directions. Gut Liver 2016;10(4):509–19.

37. Saab S. Evaluation of the impact of rehospitalization in the management of hepatic encephalopathy. Int J Gen Med 2015;8:165–73.

38. Sharma P, Sharma BC, Agrawal A, et al. Primary prophylaxis of overt hepatic encephalopathy in patients with cirrhosis: an open labeled randomized controlled trial of lactulose versus no lactulose. J Gastroenterol Hepatol 2012;27:1329–35.

39. Bajaj JS, Pinkerton SD, Sanyal AJ, et al. Diagnosis and treatment of minimal hepatic encephalopathy to prevent motor vehicle accidents: a cost-effectiveness analysis. Hepatology 2012;55:1164–71.

40. Mullen KD, Sanyal AJ, Bass NM, et al. Rifaximin is safe and well tolerated for long-term maintenance of remission from overt hepatic encephalopathy. Clin Gastroenterol Hepatol 2014;12:1390–7.e2.

41. Neff GW, Jones M, Broda T, et al. Durability of rifaximin response in hepatic encephalopathy. J Clin Gastroenterol 2012;46:168–71.

42. Mohammad RA, Regal RE, Alaniz C. Combination therapy for the treatment and prevention of hepatic encephalopathy. Ann Pharmacother 2012;46:1559–63.

43. Bajaj JS, Wade JB, Sanyal AJ. Spectrum of neurocognitive impairment in cirrhosis: implications for the assessment of hepatic encephalopathy. Hepatology 2009;50(6):2014–21.

44. Bajaj JS. Review article: the modern management of hepatic encephalopathy. Aliment Pharmacol Ther 2010;31(5):537–47.

45. Weissenborn K, Bokemeyer M, Krause J, et al. Neurological and neuropsychiatric syndromes associated with liver disease. AIDS 2005;19(Suppl 3):S93–8.

46. Kundra A, Jain A, Banga A, et al. Evaluation of plasma ammonia levels in patients with acute liver failure and chronic liver disease and its correlation with the severity of hepatic encephalopathy and clinical features of raised intracranial tension. Clin Biochem 2005;38(8):696–9.

47. Bernal W, Hall C, Karvellas CJ, et al. Arterial ammonia and clinical risk factors for encephalopathy and intracranial hypertension in acute liver failure. Hepatology 2007;46(6):1844–52.

48. Rockey DC, Vierling JM, Mantry P, et al. Randomized, double-blind, controlled study of glycerol phenylbutyrate in hepatic encephalopathy. Hepatology 2014; 59:1073–83.

49. Ventura-Cots M, Arranz JA, Simón-Talero M, et al. Safety of ornithine phenylacetate in cirrhotic decompensated patients: an open-label, dose-escalating, single-cohort study. J Clin Gastroenterol 2013;47:881–7.

50. Jover-Cobos M, Khetan V, Jalan R. Treatment of hyperammonemia in liver failure. Curr Opin Clin Nutr Metab Care 2014;17:105–10.

51. Bai M, Yang Z, Qi X, et al. l-ornithine-l-aspartate for hepatic encephalopathy in patients with cirrhosis: a meta-analysis of randomized controlled trials. J Gastroenterol Hepatol 2013;28:783–92.

52. Sundaram V, Shaikh OS. Hepatic encephalopathy: pathophysiology and emerging therapies. Med Clin North Am 2009;93:819–36.

53. Chavez-Tapia NC, Cesar-Arce A, Barrientos-Gutiérrez T, et al. A systematic review and meta-analysis of the use of oral zinc in the treatment of hepatic encephalopathy. Nutr J 2013;12:74.

54. Mukund A, Rajesh S, Arora A, et al. Efficacy of balloon-occluded retrograde transvenous obliteration of large spontaneous lienorenal shunt in patients with severe recurrent hepatic encephalopathy with foam sclerotherapy: initial experience. J Vasc Interv Radiol 2012;23:1200–6.

55. An J, Kim KW, Han S, et al. Improvement in survival associated with embolisation of spontaneous portosystemic shunt in patients with recurrent hepatic encephalopathy. Aliment Pharmacol Ther 2014;39:1418–26.

56. Clemmesen JO, Larsen FS, Kondrup J, et al. Cerebral herniation in patients with acute liver failure is correlated with arterial ammonia concentration. Hepatology 1999;29(3):648–53.

57. Tofteng F, Hauerberg J, Hansen BA, et al. Persistent arterial hyperammonemia increases the concentration of glutamine and alanine in the brain and correlates with intracranial pressure in patients with fulminant hepatic failure. J Cereb Blood Flow Metab 2006;26(1):21–7.

58. Niranjan-Azadi AM, Araz F, Patel YA, et al. Ammonia level and mortality in acute liver failure: a single-center experience. Ann Transplant 2016;21:479–83.
59. Patidar KR, Bajaj JS. Covert and overt hepatic encephalopathy: diagnosis and management. Clin Gastroenterol Hepatol 2015;13(12):2048–61.
60. Pereira K, Carrion AF, Martin P, et al. Current diagnosis and management of post-transjugular intrahepatic portosystemic shunt refractory hepatic encephalopathy. Liver Int 2015;35(12):2487–94.
61. Zuckerman DA, Darcy MD, Bocchini TP, et al. Encephalopathy after transjugular intrahepatic portosystemic shunting: analysis of incidence and potential risk factors. AJR Am J Roentgenol 1997;169:1727–31.
62. Forauer AR, McLean GK. Transjugular intrahepatic portosystemic shunt constraining stent for the treatment of refractory postprocedural encephalopathy: a simple design utilizing a Palmaz stent and Wallstent. J Vasc Interv Radiol 1998; 9:443–6.
63. Sanyal AJ, Freedman AM, Shiffman ML, et al. Portosystemic encephalopathy after transjugular intrahepatic portosystemic shunt: results of a prospective controlled study. Hepatology 1994;20(1 Pt 1):46–55.
64. Riggio O, Merlli M, Pedretti G, et al. Hepatic encephalopathy after transjugular intrahepatic portosystemic shunt: incidence and risk factors. Dig Dis Sci 1996; 41:578–84.
65. Bureau C, Garcia-Pagan JC, Otal P, et al. Improved clinical outcome using polytetrafluoroethylene-coated stents for TIPS: results of a randomized study. Gastroenterology 2004;126:469–75.
66. Yang Z, Han G, Wu Q, et al. Patency and clinical outcomes of transjugular intrahepatic portosystemic shunt with polytetrafluoroethylene-covered stents versus bare stents: a meta-analysis. J Gastroenterol Hepatol 2010;25:1718–25.
67. Riggio O, Nardelli S, Moscucci F, et al. Hepatic encephalopathy after transjugular intrahepatic portosystemic shunt. Clin Liver Dis 2012;16:133–46.
68. Riggio O, Ridola L, Lucidi C, et al. Emerging issues in the use of transjugular intrahepatic portosystemic shunt (TIPS) for management of portal hypertension: time to update the guidelines? Dig Liver Dis 2010;42:462–7.
69. Als-Nielsen B, Kjaergard L, Gluud C. Nonabsorbable disaccharides for hepatic encephalopathy. Cochrane Database Syst Rev 2000;(2):CD003044.
70. Gluud LL, Vilstrup H, Morgan MY. Nonabsorbable disaccharides for hepatic encephalopathy: a systematic review and meta-analysis. Hepatology 2016;64(3): 908–22.
71. Bai M, Qi X, Yang Z, et al. Predictors of hepatic encephalopathy after transjugular intrahepatic portosystemic shunt in cirrhotic patients: a systematic review. J Gastroenterol Hepatol 2011;26:943–51.
72. Guevara M, Baccaro ME, Ríos J, et al. Risk factors for hepatic encephalopathy in patients with cirrhosis and refractory ascites: relevance of serum sodium concentration. Liver Int 2010;30:1137–42.
73. Riggio O, Masini A, Efrati C, et al. Pharmacological prophylaxis of hepatic encephalopathy after transjugular intrahepatic portosystemic shunt: a randomized controlled study. J Hepatol 2005;42:674–9.
74. Fanelli F, Salvatori FM, Rabuffi P, et al. Management of refractory hepatic encephalopathy after insertion of TIPS: long-term results of shunt reduction with hourglass-shaped balloon-expandable stent-graft. AJR Am J Roentgenol 2009; 193:1696–702.

75. Catalina MV, Barrio J, Anaya F, et al. Hepatic and systemic haemodynamic changes after MARS in patients with acute on chronic liver failure. Liver Int 2003;23(Suppl 3):39–43.

76. Sen S, Mookerjee RP, Cheshire LM, et al. Albumin dialysis reduces portal pressure acutely in patients with severe alcoholic hepatitis. J Hepatol 2005;43:142–8.

77. Laleman W, Wilmer A, Evenepoel P, et al. Effect of the molecular adsorbent recirculating system and Prometheus devices on systemic haemodynamics and vasoactive agents in patients with acute-on-chronic alcoholic liver failure. Crit Care 2006;10:R108.

78. Bañares R, Nevens F, Larsen FS, et al. Extracorporeal albumin dialysis with the molecular adsorbent recirculating system in acute-on-chronic liver failure: the RELIEF trial. Hepatology 2013;57:1153–62.

79. Amodio P. Hepatic encephalopathy. In: Lee SS, Moreau R, editors. Cirrhosis: a practical guide to management. Chichester (England): John Wiley & Sons; 2015. p. 105–23.

80. Mcguire B, Sibae MA. Current trends in the treatment of hepatic encephalopathy. Ther Clin Risk Manag 2009;5:617–26.

81. Riggio O. Hepatic encephalopathy therapy: an overview. World J Gastrointest Pharmacol Ther 2010;1(2):54.

82. Sharma BC, Sharma P, Lunia MK, et al. A randomized, double-blind, controlled trial comparing rifaximin plus lactulose with lactulose alone in treatment of overt hepatic encephalopathy. Am J Gastroenterol 2013;108(9):1458–63.

83. Pedretti G, Calzetti C, Missale G, et al. Rifaximin versus neomycin on hyperammoniemia in chronic portal systemic encephalopathy of cirrhotics: a double-blind, randomized trial. Ital J Gastroenterol 1991;23:175–8.

84. Jiang Q, Jiang XH, Zheng MH, et al. Rifaximin versus nonabsorbable disaccharides in the management of hepatic encephalopathy: a meta-analysis. Eur J Gastroenterol Hepatol 2008;20:1064–70.

85. Hawkins RA, Jessy J, Mans AM, et al. Neomycin reduces the intestinal production of ammonia from glutamine. Adv Exp Med Biol 1994;368:125–34.

86. Morgan MH, Read AE, Speller DC. Treatment of hepatic encephalopathy with metronidazole. Gut 1982;23:1–7.

87. Shavakhi A, Hashemi H, Tabesh E, et al. Multistrain probiotic and lactulose in the treatment of minimal hepatic encephalopathy. J Res Med Sci 2014;19:703–8.

88. Dhiman RK, Rana B, Agrawal S, et al. Probiotic VSL#3 reduces liver disease severity and hospitalization in patients with cirrhosis: a randomized, controlled trial. Gastroenterology 2014;147:1327–37.e3.

89. Lunia MK, Sharma BC, Sharma P, et al. Probiotics prevent hepatic encephalopathy in patients with cirrhosis: a randomized controlled trial. Clin Gastroenterol Hepatol 2014;12:1003–8.

90. Agrawal A, Sharma BC, Sharma P, et al. Secondary prophylaxis of hepatic encephalopathy in cirrhosis: an open-label, randomized controlled trial of lactulose, probiotics, and no therapy. Am J Gastroenterol 2012;107:1043–50.

91. Zhao LN, Yu T, Lan SY, et al. Probiotics can improve the clinical outcomes of hepatic encephalopathy: an update meta-analysis. Clin Res Hepatol Gastroenterol 2015;39:674–82.

92. Manning RT, Delp M. Management of hepatocerebral intoxication. N Engl J Med 1958;258:55–62.

93. Rahimi RS, Singal AG, Cuthbert JA, et al. Lactulose vs polyethylene glycol 3350: electrolyte solution for treatment of overt hepatic encephalopathy. The HELP randomized clinical trial. JAMA Intern Med 2014;174:1727–33.

94. Laccetti M, Manes G, Uomo G, et al. Flumazenil in the treatment of acute hepatic encephalopathy in cirrhotic patients: a double blind randomized placebo controlled study. Dig Liver Dis 2000;32:335–8.
95. Lynn AM, Singh S, Congly SE, et al. Embolization of portosystemic shunts for treatment of medically refractory hepatic encephalopathy. Liver Transpl 2016; 22(6):723–31.
96. Takuma Y, Nouso K, Makino Y, et al. Clinical trial: oral zinc in hepatic encephalopathy. Aliment Pharmacol Ther 2010;32(9):1080–90.

Varices
Esophageal, Gastric, and Rectal

Thomas O.G. Kovacs, MD[a],*, Dennis M. Jensen, MD[b,c]

KEYWORDS

- Esophageal varices • Gastric varices • Rectal varices • Portal hypertension
- UGI bleed • Band ligation • Sclerotherapy • Hematochezia

KEY POINTS

- Either esophageal band ligation and/or nonselective β-blockers (propranolol, nadolol, and carvedilol) are recommended for the prevention of first hemorrhage.
- For patients presenting with acute esophageal variceal bleed, volume resuscitation, vasoactive medications (octreotide), and prophylactic antibiotics should be initiated followed by urgent upper endoscopy and endoscopic hemostasis when variceal bleeding is suspected.
- Prevention of rebleeding from esophageal varices is best accomplished by an endoscopist experienced in management of upper gastrointestinal bleeding and combination of band ligation and/or sclerotherapy and nonselective β-blockers until varices are obliterated.
- For patients with gastric variceal hemorrhage, cyanoacrylate glue injection (if available), sclerotherapy, or band ligation (if technically possible) is recommended management.
- For patients with bleeding rectal varices, endoscopic treatment includes band ligation (if technically feasible), sclerotherapy, or cyanoacrylate glue injection (if available).

INTRODUCTION

Gastrointestinal (GI) varices are abnormally dilated submucosal veins usually caused by portal hypertension that can occur throughout the digestive tract, especially the esophagus, stomach, and rectum. Sometimes they also occur at surgical anastomotic sites. Among a large Center for Ulcer Research and Education (CURE) Hemostasis Research Group cohort of approximately 1000 patients with severe

[a] Division of Digestive Diseases, David Geffen School of Medicine at UCLA, Ronald Reagan – UCLA Medical Center, Olive View-UCLA Medical Center, Sylmar, CA, USA; [b] Medicine-GI, VA Greater Los Angeles Healthcare System, Ronald Reagan – UCLA Medical Center, David Geffen School of Medicine at UCLA, CURE:DDRC, Room 318, Building 115, 11301 Wilshire Boulevard, Los Angeles, CA 90073-1003, USA; [c] Human Studies Core and GI Hemostasis Research Unit, VA/CURE Digestive Disease Research Center, Los Angeles, CA, USA
* Corresponding author.
E-mail address: TKovacs@mednet.ucla.edu

Clin Liver Dis 23 (2019) 625–642
https://doi.org/10.1016/j.cld.2019.07.005
1089-3261/19/© 2019 Elsevier Inc. All rights reserved.
liver.theclinics.com

upper GI (UGI) bleeding, gastroesophageal varices (GOVs) comprised approximately 23% of cases[1] (**Fig. 1**). Variceal hemorrhage is associated with significant morbidity and mortality, which place a major burden on health care costs.[2] The prevalence of esophageal varices (EVs) increases with the severity of liver disease (Child-Pugh class A, 43%; Child-Pugh class B, 71%; and Child-Pugh class C, 76%).[3] Approximately 50% of patients with newly diagnosed cirrhosis have GOVs. Small EVs progress to large ones at a 10% annual rate. The annual variceal hemorrhage risk for small varices is 5% and for large ones is 15%.[4] The 6-week mortality rate after an index EV bleed, however, is approximately 20%[5] but ranges from 0% among patients with Child-Pugh class A to approximately 30% among patients with Child-Pugh class C disease.[6] Red wale marks on varices in addition to variceal size and decompensated liver disease identify patients at higher risk of variceal hemorrhage[7,8].

RISK STRATIFICATION

Increased blood flow through the portosystemic collaterals due to portal hypertension leads to dilation of the submucosal venous plexus producing elevated intravariceal pressure and increased wall tension in the varices (**Fig. 2**). The mechanism of variceal rupture is best described by the Laplace law—wall tension is related to the transmural pressure x variceal radius, divided by the variceal wall thickness.

Portal pressure increments produce increased flow through the varices and increased intravariceal pressure. Randomized controlled trials (RCTs) have reported that patients with hepatic venous pressure gradient (HPVG) less than 12 mm Hg (where the normal is 3–5 mm HG) do not develop variceal hemorrhage.[9] An HPVG greater than 20 mm Hg, however, is associated with an increased risk of failure to control hemorrhage and early rebleeding and death.[10] Reducing the HPVG greater than

Causes of Severe UGI Bleeding: DEP Study UCLA & VA

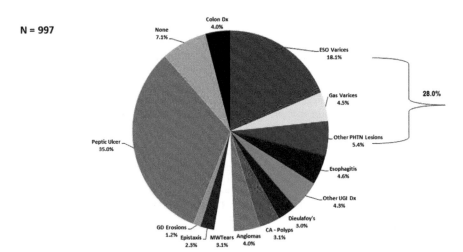

Fig. 1. Prevalence of diagnoses for severe UGI bleeding: CURE Hemostasis Research Group. CA, Cancer; Dx, Diagnoses; ESO, Esophageal; GD, Gastroduodenal; MWT, Mallory-Weiss tear; PHTN, Portal hypertension; UCLA, University of California at Los Angeles; VA, Veteran's Administration Greater Los Angeles Health Care System.

Veins of Distal Esophagus

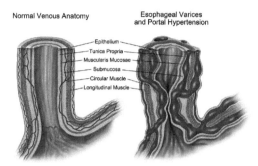

Normal Venous Anatomy

Esophageal Varices
and Portal Hypertension

Epithelium
Tunica Propria
Muscularis Mucosae
Submucosa
Circular Muscle
Longitudinal Muscle

Fig. 2. Veins of distal esophagus: normal venous anatomy and EVs with portal hypertension.

20% from baseline (by β-blockers or other drugs) decreases the risks of further bleeding and death.[11]

Esophagogastroduodenoscopy (EGD) is the gold standard for the diagnosis of esophagogastric varices and for estimating the size of the varices and finding high-risk stigmata, such as red wale marks. Endoscopy can discern whether varices are absent, small (<5 mm), medium, large (>5 mm), or giant size (>10 mm). Large or giant varices have a greater risk of bleeding due to higher wall tension. Red wale marks are another indicator of higher bleeding risk. Expense of and limited diagnostic sensitivity of current esophageal capsule endoscopy suggest it is not a useful alternative to upper endoscopy for esophagogastric variceal screening[12,13] or the detection of gastric varices.

Noninvasive tests have been used to predict the presence of esophagogastric varices, without much success, and do not correlate well with HPVG changes. Recently, in patients with compensated cirrhosis, a combination of liver stiffness (LS), measured by transient elastography (with LS <20 kPa), and platelet count (>150,000/mm^3) has been recommended as a method of identifying patients with a very low probability (<5%) of having high-risk varices.[14] Potentially, with such low scores, endoscopy could be avoided in these patients, representing approximately 20% to 25% of current screening endoscopies. These guidelines were recently validated in a large cohort of patients with hepatitis B virus–associated or hepatitis C virus–associated cirrhosis. The study showed that none of the 80 patients with LS less than 20 kPa and platelet counts greater than 150,000 had EVs requiring treatment.[15] Approximately 25% of the endoscopies could have been avoided, while missing only 1.3% of varices needing therapy.[15] Most cirrhotic patients with cirrhosis who do not meet those criteria, however, should have a screening upper endoscopy to diagnose and potentially treat esophagogastric varices.

For compensated cirrhotic patients who undergo screening endoscopy, current recommendations about esophagogastric varices include

1. If no varices are seen, screening endoscopy should be repeated every 2 years for ongoing active liver injury or every 3 years if the liver disease is quiescent.
2. If small varices are noted, endoscopy should be repeated yearly in patients with ongoing liver injury or every 2 years if the liver disease is quiescent.
3. Patients with compensated cirrhosis without varices who develop decompensation should have a repeat EGD when this occurs.[16]

There is no evidence to suggest that current medications, such as nonselective β-blockers (NSBBs), prevent the formation of EVs in patients who do not have them at baseline EGD.[17]

PREVENTION OF FIRST HEMORRHAGE IN ESOPHAGEAL VARICES

Primary prophylaxis of EV hemorrhage is indicated in patients at increased risk of bleeding. Patients with medium, large, or giant EVs; patients with small varices with red wale marks; and decompensated patients with small varices are candidates for primary prophylaxis.[7,15]

In patients with medium or large varices, meta-analyses of RCTs have shown that both NSBBs and band ligation are effective in preventing first variceal hemorrhage.[18] By consensus, either NSBBs (propranolol, nadolol, and carvedilol) or band ligation are recommended to prevent first variceal bleed in high-risk patients with EVs with medium or large varices (**Table 1**).[19]

Table 1
Prevention of first hemorrhage in cirrhotic patients: management recommendations

Therapy	Recommended Dose	Therapy Goals	Maintenance/Follow-up
EVL	• Every 4–6 wk until the eradication of varices	• Variceal eradication (no further ligation possible)	• First EGD performed 3–6 mo after eradication and every 6–12 mo thereafter
Propranolol	• 20–40 mg orally twice a day • Adjust every 2–3 d until treatment goal is achieved • Maximal daily dose: 320 mg/d in patients without ascites 160 mg/d in patients with ascites	• Resting heart rate of 55–60 beats per minute • Systolic blood pressure should not decrease <90 mm Hg • Titrate dose to reduce resting pulse to by 20%–25%	• At every outpatient visit check heart rate • Continue indefinitely • If used in combination with EVL, continue until EVs are eradicated
Nadolol	• 20–40 mg orally once a day • Adjust every 2–3 d until treatment goal is achieved • Maximal daily dose: 160 mg/d in patients without ascites 80 mg/d in patients with ascites	• Resting heart rate of 55–60 beats per minute • Systolic blood pressure should not decrease <90 mm Hg • Titrate dose to reduce resting pulse to by 20%–25%	• At every outpatient visit check heart rate • Continue indefinitely • If used in combination with EVL, continue until EVs are eradicated
Carvedilol	• Start with 6.25 mg once a day • After 3 d increase to 6.25 mg twice-daily • Maximal dose: 12.5 mg/d (except in patients with persistent arterial hypertension)	• Systolic arterial blood pressure should not decrease <90 mm Hg	• Continue indefinitely • If used in combination with EVL, continue until EVs are eradicated

Abbreviations: EV, Esophageal varices; EVL, Esophageal variceal ligation.

The potential advantages of NSBBs are low cost, no requirement for specific expertise to administer, and no need for surveillance endoscopy. Disadvantages of NSBBs include that approximately 15% to 20% of patients have absolute or relative contraindications to their use and another 15% to 20% develop side effects, such as shortness of breath, fatigue, and weakness, and need to discontinue or reduce dosage. Another major disadvantage is that patients with advanced cirrhosis and portal hypertension may respond poorly and that decreasing the pulse by 20% to 25% does not predictably reduce HPVG and the risk of bleeding in substantial proportion of patients.[19]

Advantages of band ligation are that it can be done during the initial screening endoscopy and there few contraindications. It is also well tolerated in patients.[19] Disadvantages are that sedation is required; procedural complications, such as post-banding ulcer bleeding and postbanding ulcers, may occur or bleed; and surveillance endoscopy is needed to monitor variceal obliteration and recurrence. The combination of NSBBs and band ligation was not more effective than banding alone in preventing bleeding or mortality in a RCT[20] and thus combination therapy is not usually recommended. The authors' preference based on relative patient intolerance to NSBBS and on outcomes with band ligation is for endoscopic intervention.[19]

In patients with small EVs at a high risk of bleeding, with red wale marks, and/or in decompensated cirrhotics, NSBBs are the suggested therapy.[16] For low-risk small varices, management is controversial, but limited evidence suggests that NSBBs may slow the growth of the small varices.[21] Individualization of management for primary prophylaxis is highly recommended. The main focus should be on whether high-risk varices are present and whether a patient prefers endoscopic, medical, or no therapy.

TREATMENT OF ACUTE ESOPHAGEAL VARICEAL HEMORRHAGE

Acute variceal hemorrhage is a medical emergency requiring urgent and intensive intervention. The essential treatment aims are the control of active bleeding, prevention of rebleeding, and reduction of early mortality (the main therapeutic outcome metric). All patients with variceal hemorrhage should be aggressively resuscitated to achieve hemodynamic stability and to protect the airway from aspiration, which is life threatening. Elective intubation is highly recommended in any patient with ongoing hematemesis, neurologic impairment, altered mental or respiratory disorders, or difficulty sedating with intravenous (IV) conscious sedation.

A recent RCT in patients with GI hemorrhage reported that restrictive packed red blood cell (pRBC) transfusion strategy (starting pRBC transfusion at a hemoglobin level of 7 g/dL and maintaining it at 7–9 g/dL) significantly reduced mortality compared with a liberal transfusion strategy (starting pRBC transfusion at a hemoglobin level of 9 g/dL and maintaining it at 9–11 g/dL).[22] The greatest benefit was observed in the subgroup of cirrhotic patients randomized to the restrictive transfusion protocol, who had significantly decreased early rebleeding and mortality rates. The benefits were for the Child-Pugh class A and Child-Pugh class B groups but not Child-Pugh class C.[22] This trial excluded patients with severe GI bleeding or comorbidities: active hemorrhage, severe hemodynamic compromise, and cardiac comorbidities. Therefore, the appropriate transfusion strategy needs to be carefully individualized for elderly patients with active bleeding, hypotension, and hypoperfusion and associated cardiovascular disorders, such as myocardial ischemia. In contrast, in a study of unselected patients at CURE (of no patients excluded) reported that adequate hemodynamic resuscitation and limiting red blood cell transfusions in cirrhotic patients did not increase mortality.[23] Clearly cirrhotic patient management before and after endoscopy needs to be individualized based on acute, severity of liver disease, and comorbidities.

Because cirrhotic patients with GI bleeding are at increased risk of developing bacterial infections, antibiotic prophylaxis has been demonstrated in RCTs to reduce infections, rebleeding, and mortality. Therefore, short-term (no longer than 7 days) antibiotic prophylaxis should be started in any cirrhotic patient and GI bleed. For example, IV ceftriaxone, 1 g/24 h, is the antibiotic of choice.[14]

Vasoactive medications (such as octreotide, somatostatin, vasopressin, and terlipressin) cause splanchnic vasoconstriction and can decrease portal pressure HVPG. One of these agents should be administered as an IV infusion as soon as variceal hemorrhage is suspected. A meta-analysis of 30 RCTs reported that vasoactive drug in acute EV bleeding decreased 7-day all-cause mortality and reduced transfusion requirements.[24] A selected vasoactive agent should be initiated prior to endoscopy. Octreotide is the only vasoactive medication available in the United States and a meta-analysis showed that it significantly reduced acute bleeding.[24] There were no significant differences in outcomes among patients treated with different agents—octreotide, somatostatin, or a vasopressin analog, terlipressin.[25] Vasoactive agents should be continued for 2 days to 5 days.

Currently, routine use of plasma products and platelet transfusions is not recommended. Similarly, platelet transfusions are not suggested for patients on antiplatelet medications with a normal platelet count. Although empirical, it seems reasonable to aim for an International Normalized Ratio score less than 2.0 and platelet count greater than $50,000/mm^3$ in hemodynamically unstable patients with active variceal hemorrhage. Evidence-based data are lacking to document this recommendation.

Erythromycin (250 mg IV) or metoclopramide (10 mg IV) given 30 minutes to 60 minutes before endoscopy increases gastric motility and may improve visualization during endoscopy. Clinical outcome improvements, however, have not been reported with use of these medications.

Upper endoscopy is recommended within 12 hours after presentation in cirrhotic patients with severe UGI hemorrhage once hemodynamic resuscitation has been achieved.[16] Initially, a therapeutic endoscope with a large suction channel and target irrigation is recommended. This facilitates suctioning of blood clots, target irrigation, and better visualization compared with a smaller diagnostic scope. A diagnosis of EVs as the source of a patient's UGI hemorrhage is based on the finding of a stigmata of recent hemorrhage, such as active bleeding (**Fig. 3**), a platelet plug (white nipple sign) (**Fig. 4**), or overlying clot or a combination of these, which indicates the bleeding site. Red markings on varices, veins-on-veins, or blood in the stomach and presence of varices without other potential sources of bleeding are less definitive but indicate that in the absence of other UGI findings that the EVs are the presumptive source of severe UGI hemorrhage. Red color signs or red wale marks on varices (**Fig. 5**) are predictors of higher risk for future bleeding and are not a definitive sign of recent hemorrhage.

Esophageal band ligation, first described by Van Stiegmann and Goff,[26] is the current treatment of choice for bleeding and nonbleeding EVS.

Band ligation results are excellent for most cases and provide high rates of initial hemostasis, low rates of rebleeding, few side effects, and improved survival compared with sclerotherapy. Variceal ligation with a diagnostic-sized endoscope can be used to control active variceal bleeding with bands placed over the actively bleeding varix or

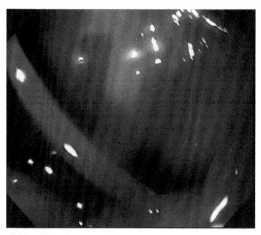

Fig. 3. Active variceal bleeding from an EV.

on the platelet plug (**Fig. 6**). The authors recommend that bands are placed distally, within 2 cm of the gastroesophageal junction (GEJ) (**Fig. 7**) and 4 cm to 6 cm proximally above the GEJ. Each bleeding and nonbleeding column of EVs should be treated similarly, with 2 bands per variceal column, placed in a spiral manner starting at the GEJ and moving proximally.

Brisk variceal hemorrhage may preclude the ability to do band ligation, either due to limited visibility or in adequate suctioning of the varix into the band housing. Endoscopic sclerotherapy is a useful alternative in such cases to control active bleeding prior to banding all varices (2 bands per column—1 distally and another proximally). The authors recommend injecting a sclerosant solution into (intravariceal) or adjacent (paraesophageal) the bleeding EV to control active bleeding. Several sclerosant solutions are available, with ethanolamine oleate (5%), polidocanol (1%–2%), and cyanoacrylate used most commonly. The authors' sclerotherapy technique through a therapeutic endoscope is to inject 1-mL to 1.5-mL aliquots per injection of

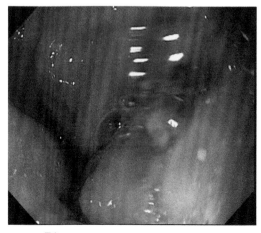

Fig. 4. Platelet plug on an EV.

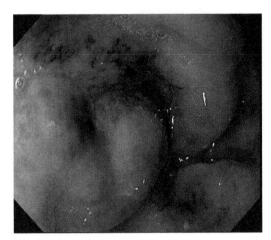

Fig. 5. Large EV with red wale marks.

ethanolamine oleate (5%) through a 25-gauge sclerotherapy needle, distal and proximal to the bleeding varix. Subsequently, all nonbleeding varices are treated with 2 bands/columns, as described previously with band ligation.

Other endoscopic modalities, such as clipping, thermal contact devices (such as multipolar coagulation or heater probe), or argon plasma coagulation, are not recommended for esophageal or gastric variceal hemostasis. These should be used for nonvariceal hemostasis.

The initial surveillance endoscopy is usually scheduled 1 week to 2 weeks after the index treatment of patients hospitalized for EV hemorrhage. Then, repeat EGDs are recommended at 4-week to 6-week intervals until all the EVs are completely obliterated. The use of a Doppler endoscopic probe (DEP) to monitor blood flow as guide to endoscopic therapy[27] improves clinical outcomes for cirrhotic patients with severe variceal bleeding. The DEP produces an audible signal related to the underlying venous blood flow of varices, allowing a distinction between arterial (higher-pitched pulsatile signal) and venous (low-pitched continuous signal) blood flow. A recent RCT of DEP monitoring in patients with severe variceal hemorrhage showed that

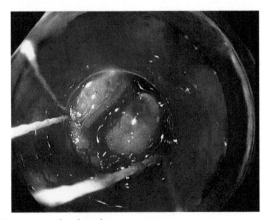

Fig. 6. Band ligation over a platelet plug.

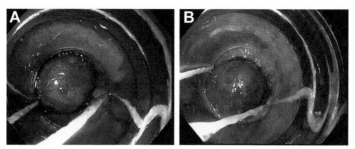

Fig. 7. Band ligation of a distal EV. (*A*) Acutely. (*B*) Follow-up band ligation.

DEP-guided endoscopic hemostasis reduced 30-day rates of rebleeding, transfusion requirement, and hospital stay.[28] Residual variceal blood flow after visually guided endoscopic therapy was strongly associated with variceal rebleeding. These improved outcomes suggest that DEP is extremely valuable in risk assessment and as a guide to completion of endoscopic treatment of patients with bleeding varices.

TREATMENT FAILURE

If variceal hemorrhage is not controlled by a combination of a vasoactive agent and endoscopic treatment, other techniques can be used as bridge to more definitive treatment. Sengstaken-Blakemore tubes have been utilized to tamponade varices. The rate of hemostasis ranges from 50% to 80%, with a rebleeding rate of approximately 50% after deflation of the balloons (usually within 24 hours).[16] Furthermore, reported serious side effects, including aspiration, esophageal ulcer formation, and esophageal perforation, occur frequently. Currently most physicians and surgeons have limited experience with tamponade tubes and their utilization should be limited.

Endoscopically placed self-expanding covered metal stents also can provide hemostasis of bleeding EVs. The stents expand inside the esophagus and tamponade the varices to produce hemostasis. The stents can be left in for up to 2 weeks (although stent retrieval is recommended after 7 days). Side effects, such as stent migration, ulcers, and rebleeding, after stent removal are less severe than for the Sengstaken-Blakemore tubes. Compared with balloon tamponade tubes, stents have been reported to have lower transfusion requirements and fewer serious adverse events but no survival advantage.[29] For patients with uncontrolled EV hemorrhage, stents may be a safer than balloon tamponade tubes and more effective bridge to definitive therapy.

Patients with persistent bleeding despite medical and endoscopic therapy should be considered for early transjugular intrahepatic portosystemic shunting (TIPS) with polytetrafluoroethylene stents.[30,31] TIPS involves the formation of a low-resistance channel between the hepatic vein and the intrahepatic portion of the portal vein using angiographic techniques. The shunt is kept open by using an expandable metal stent across it to allow blood to return to the systemic circulation. RCTs report that early TIPS (placed within 72 hours of admission) significantly decreased rates of treatment failure and mortality in Child-Pugh class B patients with active bleeding or Child-Pugh class C patients compared with standard management. Studies showing these benefits had multiple exclusion criteria, however, and therefore included only approximately 20% of the total patient group with variceal hemorrhage. The authors recommend that any patient with persistent bleeding or severe rebleeding, despite combination pharmacologic and endoscopic intervention, be considered for a TIPS. The availability of radiologists and of TIPS placement within the recommended time frame, however, may be problematic in many smaller centers. In patients with TIPS placed, vasoactive medications may be stopped. Portosystemic encephalopathy is a relative contraindication to TIPS placement, because TIPS may worsen encephalopathy.

When all other therapeutic interventions fail, shunt surgery may be a last option. Portosystemic shunts can control portal hypertension and reduce variceal rebleeding. The tradeoff, however, is the high encephalopathy rates and other perioperative surgical complications after the procedure. One RCT did report that emergency portocaval shunt surgery compared with TIPS provided improved rates of hemostasis and survival and a decreased rate of encephalopathy.[32] Distal shunts (such as splenorenal types) are reported to cause less encephalopathy than central shunts, such as portacaval or mesocaval shunts. Further studies are needed before the use of portocaval shunts after failure of combined medical and endoscopic treatment is recommended. Another problem currently is that experienced surgeons to perform emergency shunts for variceal bleeding are not available in most hospitals, including referral centers.

PREVENTION OF REBLEEDING

There is a high risk of rebleeding (60%–70% within 2 years) after a first episode of active variceal hemorrhage in high-risk patients, such as those with Child-Pugh class C cirrhosis, with accompanying mortality up to 33% on medical therapy alone. Therefore, it is critical to prevent rebleeding and appropriate treatment should be initiated while the patient is still in the hospital. This risk can be decreased to 45% by NSBB use,[33] to approximately 30% by band ligation,[34] and to approximately 25% by combining both treatments. Therefore, optimal secondary prophylactic therapy includes a combination of NSBBs (propranolol or nadolol) plus endoscopic band ligation (**Table 2**).[14] Band ligation should occur initially and within 1 week to 2 weeks of the index bleed with follow-up endoscopic surveillance and banding scheduled at 4-week to 6-week intervals until EVs are obliterated. Each EV should be banded near the GEJ and 4 cm to 6 cm above for 2 bands per variceal column. If EVs are too small to band, are scarred down, and/or have blood flow by DEP, the intravariceal sclerotherapy is recommended.[28] The authors recommend that junctional varices in a hiatal hernia be treated endoscopically similar to distal EVs.

A meta-analysis comparing band ligation or NSBBs to a combination of the 2 showed that the combined treatments were significantly more effective than either intervention alone.[35] Adding a long-acting nitrate (isosorbide mononitrate) to NSBBs decreased portal pressures further and was shown in a meta-analysis of the combination of NSBBs and nitrates compared with NSBBs to improve rebleeding and mortality while causing more side effects.[36] Reports suggest that patients with higher portal pressures respond better to NSBBs than patients with a lower HVPG.[37] Controversy exists about the safety and efficacy of NSBBs in patients with advanced liver disease, dating to a 2010 study implying that NSBBs increase mortality in patients with refractory ascites.[38] Subsequent studies, however, have not shown a harmful effect of NSBBs[39] if they are carefully titrated, and doses of propranolol over 160 mg/d or of nadolol over 80 mg/d are avoided.[40] NSBBs may not be appropriate in patients with hemodynamic instability or renal dysfunction. Current guidelines recommend a combination of band ligation and NSBBs for the prevention of recurrent variceal bleeding even in patients who bled while receiving primary prophylaxis with band ligation or NSBBs alone. If a patient is unable to tolerate NSBBs, band ligation alone is suggested, although TIPS may be a useful alternative, especially if the patient has

Table 2
Prevention of recurrent esophageal variceal hemorrhage: management recommendations

Therapy	Recommended Dose	Therapy Goals	Maintenance/Follow-up
EVL	• Every 4–6 wk until the eradication of varices	• Variceal eradication (no further ligation possible)	• First EGD performed 3–6 mo after eradication and every 6–12 mo thereafter
Propranolol	• 20–40 mg orally twice a day • Adjust every 2–3 d until treatment goal is achieved • Maximal daily dose: 320 mg/d in patients without ascites 160 mg/d in patients with ascites	• Resting heart rate of 55–60 beats per minute • Systolic blood pressure should not decrease <90 mm Hg • Reduction of resting pulse by 20%–25%	• At every outpatient visit check heart rate • Continue indefinitely, or if used in combination with EVL, until EVs are eradicated
Nadolol	• 20–40 mg orally once a day • Adjust every 2–3 d until treatment goal is achieved • Maximal daily dose: 160 mg/d in patients without ascites 80 mg/d in patients with ascites	• Reduction of resting pulse by 20%–25% • Resting heart rate of 55–60 beats per minute • Systolic blood pressure should not decrease <90 mm Hg	• At every outpatient visit check heart rate • Continue indefinitely or, if used in combination with EVL, until EVs are eradicated

A combination of EV ligation and either propranolol or nadolol is recommended.
Abbreviations: EV, Esophageal varices; EVL, Esophageal variceal ligation.

difficult-to-treat ascites.[16] Carvedilol has been compared with both band ligation alone and combined NSBBS and nitrates but not to the combination of banding and NSBBS. Therefore, carvedilol cannot be recommended for secondary prophylaxis at this time.

TIPS is the recommended rescue treatment in patients with recurrent bleeding despite combination therapy with band ligation and NSBBs. An RCT reported that TIPS (with covered stents) significantly reduced rebleeding compared with endoscopic hemostasis and NSBBs (0% vs 29%). TIPs, however, did not improve survival and increased early encephalopathy.[41] If TIPS is placed successfully, band ligation and NSBBs can be discontinued. HPVG responders (defined as an HPVG reduction <12 mm Hg or >20% decrease from baseline) have the lowest rebleeding rates. Therefore, HPVG measurement and monitoring during therapy are an ideal strategy in centers where available. Currently in the United States, HPVG is not available in most medical centers and is not the standard of care for secondary (or primary) management.[19]

GASTRIC VARICES

Gastric varices are less prevalent than EVs and occur in approximately 20% of cirrhotic patients. Sarin and colleagues'[42] classification of gastric varices includes GOV type 1, EVs extending below the GEJ along the lesser curve (most common—75% of all gastric varices); GOV type 2 , EVs extending into the stomach along the greater curve into the fundus (**Fig. 8**); isolated gastric varix type 1 (IGV1), isolated in the fundus; and isolated

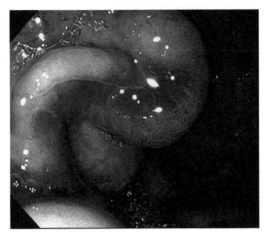

Fig. 8. Gastric varix in the fundus.

gastric varix type 2, located elsewhere in the stomach (body, antrum, or pylorus). Bleeding risk is associated with localization (IGV1> GOV2> GOV1), large size, presence of red color signs, and severity of hepatic disease. Gastric varices bleed less often than EVs but have a higher mortality due to the severity of the hemorrhage and response to medical and endoscopic therapies. Because fundic varices occur more frequently with portal or splenic vein thrombosis, especially in the context of malignancy or pancreatitis, radiologic imaging should be done to exclude venous thrombosis. Gastric varices are best diagnosed at endoscopy in resuscitated patients because they may not be seen on EGD in hypovolemic patients.

The guidelines for the management of gastric varices are much less evidence based than for EVs.

PREVENTION OF FIRST HEMORRHAGE FROM GASTRIC VARICES

To date, there has been only 1 RCT published on the primary prevention of gastric varices. It compared NSSBs, endoscopic cyanoacrylate glue injection, and observation of patients with large GOV2 and IGV1 varices. The glue group had decreased bleeding (10%) compared with the NSSBs group (38%) and observation group (53%). There was significantly better survival of the glue group (93%) compared with the observation group (74%) but not significantly better than the NSBBs group (83%).[43] Prevention of first hemorrhage from GOV1 varices has not been reported yet. GOV1 varices usually are managed based on the EV guidelines.[16]

Current recommendations for primary prophylaxis of gastric variceal bleeding are based on limited data but include for GOV2 and IGV1 varices—NSBBs may be used, and for GOV1 varices—follow the EVs guidelines. Neither TIPS nor balloon-occluded retrograde transvenous obliteration (BRTO) is recommended for preventing the first bleed in patients with fundic varices.

TREATMENT OF ACUTE HEMORRHAGE FROM GASTRIC VARICES

The initial management of patients with gastric variceal hemorrhage is similar to that of esophageal bleeding. Rudiments are airway protection, hemodynamic and volume resuscitation, blood transfusion (the authors recommended based on CURE studies of hemoglobin to ≥ 8 g)[23] and treatment of severe coagulopathies, admission to a monitored care area, vasoactive medications, and antibiotics prior to upper endoscopy. The definitive diagnosis of acute gastric variceal hemorrhage is based on the endoscopic findings of active bleeding, a platelet plug, or a clot overlying a gastric varix. A meta-analysis of endoscopic therapy showed that both band ligation and cyanoacrylate injection provided similar initial hemostasis rates, with significantly less rebleeding in the cyanoacrylate group.[44] The investigators of this Cochrane review, however, cautioned about their findings for all-cause and bleeding-related mortality, failure of intervention, adverse events, and control of bleeding because of the very low quality of the available studies and their results. Band ligation has a limited application in the treatment of gastric varices, because only small varices ($\leq$1 cm) can be effectively banded and adjacent varices need to be banded to prevent early rebleeding. Cyanoacrylate used in most clinical trials has been N-butyl-2-cyanoacrylate. Another glue, 2-octyl cyanoacrylate, which has a longer polymerization time, has also been reported to produce beneficial outcomes in acute gastric variceal hemorrhage.[45] Neither of these glues is Food and Drug Administration approved for treating gastric varices in the United States. Although glue injection is widely recommended as the treatment of choice for gastric variceal bleeding, endoscopic therapeutic skill and experience are required. Several major complications are reported, including stroke, pulmonary embolism, paraplegia, gastric ulcers and ulcer hemorrhage, and portal and splenic vein thrombosis. Combined glue injection and band ligation for gastric variceal hemorrhage has been advocated[46] but cannot be recommended at present because data from evidence-based studies, such as RCTs, are not available.

As described previously for EVs, DEP monitoring in gastric variceal bleeding can also significantly reduce rates of rebleeding, transfusion requirements, and duration of hospitalization.[28] Furthermore, residual blood flow after endoscopic therapy corelates closely with rebleeding.[28] Other endoscopic approaches, such as endoscopic ultrasound (EUS)–guided insertion of coils and/or cyanoacrylate, show promise. Studies in gastric variceal hemorrhage patients have reported that EUS-guided coil and glue injection reduced bleeding rates, transfusions, and mortality compared with glue injection.[47] No confirmatory larger studies or RCTs have been reported to confirm or expand these results.

For patients with uncontrolled gastric variceal bleeding despite endoscopic therapy, balloon tamponade with a Linton-Nachlas or Sengstaken-Blakemore tube may be a temporary bridge to more definitive intervention. If available, the Linton tube with its larger gastric balloon (500 mL), is recommended.

TIPS may be effective in some patients with continued bleeding from gastric varices. TIPS has not been compared in an RCT to either glue injection or band ligation for acute gastric variceal hemorrhage. TIPS should be considered early for bleeding fundic varices, which often are associated with early rebleeding after endoscopic or medical therapy.

The authors recommend that if bleeding occurs from GOV1 varices, either band ligation, if feasible, or glue injection be used for endoscopic hemostasis. If that fails or is unavailable, TIPS should be used for fundic varices (GOV2 or IGV1).[16]

PREVENTION OF REBLEEDING FROM GASTRIC VARICES

For patients who had index bleeding from GOV1 varices, a combination of endoscopic treatment (band ligation or cyanoacrylate injection) and NSBBs is the recommended therapy, as for EVs.[16] For patients with fundic gastric varices, repeated cyanoacrylate injection can reduce rebleeding and mortality compared with NSBBs[48] Combination therapy with glue injection and NSBBs did not improve outcomes in comparison to injection alone in fundic variceal patients.[49]

An RCT of patients with GOV1 and GOV2 varices showed that TIPS was associated with lower early rebleeding (11% vs 38%) and transfusion needs, compared with glue injection. There was no benefit, however, in initial hemostasis or survival and there was a higher rate of encephalopathy after TIPS.[50]

Patients with gastric fundic varices and gastro-splenorenal collaterals also can be managed with BRTO. This intervention is performed using angiographic techniques and includes retrograde cannulation of the left renal vein by the jugular or femoral vein, followed by balloon occlusion and slow infusion of sclerosant and/or coils to obliterate the gastro-splenorenal collateral and fundic varices.[51] Compared with TIPS, BRTO does not divert portal blood flow away from the liver but may increase portal pressure, potentially promoting EV bleeding and exacerbating ascites.[8] When BRTO was compared with TIPS in patients with acutely bleeding gastric varices, the BRTO group had significantly less rebleeding (9% vs 20%) at 1 year, but there was no survival advantage.[52] A recent retrospective study of patients with gastric variceal bleeding reported that BRTO improved rates of early hemostasis, rebleeding, and survival compared with TIPS.[53]

In summary, combination therapy with NSBBs and endoscopic hemostasis (band ligation or glue injection) is recommended for prevention of rebleeding in patients with GOV1 varices. TIPS or BRTO is recommended for patients with prior GOV2 or IGV1 variceal hemorrhage to reduce rebleeding.[16]

Rectal Varices

Rectal varices are defined as dilated rectal veins that originate at least 4 cm above the anal verge and are distinct from internal hemorrhoids and do not extend to the dentate line.[54] They originate from portosystemic anastomosis between the superior hemorrhoidal veins and the middle or inferior hemorrhoidal veins. The prevalence of rectal varices varies between 40% and 56% in cirrhotic patients and increases to 63% to 94% in patients with extrahepatic portal vein obstruction.[55] Clinically severe bleeding is uncommon, occurring in 0.5% to 5% of cirrhotic patients.[56] There are no established management guidelines to treat rectal variceal hemorrhage. Colonoscopy and flexible sigmoidoscopy are the main methods for diagnosing the presence of rectal varices, and these are best visualized in both retroflexed and end-on views in hemodynamically resuscitated patients (**Fig. 9**). Endoscopic band ligation is the

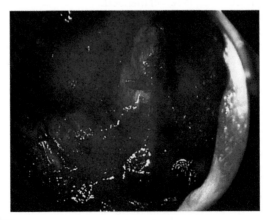

Fig. 9. Rectal varices.

recommended treatment modality. Sclerotherapy or glue injection can be utilized also, but rebleeding rates are high. Sclerotherapy is associated with frequent postinjection ulcer formation and glue is associated with an embolization rate of up to 4.3%.[55] EUS-guided coil and glue injection also may be useful in large bleeding rectal varices, which cannot be treated with band ligation. Subsequently, TIPS and BRTO are possible options, but the optimal management of rectal varices is currently uncertain.

SUMMARY

Despite current guidelines for the optimal management of variceal hemorrhage, morbidity and mortality related to bleeding are still substantial, especially in poor-risk cirrhotic patients. Although advances in medical, endoscopic, and radiologic interventions have improved patient outcomes by preventing the first bleed, treating acute hemorrhage, and preventing rebleeding, further innovations are needed to lessen the dire consequences of variceal hemorrhage in patients with decompensated liver disease.

ACKNOWLEDGMENTS

The research studies included in this article from the CURE: Digestive Diseases Research Center-Human Studies Core of Dennis M. Jensen, MD, were funded by grants from the VA Research Service (VA Clinical Merit Review CLIN-013–07F) and the NIH-NIDDK grant (P30 DK041301) to CURE: Digestive Diseases Research Center–Human Studies Core.

REFERENCES

1. Kovacs TO, Jensen DM. Gastrointestinal hemorrhage. In: Goldman L, Schafer A, editors. Goldman-cecil medicine. 25th edition. Elsevier Saunders; 2016. p. 879–84.
2. Gralnek IAM, Jensen DM, Kovacs TOG, et al. The economic impact of esophageal variceal hemorrhage: cost-effectiveness implications of endoscopic therapy. Hepatology 1999;29:44–50.
3. Kovalak M, Lake J, Mattek N, et al. Endoscopic screening for varices in cirrhotic patients: data from a national endoscopic database. Gastrointest Endosc 2007; 65:82–8.
4. North Italian Endoscopic Club for the Study and Treatment of Esophageal Varices. Prediction of the first variceal hemorrhage in patients with cirrhosis of the liver and esophageal varices. A prospective multicenter study. N Engl J Med 1988;319:983–9.
5. Amitrano L, Guardascione MA, Manguso F, et al. The effectiveness of current acute variceal bleed treatments in unselected cirrhotic patients: refining short-term prognosis and risk factors. Am J Gastroenterol 2012;107:1872–8.
6. Bosch J, Thabut D, Albillos A, et al. Recombinant factor VIIa for variceal bleeding in patients with advanced cirrhosis: a randomized controlled trial. Hepatology 2008;47:1604–14.
7. Jensen DM. Endoscopic screening for varices in cirrhosis: findings, implications, and outcomes. Gastroenterology 2002;122:1620–30.
8. Park JK, Saab S, Kee ST, et al. Balloon-occluded retrograde transvenous obliteration (BRTO) for treatment of gastric varices: review and Meta-analysis. Dig Dis Sci 2015;60:1543–53.

9. Groszmann RJ, Bosch J, Grace ND, et al. Hemodynamic events in a prospective randomized trial ofpropranolol versus placebo in the prevention of a first variceal hemorrhage. Gastroenterology 1990;99:1401–7.

10. Abraldes JG, Villanueva C, Banares R, et al, Spanish Cooperative Group for Portal Hypertension and Variceal Bleeding. Hepatic venous pressure gradient and prognosis in patients with acute variceal bleeding treated with pharmacologic and endoscopic therapy. J Hepatol 2008;48:229–36.

11. D'Amico G, Garcia-Pagan JC, Luca A, et al. Hepatic vein pressure gradient reduction and prevention of variceal bleeding in cirrhosis: a systematic review. Gastroenterology 2006;131:1611–24.

12. McCarty TR, Afinogenova Y, Njei B. Use of wireless capsule endoscopy for the diagnosis and grading of esophageal varices in patients with portal hypertension: a systematic review and meta-analysis. J Clin Gastroenterol 2017;51:174–82.

13. Chavalitdhamrong D, Jensen DM, Singh B, et al. Capsule endoscopy is not as accurate as esophagogastroduodenoscopy in screening cirrhotic patients for varices. Clin Gastroenterol Hepatol 2012;10:254–8.

14. De Franchis R, Baveno VI Faculty. Expanding consensus in portal hypertension. Report of the Baveno VI Consensus workshop: stratifying risk and individualizing care for portal hypertension. J Hepatol 2015;63:743–52.

15. Thabut D, Bureau C, Layese R, et al. Validation of Baveno VI criteria for screening and surveillance of esophageal varices in patients with compensated cirrhosis and a sustained response to antiviral therapy. Gastroenterology 2019;156: 997–1009.

16. Garcia-Tsao G, Abraldes J, Berzigotti A, et al. Portal hypertensive bleeding in cirrhosis: risk stratification, diagnosis, and management: 2016 practice guidance by the American Association for the Study of Liver diseases. Hepatology 2017;65: 310–35.

17. Groszmann RJ, Garcia-Tsao G, Bosch J, et al. Beta-blockers to prevent gastroesophageal varices in patients with cirrhosis. N Engl J Med 2005;353:2254–61.

18. Gluud LL, Krag A. Band ligation versus beta-blockers for primary prevention in oesophageal varices in adults. Cochrane Database Syst Rev 2012;(8):CD004544.

19. Jutabha R, Jensen DM, Martin P, et al. Randomized study comparing banding and propranolol to prevent initial variceal hemorrhage in cirrhotics with high-risk esophageal varices. Gastroenterology 2005;128:870–81.

20. Sarin SK, Wadhawan M, Agarwal SR, et al. Endoscopic variceal ligation plus propranolol versus endoscopic band ligation alone in primary prophylaxis of variceal bleeding. Am J Gastroenterol 2005;100:797–804.

21. Bhardwaj A, Kedarisetty CK, Vashishtha C, et al. Carvedilol delays the progression of small oesophageal varices in patients with cirrhosis: a randomized placebo-controlled trial. Gut 2017;66:1838–43.

22. Villanueva C, Colomo A, Bosch A, et al. Transfusion strategies for acute upper gastrointestinal bleeding. N Engl J Med 2013;368:11–21.

23. Jensen DM, Markovic D, Jensen ME, et al. Red cell transfusions do not increase 30 day mortality rates for unselected patients with severe UGI hemorrhage. Gastroenterology 2015;148:154.

24. Wells M, Chande N, Adams P, et al. Met-analysis: vasoactive medications for the management of acute variceal bleeds. Aliment Pharmacol Ther 2012;35: 11267–78.

25. Seo YS, Park SY, Kim MY, et al. Lack of difference among terlipressin, somatostatin and octreotide in the control of acute gastroesophageal variceal hemorrhage. Hepatology 2014;60:954–63.

26. Van Stiegman G, Goff JS. Endoscopic esophageal varix ligation: preliminary clinical experience. Gastrointest Endosc 1988;34:113–7.
27. Jensen DM, Kovacs TOG, Ohning CV, et al. Doppler endoscopic probe monitoring for blood flow improves risk stratification and outcomes of patients with severe non-variceal UGI hemorrhage. Gastroenterology 2017;152:1310–8.
28. Jensen DM, Jensen ME, Markovic D, et al. Doppler endoscopic probe improves outcomes of severe UGI hemorrhage from varices and other portal hypertension lesions. Gastroenterology 2018;154(Supplement 1):5529–30.
29. Escorsell A, Pavel O, Cardenas A, et al. Esophageal balloon tamponade versus esophageal stent in controlling acute refractory variceal bleeding: a multicenter randomized, controlled trial. Hepatology 2016;63:1957–67.
30. Garcia-Pagan JC, Caca K, Bureau C, et al. Early use of TIPS in patients with cirrhosis and variceal bleeding. N Engl J Med 2010;362:2370–9.
31. Thabut D, Pauwels A, Carbonell N, et al. Cirrhotic patients with portal hypertension-related bleeding and an indication for early-TIPS: a large multicentre audit with real-life results. J Hepatol 2018;68:73–81.
32. Oroff MJ, Hye R, Wheeler HO, et al. Randomized trials of endoscopic therapy and transjugular intrahepatic portosystemic shunt versus portocaval shunt for emergency and elective treatment of bleeding gastric varices in cirrhosis. Surgery 2015;157:1028–45.
33. Bernard B, Lebrec D, Mathurin P, et al. Beta-adrenergic antagonists in the prevention of gastrointestinal rebleeding in patients with cirrhosis: a meta-analysis. Hepatology 1997;25:63–70.
34. Thiele M, Krag A, Rohde U, et al. Meta-analysis: banding ligation and medical interventions for the prevention of rebleeding from oesophageal varices. Aliment Pharmacol Ther 2012;35:1155–65.
35. Puente A, Hernadez-Gea V, Graupera I, et al. Drugs plus ligation to prevent rebleeding in cirrhosis: an updated systematic review. Liver Int 2014;34:823–33.
36. Gluud LL, Langholz E, Krag A. Met-analysis: isosorbide -mononitrate alone or with either beta-blockers or endoscopic therapy of oesophageal varices. Aliment Pharmacol Ther 2010;32:859–71.
37. Villanueva C, Albillos A, Genesca J, et al. Development of hyperdynamic circulation and response to B-blockers in compensated cirrhosis with portal hypertension. Hepatology 2016;63:197–206.
38. Serste T, Melot C, Francoz C, et al. Deleterious effects of beta-blockers on survival in patients with cirrhosis and refractory ascites. Hepatology 2010;52:1017–22.
39. Facciorusso A, Roy S, Livadas S, et al. Nonselective beta-blockers do not affect survival in cirrhotic patients with ascites. Dig Dis Sci 2018;63:1737–46.
40. Moctezuma-Velazquez C, Kalainy S, Abraldes JG. Beta-blockers in patients with advanced liver disease: has the dust settled? Liver Transpl 2017;23:1058–69.
41. Holster IL, Tjwa ET, Moelker A, et al. Covered transjugular intrahepatic portosystemic shunt versus endoscopic therapy + beta-blocker for prevention of variceal rebleeding. Hepatology 2016;63:581–9.
42. Sarin SK, Lahoti D, Saxena SP, et al. Prevalence, classification and natural history of gastric varices: a long-term follow-up study in 568 portal hypertension patients. Hepatology 1992;16:1343–9.
43. Mishra SR, Sharma BC, Kumar A, et al. Primary prophylaxis of gastric variceal bleeding comparing cyanoacrylate injection and beta-blockers: a randomized controlled trial. J Hepatol 2011;54:1161–7.

44. Rios CE, Seron P, Gisbert JP, et al. Endoscopic injection of cyanoacrylate glue versus other endoscopic procedures for acute bleeding gastric varices in people with portal hypertension. Cochrane Database Syst Rev 2015;(5):CD010180.
45. Kahloon A, Chalasani N, DeWitt J, et al. Endoscopic therapy with 2- octyl-cyanoacrylate for the treatment of gastric varices. Dig Dis Sci 2014;59:2178–83.
46. Mansour L, Ei-Kalla F, El-Bassat H, et al. Randomized controlled trial of scleroligation versus band ligation alone for eradication of gastroesophageal varices. Gastrointest Endosc 2017;86:307–15.
47. Bhat YM, Weilert F, Fredrick RT, et al. EUS-guided treatment of gastric fundal varices with combined injection of coils and cyanoacrylate glue: a large U.S. experience over 6 years (with video). Gastrointest Endosc 2016;83:1164–72.
48. Mishra SR, Chander SB, Kumar A, et al. Endoscopic cyanoacrylate injection versus beta-blocker for secondary prophylaxis of gastric variceal bleed: a randomised controlled trial. Gut 2010;59:729–35.
49. Hung HH, Chang CJ, Hou MC, et al. Efficacy of non-selective beta-blockers as adjunct to endoscopic prophylaxis for gastric variceal bleeding: a randomized controlled trial. J Hepatol 2012;56:1025–32.
50. Lo GH, Liang HL, Chen WC, et al. A prospective randomized controlled trial of transjugular intrahepatic portosystemic shunt versus cyanoacrylate injection in the prevention of gastric variceal rebleeding. Endoscopy 2007;39:679–85.
51. Saad WE. Endovascular management of gastric varices. Clin Liver Dis 2014;18: 829–51.
52. Lee SJ, Kim SU, Kim MD, et al. Comparison of treatment outcomes between balloon-occluded retrograde transvenous obliteration and transjugular intrahepatic portosystemic shunt for gastric variceal bleeding hemostasis. J Gastroenterol Hepatol 2017;32:1487–94.
53. Gimm G, Chang Y, Kim H-C, et al. Balloon-occluded retrograde transvenous obliteration versus transjugular intrahepatic portosystemic shunt for the management of gastric variceal bleeding. Gut Liver 2018;12:704–13.
54. Ganguly S, Sarin SK, Bhatia V, et al. The prevalence and spectrum of colonic lesions in patients with cirrhotic and non-cirrhotic portal hypertension. Hepatology 1995;21:1226–31.
55. Al Khalloufi K, Laiyemo AO. Management of rectal varices in portal hypertension. World J Hepatol 2015;7:2992–8.
56. Shudo R, Yazaki Y, Sakurai S, et al. Clinical study comparing bleeding and non-bleeding rectal varices. Endoscopy 2002;34:189–94.

An Update
Portal Hypertensive Gastropathy and Colopathy

Don C. Rockey, MD

KEYWORDS

- Cirrhosis • Hemorrhage • Bleeding • Pressure • Portal hypertension

KEY POINTS

- Portal hypertensive gastropathy and portal hypertensive colopathy are common in patients with cirrhosis and portal hypertension.
- Diagnosis of portal hypertensive gastropathy and portal hypertensive colopathy is endoscopic, and grading systems to categorize severity are suboptimal.
- For portal hypertensive gastropathy, the best grading system seems to be simply "mild" and "severe".
- Treatment of acute bleeding owing to portal hypertensive gastropathy and portal hypertensive colopathy is initially pharmacologic to lower portal pressure.
- When needed, chronic therapy is typically with nonselective beta-blockers. Again, specific endoscopic therapies and more aggressive lowering of portal pressure with transjugular intrahepatic portosystemic shunt may be effective in some patients.

INTRODUCTION AND DEFINITION

Portal hypertensive gastropathy (PHG) and colopathy (PHC) are commonly found in patients with sinusoidal portal hypertension. However, PHG and PHC may also occur in patients with presinusoidal and postsinusoidal diseases such as portal vein thrombosis, schistosomiasis, veno-occlusive disease, and cardiac failure, all of which may also cause increased portal pressure.

The cause of PHG and PHC is poorly understood; however, it is presumed that portal hypertension in these patients likely causes hemodynamic and mucosal changes in the entire gastrointestinal (GI) tract. The mucosal changes associated with PHG and PHC include inflammatory changes and a primary histopathologic lesion characterized by vascular ectasia (**Table 1**). PHG and PHC are defined endoscopically, and indeed, these entities are closely tied to their endoscopic appearance

D.C. Rockey was supported by the NIH (Research Grant R01 DK 113159).

Disclosure of Conflicts: The author certifies that he has no financial arrangements (eg, consultancies, stock ownership, equity interests, patent-licensing arrangements, research support, major honoraria, etc.) pertinent to this work.

Department of Medicine, Medical University of South Carolina, 96 Jonathan Lucas Street, Suite 803, Charleston, SC 29425, USA

E-mail address: rockey@musc.edu

Table 1
Key features of PHG and PHC

Features	PHG	PHC
Pathology	Dilated capillaries and venules No inflammation	Edema and capillary dilatation Lymphocytes and plasma cells
Endoscopic characteristics	Classic mosaic pattern and red spots	Vascular ectasias Nonspecific mucosal changes
Differential diagnosis	GAVE Inflammatory gastritis Nonspecific inflammation	Idiopathic vascular ectasia Nonspecific inflammation
Treatment	Iron replacement therapy Transfusions Portal pressure reducing pharmacologic agents	Iron replacement therapy[a] Transfusions Portal pressure reducing pharmacologic agents APC, sclerotherapy, ligation
Salvage treatment	TIPS/shunt surgery APC Liver transplantation	TIPS/shunt surgery Liver transplantation

Current practice is largely based on case and case series reports.

Abbreviations: APC, argon plasma coagulation; GAVE, gastric antral vascular ectasia; TIPS, transjugular intrahepatic portosystemic shunting.

[a] There are insufficient data for standard recommendations in PHC bleeding.

Adapted from Urrunaga NH, Rockey DC. Portal hypertensive gastropathy and colopathy. Clin Liver Dis 2014;18(2):389-406; with permission.

as a mosaic-like pattern called snakeskin mucosa with or without red spots.[1] It should also be noted that the term portal hypertensive enteropathy is used to describe changes in the small bowel that are similar to those in the stomach.[2,3] PHC is perhaps less well-characterized than PHG and can be reflected by erythema of the colonic mucosa, vascular lesions including cherry red spots, telangiectasias, or angiodysplasia-like lesions.

PHG and PHC most often lead to chronic GI bleeding. However, they may also present with acute GI bleeding, and in 1 study PHG accounted for some 10% of all causes of upper GI bleeding.[4] Both disorders are very often confused with other diseases that can present similarly, in particular with other types of inflammatory mucosal disorders causing similar appearing lesions (ie, irritant or inflammatory gastritis or colitis). A high index of suspicion is required to make a timely and accurate diagnosis and to institute specific treatment.

PATHOGENESIS OF PORTAL HYPERTENSIVE GASTROPATHY AND COLOPATHY

Although the pathogenesis of PHG is poorly understood, a unifying theme is that the presence of some degree of portal hypertension seems to be essential. It should be noted that, although proposed, a direct correlation between the degree of portal hypertension and the severity of PHG has not been well-documented.[5,6] Perhaps the best evidence that portal hypertension is required as part of the pathogenesis are studies that demonstrate improvement of PHG after shunt surgery or transjugular intrahepatic portosystemic shunt (TIPS).[7,8]

It has been suggested that the pathogenesis of PHG and PHC requires some form of local injury to the mucosa. This notion is supported by histologic findings typical in PHG, such as dilatation of capillaries and venules in the mucosa and submucosa without significant inflammation[9] (see **Table 1**). There also seem to be abnormalities in the mucosal microcirculation in PHG.[10–12] Two specific factors that have gained considerable attention include (1) hypoxia and (2) inflammation, which may or may not be interrelated. Hypoxia seems to be related to the dysregulation of the mucosal microcirculation (particularly in PHG).[10] This abnormality in turn may lead to epithelial cell injury and set up a milieu in which there is overproduction of oxygen free radicals, nitric oxide, tumor necrosis factor-α, endothelin-1, prostaglandins, and/or other factors that cause cell injury.[10,13–17] Tumor necrosis factor-α, an inflammatory cytokine, seems to be prominent. Further, because of these changes and injury to the epithelium, it has been proposed that the abnormal mucosa in PHG and PHC is unable to repair normally and thus may be predisposed to bleeding.[18] However, the precise mechanism of bleeding remains unclear.

The pathogenesis of PHC is likely similar to that of PHG in that portal hypertension seems to be essential.[19] Evaluation of the colonic mucosa has demonstrated that vessels are dilated (including both small and large vessels), with an increased mean cross-sectional vascular area, and thickness of the capillary wall (ie, in patients with cirrhosis compared with those without cirrhosis or PHC and/or rectal varices).[20] Dilated and congested capillaries as well as capillaries with irregular thickening of the wall are typical.[21] Colonic mucosal edema and capillary dilation and evidence of inflammation (manifest by lymphocytes and plasma cells in the lamina propria) is typical, and may resemble chronic colitis.

It has also been proposed for both PHG and PHC that dysregulation of nitric oxide synthase may be involved,[22] leading to local changes in mucosal blood flow. It has been proposed that excess nitric oxide generated by an increased expression of inducible nitric oxide synthase leads to the vascular and hemodynamic changes seen in portal hypertensive mucosal lesions.

PORTAL HYPERTENSIVE GASTROPATHY
Epidemiology

The prevalence of PHG in patients with cirrhosis varies greatly, from 20% to 98%.[6,23–27] The cause of this variation is likely multifactorial, and is a result of (1) variation in endoscopic descriptions, (2) reports in different populations of patients, and (3) the lack of uniform diagnostic criteria and classification. Although it has been proposed that PHG is more prevalent in patients with advanced liver disease,[5,25,26,28] available data suggest that it remains "mild" in most patients.[26] Although it has also been speculated that that the prevalence of PHG may increase during esophageal variceal obliteration,[24] weak data support this possibility.

Clinical Findings

PHG typically presents in patients with symptoms related to chronic GI bleeding and chronic blood loss, often manifest as iron deficiency anemia. Data characterizing the frequency of chronic bleeding from PHG are old and the prevalence has been reported in from 3% to 60% of patients.[23,29,30] The definition of chronic bleeding varies, but is most often taken to be a decrease in hemoglobin of 2 g/dL within a 6-month time period without evidence of overt bleeding and nonsteroidal anti-inflammatory drug use.[31]

Acute GI hemorrhage occurs less commonly than chronic bleeding. The prevalence of acute GI bleeding from PHG in patients with cirrhosis has been reported to be between 2% and 12%.[4,25,32] In a recent study of patients with cirrhosis and acute upper GI bleeding, approximately 10% of patients had PHG,[4] consistent with the idea that

PHG can lead to acute bleeding, although it is not as common as other forms of bleeding. The diagnosis of acute hemorrhage from PHG is made when active hemorrhage from PHG lesions is visualized or in the setting of endoscopic PHG without another likely source of bleeding. It should be emphasized that caution is urged before assigning bleeding to PHG in patients with trivial lesions (as discussed elsewhere in this article).

Differential Diagnosis

The diagnosis of PHG is typically made at the time of endoscopy, in the appropriate clinical setting. Endoscopic features of PHG include a typical snakeskin mosaic pattern, flat or bulging red marks, or red spots resembling vascular ectasias found in the stomach (**Fig. 1**). The most common location for PHG is the fundus and body of the stomach (ie, proximal).[33,34]

The differential diagnosis of PHG includes several entities, which the endoscopist must be cognizant of. Perhaps the major distinction is with gastric antral vascular ectasia (GAVE) or watermelon stomach. GAVE also presents with flat red spots, but typically without the mosaic pattern[35] and GAVE often (but not always) appears endoscopically as streaks of erythema, appearing to emanate from the pylorus—appearing like a watermelon rind—thus, the name watermelon stomach. Importantly, GAVE is usually located in the distal stomach (antrum). Thus, the location of the lesions (PHG—proximal stomach vs GAVE—distal stomach) may help to distinguish these

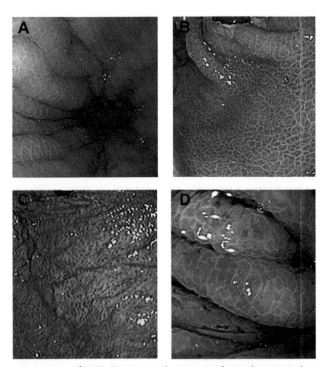

Fig. 1. Endoscopic images of PHG. For comparison, normal gastric mucosa is seen in (*A*), and mild PHG is visualized in (*B, C*). Severe PHG is seen in (*D*), including evidence of bleeding. (*From* Urrunaga NH, Rockey DC. Portal hypertensive gastropathy and colopathy. Clin Liver Dis 2014;18(2):389-406; with permission.)

disorders. However, there is overlap in the location of the lesions, and red spots can coalesce throughout the entire stomach (proximal and distal), leading to diffuse gastric vascular ectasia. When the endoscopic diagnosis is in question, biopsy and histologic assessment of the mucosa should be considered (biopsy in the absence of severe coagulopathy is generally considered to be safe). The histologic findings of GAVE are usually distinct from PHG and include vascular ectasia, spindle cell proliferation and fibrin thrombi, and fibrohyalinosis.[36]

Although the distinction between GAVE and PHG may be difficult in some situations, it is important because the treatments are typically different. It should also be noted that acute bleeding in patients with cirrhosis from GAVE is much less common than bleeding from PHG.[4] GAVE is also identified in patients with a diverse array of other diseases, including chronic renal failure, bone marrow transplantation, and autoimmune and connective tissue diseases, including scleroderma, atrophic gastritis, pernicious anemia, and sclerodactyly.[35,37] The major treatment issue (see also the Treatment section) is that, despite scattered reports, GAVE does not seem to be caused by portal hypertension and thus does not respond to treatments aimed at portal hypertension.[7,38] The primary mode of treatment for GAVE lesions is with endoscopic ablative methods (most often thermal) and not beta-blockers or TIPS.

It should also be mentioned that that the diagnosis of PHG may be made with capsule endoscopy; in 1 study, it was shown to have a sensitivity of 74% and specificity of 83% when compared with EGD.[39] Another study of 119 patients showed that the sensitivity of capsule endoscopy for the detection of PHG was 69% and the specificity was 99%.[40] However, the diagnostic yield in the gastric body was significantly greater than in the fundus (100% vs 48%, respectively). These data suggest that the role of capsule endoscopy is likely more important in the assessment of small bowel enteropathy than PHG.[41]

Nonendoscopic modalities with which to make a diagnosis of PHG include MRI and computed tomography scans.[42,43] With a computed tomography scan, PHG can be identified via enhancement of the inner layer of the gastric walls, which may reflect gastric congestion. In a study of 32 patients, 10 had PHG and 22 did not.[42] MRI has been used in patients with portal hypertension to examine collateral veins, including the left gastric, paraesophageal, and azygos veins.[43] However, in 57 patients the mean diameters of these veins were not different in patients with and without PHG, suggesting that this technique is not ready for clinical use.

PHG is typically classified based on how severe the lesion seem to be at the time of endoscopy. Most experts and societies are now recommending a 2-category classification system to describe the severity of the lesion, that is, mild and severe.[44,45] A 3-category system has also been proposed,[1,46] although this system is problematic because it introduces substantial variation in grading. PHG should be classified as mild when the only change consists of a snakeskin mosaic pattern and should be classified as severe when there is active bleeding and/or flat or bulging red or black-brown spots. The 2-category classification system has significantly better reproducibility.[47,48] It is intuitively expected that patients with more advanced appearing PHG lesions have a greater chance of acute or chronic bleeding than those with less severe lesions.[25,49]

Treatment

Treatment of PHG is difficult, primarily because there is such a wide variety of presentation of the disorder. In most situations, treatment recommendations are targeted according to specific features of the patient's presentation and moreover will vary based on the severity of symptoms (especially bleeding) (**Fig. 2**).

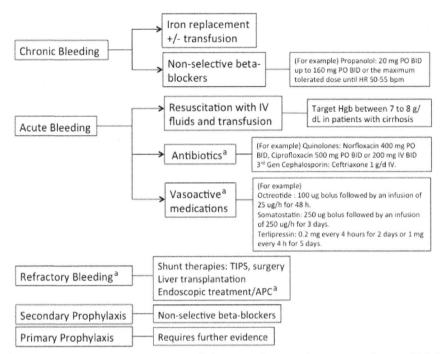

Fig. 2. PHG management. Recommended approaches to therapy are shown. PHC is managed similarly. [a] Based on available studies. Further evidence and research is needed. (*Adapted from* Urrunaga NH, Rockey DC. Portal hypertensive gastropathy and colopathy. Clin Liver Dis 2014;18(2):389-406; with permission.)

Primary Prophylaxis

It is extremely common to identify PHG during endoscopic screening for esophageal varices in patients with cirrhosis or during endoscopy for other reasons. Further, often times the patient is entirely asymptomatic without any evidence of chronic (or acute) bleeding. Thus, the question of primary prophylaxis to prevent GI bleeding in patients with PHG has been raised.[29,50] However, this topic has not been assessed rigorously enough to make evidence-based recommendations. In patients with trivial PHG, there is no evidence to support the use of primary prophylaxis with nonselective beta-blockers. In patients with varices, nonselective beta-blockers should be used (even if varices are small), because there is evidence that nonselective beta-blockers may delay the progression of small to large varices.[51] In patients with severe PHG and no varices, prophylaxis with nonselective β-blockers should be considered. However, this recommendation is largely empiric.

Chronic Bleeding

Patients with PHG may present with iron deficiency anemia, consistent with chronic blood loss. First, it is important to emphasize that other causes of iron deficiency anemia be excluded.[52] Although fecal blood levels can be measured,[53] the diagnosis of PHG in patients with cirrhosis and iron deficiency anemia should be considered a diagnosis of exclusion. Iron replacement therapy should be started in all patients with iron deficiency anemia owing to PHG; oral preparations are preferred, but intravenous iron may be used.

In patients with severe chronic bleeding owing to PHG, nonselective beta-blockers may be effective. One study demonstrated a decrease in gastric mucosal perfusion in patients with PHG, suggesting a putative mechanism of action.[54] A double-blind, placebo-controlled cross-over trial that included 22 patients with nonbleeding PHG who received either propanol (160 mg/d of long-acting propanol) or placebo for 6 weeks[55] showed that PHG improved in 9 patients after propranolol compared with only 3 after placebo. Another randomized control trial of 54 patients with cirrhosis and acute and/or chronic bleeding from severe PHG revealed that bleeding was less in the propranolol group at 12 months compared with control (38% vs 65%) and at 30 months (7% vs 52%).[29] In 77 patients with esophageal varices who were randomized to band ligation alone (40 patients) or combined with propranolol (37 patients), it was found that PHG developed less frequently in patients who received propranolol than in patients who received only banding.[56] Therefore, in patients with severe PHG, iron supplementation and propranolol (propranolol up to 160 mg by mouth 2 times per day or to the maximum tolerated dose with goal heart rate of 50–55 bpm) should be started.

Acute Bleeding

In patients with acute bleeding, it is important first to make a clear diagnosis of PHG by excluding other causes of bleeding. In patients with upper GI bleeding, the differential diagnosis includes bleeding varices (which account for approximately two-thirds of the lesions in these patients)[4] as well as other causes of bleeding such as ulcerative processes and even malignancy. The management of acute bleeding includes the typical measures such as volume resuscitation and aggressive and early generalized support. Blood transfusion should be performed with the goal to maintain the hemoglobin level between 7 and 8 g/dL; in addition, antibiotics and a proton pump inhibitor are recommended. The routine use of nasogastric lavage is not currently recommended in patients with any form of upper GI bleeding—whether in cirrhosis or not.[57] In the United States, octreotide should be used empirically in patients with known cirrhosis, although its effectiveness in patients with PHG is unclear (as discussed elsewhere in this article).

The treatment of acute bleeding for PHG is typically pharmacologic and focused on reduction of portal pressure. In a study of 68 patients comparing octreotide, vasopressin, and omeprazole, octreotide controlled bleeding in 100% of patients. Of note, omeprazole and vasopressin alone controlled bleeding in 64% and 59% of patients, respectively.[58] In another study of 26 patients with cirrhosis, somatostatin led to the cessation of acute bleeding from PHG, with a rate of relapse of 11.5%.[59] A double-blind, randomized, multicenter study of terlipressin in 68 patients with bleeding esophageal varices and PHG revealed that more patients receiving a higher dose (1 mg/4 h) stopped bleeding and had less recurrence than patients receiving control; however, methodologic problems limited the differentiation of PHG from varices.[60] Vasopressin may decrease gastric mucosal perfusion in patients with PHG,[61] but is not generally used in patients with cirrhosis any longer because of the concern about vascular-related side effects. The use of beta-blockers has been evaluated in small numbers of patients with acute PHG bleeding. For example, in 1 small study of 14 patients with acute PHG bleeding who were treated with propranolol, bleeding was controlled within 3 days in 13 of 14 patients (93%).[55] Although these data are intriguing, it is not clear whether nonselective beta-blockers would be expected to have acute effects; thus, parenteral vasoactive drugs are preferable acutely.

Endoscopic treatment for acute bleeding secondary to PHG is reserved for situations in which a single or a limited number of lesions are identified, in which case argon plasma coagulation (APC) or coagulation therapy may be considered depending on the lesions identified.

Refractory Bleeding

Refractory bleeding despite iron and nonselective beta-blocker therapy (ie, refractory iron deficiency anemia, transfusion-dependent, or acute on chronic bleeding[62] owing to PHG) is problematic. Additionally, in patients with acute GI bleeding secondary to PHG, failure of medical treatment should be considered when there is recurrent hematemesis (after ≥2 hours of treatment with vasoactive medications), or a 3-g decrease in hemoglobin in the absence of transfusion/an inadequate hemoglobin increase after transfusion.[31] In these clinical scenarios, rescue therapies such as TIPS may be considered.[31] Surgical shunts may be considered in patients with well-preserved liver function or in those with noncirrhotic portal hypertension because they have been shown to improve gastric mucosal lesions and decreased the number of transfusions.[63,64] TIPS is attractive in severe PHG bleeding because it has been shown to improve the endoscopic appearance of lesions within 6 to 12 weeks and led to decreased transfusion requirements.[7,8,65,66]

APC is attractive as a potential therapy for PHG because of its ease of application. However, it is difficult and not practical for those with a large area of stomach involved. Nonetheless, APC was shown, in a group of 11 patients with bleeding from PHG, to lead to a decrease in transfusion requirements in 81% of patients (it should be noted that these were highly selected patients and APC of ≥80% of the involved mucosal surface at 30–40 W and 1.5–2 L/min of AP flow every 2–4 weeks was used).[67] More recently, a hemostatic powder formulation has been found to provide at least temporizing control of bleeding.[68]

Of course, liver transplantation decreases portal pressure and is effective for treatment of refractory PHG. However, transplantation is most appropriate for patients with decompensated liver disease.[69]

Secondary Prevention

Secondary prophylaxis of bleeding in PHG should be undertaken with a nonselective beta-blocker,[29,31] although again, the data supporting the effectiveness of this approach are limited.

PORTAL HYPERTENSIVE COLOPATHY
Epidemiology

PHC mimics PHG in a number of ways, but also has some differences. Although both disorders are a result of portal hypertension, PHC seems to be more heterogenous and has been variably associated with vascular ectasias, anorectal or colonic varices, hemorrhoids, and even nonspecific inflammatory changes.[20,21,70,71] Although PHC is likely common in patients with portal hypertension, bleeding from PHC seems to be uncommon.

The prevalence of PHC in patients with cirrhosis is highly variable, ranging from 3% to 71%.[20,71–73] The variation in prevalence is undoubtedly related to exactly which mucosal lesions are considered to be consistent with PHC, as well as selection bias in published studies. For example, in a relatively recent study in which the prevalence of PHC was reported to be 71%, a variety of lesions were considered to be consistent with PHC—including red spots.[71] Additionally, only patients with a previous history of esophageal varices were included, likely increasing the likelihood of portal hypertension and its associated abnormalities. The presence of rectal or colonic varices also varies widely, being reported in from 4% to 40% of patients.[72,74,75] Bleeding from PHC is uncommon, reported to be between 0% and 9%.[72,75–77] The reason for the wide variation in reported bleeding rates is similar to that for prevalence estimates, and is due any of the following: variation in patient selection, lack of a clear classification system as to what constitutes PHC, as well as interobserver variability among endoscopists as to endoscopy findings consistent with PHC.

Some studies have reported that PHC is associated with certain clinical features—such as decreased platelet counts,[78] more advanced end-stage liver disease,[19,78] gastric varices,[72] and a higher portal pressure.[19,79] However, other studies have failed to find that PHC is associated with the severity of liver disease,[75] portal pressure,[76,80] or gastroesophageal varices.[71,75,77] Currently, similar to PHG, there simply are not enough robust data from studies of patients with PHC from which to draw clear conclusions.

Clinical Findings

In general, PHC may present in a fashion similar to PHG—that is, with evidence of chronic blood loss (ie, iron deficiency anemia), or with acute bleeding, in the colon, manifest as hematochezia or bright red blood per rectum.[70]

Differential Diagnosis

As with PHG, the diagnosis of PHC is made by endoscopy. Patients with cirrhosis and hematochezia may bleed from any number of typical lower GI sources.[81] Thus, a diagnostic evaluation of the colonic mucosa should generally be performed expeditiously in patients with hematochezia or bright red blood per rectum. In patients with aggressive hematochezia and/or significant alterations in vital signs, an upper GI source should always be considered.[4]

Typical PHC lesions have been described as slightly raised reddish lesions less than 10 mm in diameter on an otherwise normal appearing mucosa.[20] However, considerable variation exists.

Rectal varices in patients with portal hypertension bear mention because these lesions can be confused with PHC. Typical portal hypertensive varices are prominent in the submucosa and are proximal to the pectinate line. These veins were different from normal rectal veins because of their greater diameter and tortuosity (measuring ≥3–6 mm in diameter). Additionally, colonic varices should be differentiated from hemorrhoids, especially before surgical excision, and angiography may be considered.[82]

The endoscopic appearance of PHC can be sometimes difficult to differentiate from angiodysplasia of the colon secondary to degenerative changes. Other noninflammatory and inflammatory etiologies of bleeding such as ischemia, radiation changes, and hereditary hemorrhagic telangiectasia are also in the differential diagnosis. Biopsy may or may not be helpful in differentiation of PHC from these other lesions.[21]

Classification

Currently, there is no ideal classification system for grading the severity of mucosal abnormalities in patients with PHC. Several classifications have been proposed. Initially, a histologic criteria for the vascular lesions typical of PHC included 2 types of lesions[20] including a so-called early lesion, which was characterized by a moderately dilated, tortuous, thin-walled, and endothelial-lined vein and venule appearance in the submucosa. In contrast, a so-called late-stage lesion had progressively more dilated submucosal veins and dilated and tortuous venules and capillaries in the mucosa. Another endoscopic grading system of typical vascular ectasias, or diffuse red spots included types 1, 2, or 3 lesions as follows: type 1, a flat, fernlike vascular lesion (spider-like lesion); type 2, a flat or slightly elevated red lesion less than 10 mm in diameter or a cherry red lesion; and type 3, a slightly elevated submucosal tumor-like lesion with a central red color and depression. A further study proposed a 3-grade classification system as follows: grade 1, characterized by erythema of the colonic mucosa; grade 2, erythema of the colonic mucosa with a mosaic-like pattern; and grade 3, vascular lesions in the colon including cherry red spots, telangiectasias, or angiodysplasia-like lesions.[83] In aggregate, classification of the severity of lesions in PHC is difficult and thus it is this author's practice to simply carefully describe the visualized lesions.

Treatment

Few data exist about the treatment of PHC. Thus, treatment is largely guided by local expertise and experience. As with PHG, for patients with chronic bleeding and iron deficiency anemia, treatment should be supportive and include iron therapy, either oral or parenteral.

In an animal study of rats using a PHC model, propranolol and octreotide improved typical PHC changes in colonic mucosa (including mucosal edema, hyperemia and hemorrhage), although the effects of octreotide were found to be more prominent than with propanolol.[84] In patients with lower GI bleeding secondary to PHC, treatment with long-acting octreotide or beta-blockers has been reported to be effective.[1,83,85] The risk of bleeding from PHC in patients with portal hypertension who are taking beta-blockers may also be decreased.[83] Given the known effects of nonselective beta-blockers on portal pressure, it is reasonable to institute beta-blocker therapy as tolerated to achieve a resting heart rate of 50 to 55 bpm.

In patients with acute bleeding, pharmacologic therapies should be attempted (octreotide/terlipressin), although evidence of their effectiveness is limited. Octreotide has been reported to be effective in isolated patients with severe bleeding from PHC.[86] Nonselective beta-blockers should be started as soon as is possible. Depending on the severity of the bleeding and the number of vascular lesions present, local therapies such as APC may be effective. Other local therapies with sclerosis or band ligation, or even coil embolization, may be attempted.[70,87] Cryotherapy[88] or even hemostatic powder[68] may be effective. Again, such treatments largely depend on local experience and expertise.

As for PHG, in patients with refractory bleeding that does not respond to vasoactive medications or beta-blockers, TIPS may be used as a rescue therapy for PHC — although data are limited largely to case reports.[70,89,90] Other reports suggest that the use of TIPS may effectively control bleeding owing to portal hypertensive anorectal and/or colonic varices.[91] It should be noted that before performing TIPS in this setting, it is critical to ensure that bleeding is portal hypertensive in etiology.

Prophylaxis

There are no data with which to guide recommendations about secondary prophylaxis of bleeding owing to PHC. In patients with an indication for nonselective beta-blockers, these should be used. If local measures (banding, sclerotherapy, APC, and so on) are used, ongoing surveillance is indicated.

SUMMARY

PHG and PHC typically cause chronic GI bleeding. When they cause acute GI bleeding, careful attention to the differential diagnosis is essential. The pathogenesis of PHG and PHC is incompletely understood, but seems to be closely tied to portal hypertension and local changes in vascular blood flow in the intestinal mucosa. The diagnosis for both of these disorders is endoscopic and it is important to recognize that the differential diagnosis may be difficult. The management of PHG and PHC depends on individual patient factors; for acute bleeding, hemodynamic stabilization with intravenous fluids, intravenous antibiotics, and blood transfusion as needed are indicated. Pharmacologic therapy to decrease portal pressure followed by nonselective beta-blockers as soon as the patient is hemodynamically stable are appropriate. In patients with chronic bleeding, therapy with beta-blockers and iron replacement is recommended. Patients with refractory bleeding from either PHG or PHC represent difficult clinical challenges and are best managed on an individual basis. TIPS or shunt procedures may be appropriate in some situations. Liver transplantation decrease portal hypertension in patients with cirrhosis and is highly effective at decreasing the portal pressure.

REFERENCES

1. Urrunaga NH, Rockey DC. Portal hypertensive gastropathy and colopathy. Clin Liver Dis 2014;18(2):389–406.
2. Menchen L, Ripoll C, Marin-Jimenez I, et al. Prevalence of portal hypertensive duodenopathy in cirrhosis: clinical and haemodynamic features. Eur J Gastroenterol Hepatol 2006;18(6):649–53.
3. Higaki N, Matsui H, Imaoka H, et al. Characteristic endoscopic features of portal hypertensive enteropathy. J Gastroenterol 2008;43(5):327–31.
4. Lyles T, Elliott A, Rockey DC. A risk scoring system to predict in-hospital mortality in patients with cirrhosis presenting with upper gastrointestinal bleeding. J Clin Gastroenterol 2014;48(8):712–20.
5. Iwao T, Toyonaga A, Oho K, et al. Portal-hypertensive gastropathy develops less in patients with cirrhosis and fundal varices. J Hepatol 1997;26(6):1235–41.
6. Sarin SK, Sreenivas DV, Lahoti D, et al. Factors influencing development of portal hypertensive gastropathy in patients with portal hypertension. Gastroenterology 1992;102(3):994–9.
7. Kamath PS, Lacerda M, Ahlquist DA, et al. Gastric mucosal responses to intrahepatic portosystemic shunting in patients with cirrhosis. Gastroenterology 2000; 118(5):905–11.
8. Mezawa S, Homma H, Ohta H, et al. Effect of transjugular intrahepatic portosystemic shunt formation on portal hypertensive gastropathy and gastric circulation. Am J Gastroenterol 2001;96(4):1155–9.
9. McCormack TT, Sims J, Eyre-Brook I, et al. Gastric lesions in portal hypertension: inflammatory gastritis or congestive gastropathy? Gut 1985;26(11):1226–32.
10. Albillos A, Colombato LA, Enriquez R, et al. Sequence of morphological and hemodynamic changes of gastric microvessels in portal hypertension. Gastroenterology 1992;102(6):2066–70.
11. Cubillas R, Rockey DC. Portal hypertensive gastropathy: a review. Liver Int 2010; 30(8):1094–102.
12. Ma C, Chen CH, Liu TC. The spectrum of gastric pathology in portal hypertension-An endoscopic and pathologic study of 550 cases. Pathol Res Pract 2016;212(8):704–9.
13. Lopez-Talavera JC, Merrill WW, Groszmann RJ. Tumor necrosis factor alpha: a major contributor to the hyperdynamic circulation in prehepatic portal-hypertensive rats. Gastroenterology 1995;108(3):761–7.

14. Kaviani A, Ohta M, Itani R, et al. Tumor necrosis factor-alpha regulates inducible nitric oxide synthase gene expression in the portal hypertensive gastric mucosa of the rat. J Gastrointest Surg 1997;1(4):371–6.

15. Migoh S, Hashizume M, Tsugawa K, et al. Role of endothelin-1 in congestive gastropathy in portal hypertensive rats. J Gastroenterol Hepatol 2000;15(2):142–7.

16. Kawanaka H, Tomikawa M, Jones MK, et al. Defective mitogen-activated protein kinase (ERK2) signaling in gastric mucosa of portal hypertensive rats: potential therapeutic implications. Hepatology 2001;34(5):990–9.

17. Kinjo N, Kawanaka H, Akahoshi T, et al. Significance of ERK nitration in portal hypertensive gastropathy and its therapeutic implications. Am J Physiol Gastrointest Liver Physiol 2008;295(5):G1016–24.

18. Perini RF, Camara PR, Ferraz JG. Pathogenesis of portal hypertensive gastropathy: translating basic research into clinical practice. Nat Clin Pract Gastroenterol Hepatol 2009;6(3):150–8.

19. Yamakado S, Kanazawa H, Kobayashi M. Portal hypertensive colopathy: endoscopic findings and the relation to portal pressure. Intern Med 1995;34(3):153–7.

20. Naveau S, Bedossa P, Poynard T, et al. Portal hypertensive colopathy. A new entity. Dig Dis Sci 1991;36(12):1774–81.

21. Misra V, Misra SP, Dwivedi M, et al. Colonic mucosa in patients with portal hypertension. J Gastroenterol Hepatol 2003;18(3):302–8.

22. Ohta M, Kaviani A, Tarnawski AS, et al. Portal hypertension triggers local activation of inducible nitric oxide synthase gene in colonic mucosa. J Gastrointest Surg 1997;1(3):229–35.

23. Primignani M, Carpinelli L, Preatoni P, et al. Natural history of portal hypertensive gastropathy in patients with liver cirrhosis. The New Italian Endoscopic Club for the study and treatment of esophageal varices (NIEC). Gastroenterology 2000; 119(1):181–7.

24. Thuluvath PJ, Yoo HY. Portal hypertensive gastropathy. Am J Gastroenterol 2002; 97(12):2973–8.

25. Merli M, Nicolini G, Angeloni S, et al. The natural history of portal hypertensive gastropathy in patients with liver cirrhosis and mild portal hypertension. Am J Gastroenterol 2004;99(10):1959–65.

26. Fontana RJ, Sanyal AJ, Mehta S, et al. Portal hypertensive gastropathy in chronic hepatitis C patients with bridging fibrosis and compensated cirrhosis: results from the HALT-C trial. Am J Gastroenterol 2006;101(5):983–92.

27. Fontana RJ, Sanyal AJ, Ghany MG, et al. Development and progression of portal hypertensive gastropathy in patients with chronic hepatitis C. Am J Gastroenterol 2011;106(5):884–93.

28. D'Amico G, Montalbano L, Traina M, et al. Natural history of congestive gastropathy in cirrhosis. The Liver Study Group of V. Cervello hospital. Gastroenterology 1990;99(6):1558–64.

29. Perez-Ayuso RM, Pique JM, Bosch J, et al. Propranolol in prevention of recurrent bleeding from severe portal hypertensive gastropathy in cirrhosis. Lancet 1991; 337(8755):1431–4.

30. Sarin SK, Shahi HM, Jain M, et al. The natural history of portal hypertensive gastropathy: influence of variceal eradication. Am J Gastroenterol 2000;95(10): 2888–93.

31. de Franchis R, Baveno VF. Revising consensus in portal hypertension: report of the Baveno V consensus workshop on methodology of diagnosis and therapy in portal hypertension. J Hepatol 2010;53(4):762–8.

32. Gostout CJ, Viggiano TR, Balm RK. Acute gastrointestinal bleeding from portal hypertensive gastropathy: prevalence and clinical features. Am J Gastroenterol 1993;88(12):2030–3.
33. Cales P, Pascal JP. Gastroesophageal endoscopic features in cirrhosis: comparison of intracenter and intercenter observer variability. Gastroenterology 1990; 99(4):1189.
34. Vigneri S, Termini R, Piraino A, et al. The stomach in liver cirrhosis. Endoscopic, morphological, and clinical correlations. Gastroenterology 1991;101(2):472–8.
35. Gostout CJ, Viggiano TR, Ahlquist DA, et al. The clinical and endoscopic spectrum of the watermelon stomach. J Clin Gastroenterol 1992;15(3):256–63.
36. Payen JL, Cales P, Voigt JJ, et al. Severe portal hypertensive gastropathy and antral vascular ectasia are distinct entities in patients with cirrhosis. Gastroenterology 1995;108(1):138–44.
37. Ingraham KM, O'Brien MS, Shenin M, et al. Gastric antral vascular ectasia in systemic sclerosis: demographics and disease predictors. J Rheumatol 2010;37(3): 603–7.
38. Spahr L, Villeneuve JP, Dufresne MP, et al. Gastric antral vascular ectasia in cirrhotic patients: absence of relation with portal hypertension. Gut 1999;44(5): 739–42.
39. de Franchis R, Eisen GM, Laine L, et al. Esophageal capsule endoscopy for screening and surveillance of esophageal varices in patients with portal hypertension. Hepatology 2008;47(5):1595–603.
40. Aoyama T, Oka S, Aikata H, et al. Small bowel abnormalities in patients with compensated liver cirrhosis. Dig Dis Sci 2013;58(5):1390–6.
41. De Palma GD, Rega M, Masone S, et al. Mucosal abnormalities of the small bowel in patients with cirrhosis and portal hypertension: a capsule endoscopy study. Gastrointest Endosc 2005;62(4):529–34.
42. Ishihara K, Ishida R, Saito T, et al. Computed tomography features of portal hypertensive gastropathy. J Comput Assist Tomogr 2004;28(6):832–5.
43. Erden A, Idilman R, Erden I, et al. Veins around the esophagus and the stomach: do their calibrations provide a diagnostic clue for portal hypertensive gastropathy? Clin Imaging 2009;33(1):22–4.
44. Spina GP, Arcidiacono R, Bosch J, et al. Gastric endoscopic features in portal hypertension: final report of a consensus conference, Milan, Italy, September 19, 1992. J Hepatol 1994;21(3):461–7.
45. de Franchis R. Updating consensus in portal hypertension: report of the Baveno III Consensus Workshop on definitions, methodology and therapeutic strategies in portal hypertension. J Hepatol 2000;33(5):846–52.
46. Tanoue K, Hashizume M, Wada H, et al. Effects of endoscopic injection sclerotherapy on portal hypertensive gastropathy: a prospective study. Gastrointest Endosc 1992;38(5):582–5.
47. Yoo HY, Eustace JA, Verma S, et al. Accuracy and reliability of the endoscopic classification of portal hypertensive gastropathy. Gastrointest Endosc 2002; 56(5):675–80.
48. de Macedo GF, Ferreira FG, Ribeiro MA, et al. Reliability in endoscopic diagnosis of portal hypertensive gastropathy. World J Gastrointest Endosc 2013;5(7): 323–31.
49. Stewart CA, Sanyal AJ. Grading portal gastropathy: validation of a gastropathy scoring system. Am J Gastroenterol 2003;98(8):1758–65.
50. Munoz SJ. Propranolol for portal hypertensive gastropathy: another virtue of beta-blockade? Hepatology 1992;15(3):554–6.

51. Merkel C, Marin R, Angeli P, et al. A placebo-controlled clinical trial of nadolol in the prophylaxis of growth of small esophageal varices in cirrhosis. Gastroenterology 2004;127(2):476–84.
52. Rockey DC, Cello JP. Evaluation of the gastrointestinal tract in patients with iron-deficiency anemia. N Engl J Med 1993;329:1691–5.
53. Ahlquist DA, McGill DB, Schwartz S, et al. Fecal blood levels in health and disease. A study using HemoQuant. N Engl J Med 1985;312:1422–8.
54. Shigemori H, Iwao T, Ikegami M, et al. Effects of propranolol on gastric mucosal perfusion and serum gastrin level in cirrhotic patients with portal hypertensive gastropathy. Dig Dis Sci 1994;39(11):2433–8.
55. Hosking SW, Kennedy HJ, Seddon I, et al. The role of propranolol in congestive gastropathy of portal hypertension. Hepatology 1987;7(3):437–41.
56. Lo GH, Lai KH, Cheng JS, et al. The effects of endoscopic variceal ligation and propranolol on portal hypertensive gastropathy: a prospective, controlled trial. Gastrointest Endosc 2001;53(6):579–84.
57. Rockey DC, Ahn C, de Melo SW Jr. Randomized pragmatic trial of nasogastric tube placement in patients with upper gastrointestinal tract bleeding. J Investig Med 2017;65(4):759–64.
58. Zhou Y, Qiao L, Wu J, et al. Comparison of the efficacy of octreotide, vasopressin, and omeprazole in the control of acute bleeding in patients with portal hypertensive gastropathy: a controlled study. J Gastroenterol Hepatol 2002;17(9):973–9.
59. Kouroumalis EA, Koutroubakis IE, Manousos ON. Somatostatin for acute severe bleeding from portal hypertensive gastropathy. Eur J Gastroenterol Hepatol 1998;10(6):509–12.
60. Bruha R, Marecek Z, Spicak J, et al. Double-blind randomized, comparative multicenter study of the effect of terlipressin in the treatment of acute esophageal variceal and/or hypertensive gastropathy bleeding. Hepatogastroenterology 2002;49(46):1161–6.
61. Iwao T, Toyonaga A, Shigemori H, et al. Vasopressin plus oxygen vs vasopressin alone in cirrhotic patients with portal-hypertensive gastropathy: effects on gastric mucosal haemodynamics and oxygenation. J Gastroenterol Hepatol 1996;11(3):216–22.
62. Rockey DC, Hafemeister AC, Reisch JS. Acute on chronic gastrointestinal bleeding: a unique clinical entity. J Investig Med 2017;65(5):892–8.
63. Soin AS, Acharya SK, Mathur M, et al. Portal hypertensive gastropathy in noncirrhotic patients. The effect of lienorenal shunts. J Clin Gastroenterol 1998;26(1):64–7 [discussion: 68].
64. Orloff MJ, Orloff MS, Orloff SL, et al. Treatment of bleeding from portal hypertensive gastropathy by portacaval shunt. Hepatology 1995;21(4):1011–7.
65. Urata J, Yamashita Y, Tsuchigame T, et al. The effects of transjugular intrahepatic portosystemic shunt on portal hypertensive gastropathy. J Gastroenterol Hepatol 1998;13(10):1061–7.
66. Vignali C, Bargellini I, Grosso M, et al. TIPS with expanded polytetrafluoroethylene-covered stent: results of an Italian multicenter study. AJR Am J Roentgenol 2005;185(2):472–80.
67. Herrera S, Bordas JM, Llach J, et al. The beneficial effects of argon plasma coagulation in the management of different types of gastric vascular ectasia lesions in patients admitted for GI hemorrhage. Gastrointest Endosc 2008;68(3):440–6.
68. Smith LA, Morris AJ, Stanley AJ. The use of hemospray in portal hypertensive bleeding; a case series. J Hepatol 2014;60(2):457–60.

69. DeWeert TM, Gostout CJ, Wiesner RH. Congestive gastropathy and other upper endoscopic findings in 81 consecutive patients undergoing orthotopic liver transplantation. Am J Gastroenterol 1990;85(5):573–6.

70. Kozarek RA, Botoman VA, Bredfeldt JE, et al. Portal colopathy: prospective study of colonoscopy in patients with portal hypertension. Gastroenterology 1991; 101(5):1192–7.

71. Guimaraes RA, Perazzo H, Machado L, et al. Prevalence, variability, and outcomes in portal hypertensive colopathy: a study in patients with cirrhosis and paired controls. Gastrointest Endosc 2015;82(3):469–76.e2.

72. Misra SP, Dwivedi M, Misra V. Prevalence and factors influencing hemorrhoids, anorectal varices, and colopathy in patients with portal hypertension. Endoscopy 1996;28(4):340–5.

73. Zaman A, Hapke R, Flora K, et al. Prevalence of upper and lower gastrointestinal tract findings in liver transplant candidates undergoing screening endoscopic evaluation. Am J Gastroenterol 1999;94(4):895–9.

74. Rabinovitz M, Schade RR, Dindzans VJ, et al. Colonic disease in cirrhosis. An endoscopic evaluation in 412 patients. Gastroenterology 1990;99(1):195–9.

75. Bresci G, Parisi G, Capria A. Clinical relevance of colonic lesions in cirrhotic patients with portal hypertension. Endoscopy 2006;38(8):830–5.

76. Chen LS, Lin HC, Lee FY, et al. Portal hypertensive colopathy in patients with cirrhosis. Scand J Gastroenterol 1996;31(5):490–4.

77. Ganguly S, Sarin SK, Bhatia V, et al. The prevalence and spectrum of colonic lesions in patients with cirrhotic and noncirrhotic portal hypertension. Hepatology 1995;21(5):1226–31.

78. Ito K, Shiraki K, Sakai T, et al. Portal hypertensive colopathy in patients with liver cirrhosis. World J Gastroenterol 2005;11(20):3127–30.

79. Diaz-Sanchez A, Nunez-Martinez O, Gonzalez-Asanza C, et al. Portal hypertensive colopathy is associated with portal hypertension severity in cirrhotic patients. World J Gastroenterol 2009;15(38):4781–7.

80. Wang TF, Lee FY, Tsai YT, et al. Relationship of portal pressure, anorectal varices and hemorrhoids in cirrhotic patients. J Hepatol 1992;15(1–2):170–3.

81. Schmulewitz N, Fisher DA, Rockey DC. Early colonoscopy for acute lower GI bleeding predicts shorter hospital stay: a retrospective study of experience in a single center. Gastrointest Endosc 2003;58(6):841–6.

82. Leone N, Debernardi-Venon W, Marzano A, et al. Portal hypertensive colopathy and hemorrhoids in cirrhotic patients. J Hepatol 2000;33(6):1026–7.

83. Bini EJ, Lascarides CE, Micale PL, et al. Mucosal abnormalities of the colon in patients with portal hypertension: an endoscopic study. Gastrointest Endosc 2000;52(4):511–6.

84. Aydede H, Sakarya A, Erhan Y, et al. Effects of octreotide and propranolol on colonic mucosa in rats with portal hypertensive colopathy. Hepatogastroenterology 2003;50(53):1352–5.

85. Branco JC, Carvalho R, Alberto SF, et al. Long-acting octreotide is effective in the treatment of portal hypertensive colopathy. Gastroenterol Hepatol 2017;40(8): 536–7.

86. Yoshie K, Fujita Y, Moriya A, et al. Octreotide for severe acute bleeding from portal hypertensive colopathy: a case report. Eur J Gastroenterol Hepatol 2001; 13(9):1111–3.

87. Richon J, Berclaz R, Schneider PA, et al. Sclerotherapy of rectal varices. Int J Colorectal Dis 1988;3(2):132–4.

88. Patel J, Parra V, Kedia P, et al. Salvage cryotherapy in portal hypertensive gastropathy. Gastrointest Endosc 2015;81(4):1003.

89. Balzer C, Lotterer E, Kleber G, et al. Transjugular intrahepatic portosystemic shunt for bleeding angiodysplasia-like lesions in portal-hypertensive colopathy. Gastroenterology 1998;115(1):167–72.

90. Ozgediz D, Devine P, Garcia-Aguilar J, et al. Refractory lower gastrointestinal bleeding from portal hypertensive colopathy. J Am Coll Surg 2008;207(4):613.

91. Fantin AC, Zala G, Risti B, et al. Bleeding anorectal varices: successful treatment with transjugular intrahepatic portosystemic shunting (TIPS). Gut 1996;38(6): 932–5.

Ascites and Hepatorenal Syndrome

Danielle Adebayo, BSc (Hons), MBBS, MRCP[1], Shuet Fong Neong, MBBS, MRCP[1],
Florence Wong, MBBS, MD, FRACP, FRCPC*

KEYWORDS

- Cirrhosis • Ascites • Acute kidney injury • Hepatorenal syndrome

KEY POINTS

- It is important to establish adherence to sodium restriction and compliance with diuretic therapy before making a diagnosis of refractory ascites (RA), which has a poor prognosis with a 1-year median survival of 50%.
- Large-volume paracentesis can be safely performed at the bedside, the frequency of which can be estimated by calculating the daily net sodium balance, and should be accompanied by albumin replacement to prevent paracentesis-induced circulatory dysfunction.
- Transjugular intrahepatic portosystemic shunt may be considered in selected patients with RA.
- Liver transplant (LT) remains the definitive treatment of RA and HRS, therefore eligible candidates should be identified early and referred for LT evaluation.
- Patients with liver dysfunction and HRS or chronic kidney disease who are dialysis dependent for 6 weeks or longer should be considered for simultaneous liver and kidney transplant.

NATURAL HISTORY OF CIRRHOSIS AND PORTAL HYPERTENSION

Portal hypertension is a major prognostic factor for clinical decompensation in patients with cirrhosis,[1] who usually remain asymptomatic during the compensated stage. When the portal pressure, as measured by the hepatic venous pressure gradient (HVPG), exceeds 10 mm Hg, clinically significant portal hypertension (CSPH) occurs.[1] The most common manifestations of CSPH are ascites and gastroesophageal varices.[1,2] Other complications, such as spontaneous bacterial peritonitis

Disclosures: Dr D. Adebayo and Dr S.F. Neong have nothing to declare. Dr F. Wong is a consultant for Mallinckrodt Pharmaceuticals and Sequana Medical Inc.
Division of Gastroenterology, Department of Medicine, Toronto General Hospital, University of Toronto, 200 Elizabeth Street, Room 222, 9th floor, Eaton Wing, Toronto, Ontario M5G2C4, Canada
[1] Dr D. Adebayo and Dr S.F. Neong are equal first authors.
* Corresponding author.
E-mail address: florence.wong@utoronto.ca

(SBP), variceal bleeding, and hepatorenal syndrome (HRS), occur as the severity of portal hypertension increases.[1,2] **Fig. 1** shows the natural history of the development of portal hypertension and the clinical manifestations of CSPH as the severity of portal hypertension progresses. This article expands the current understanding of the natural history and pathophysiology of ascites and HRS as well as the management of these significant complications of portal hypertension.

PATHOPHYSIOLOGY

Refractory ascites (RA), defined as ascites that is not easily mobilized because of ineffectiveness of diuretic therapy and sodium restriction or adverse events from diuretics, and HRS share some common pathophysiologic mechanisms. For many years, splanchnic vasodilatation resulting in effective central hypovolemia and subsequent activation of vasoconstrictor systems, resulting in systemic circulatory dysfunction, was thought to underpin the development of these complications.[3,4] However, it is now clear that, in addition to this, systemic inflammation also plays an important role in the development of ascites, renal dysfunction, and other complications associated with portal hypertension.[4,5] These complications are discussed further later and summarized in **Fig. 2**.

Peripheral Arterial Vasodilatation and Systemic Circulatory Dysfunction

According to the peripheral arterial vasodilatation hypothesis, the structural changes and architectural distortion associated with cirrhosis lead to an increase in intrahepatic vascular resistance. Furthermore, there is an increase in sheer stress on the splanchnic vessels from the obstruction to portal flow. Both of these factors trigger an increased production of vasoactive substances, with the most important being the vasodilator nitric oxide. Together with decreased degradation of these vasodilators in the diseased liver, this results in splanchnic vasodilatation. The consequent increased splanchnic inflow and increased intrahepatic vascular resistance lead to the development of portal hypertension.[5,6] Some of these splanchnic vasodilators are transferred to the systemic circulation via portosystemic shunts, which open as

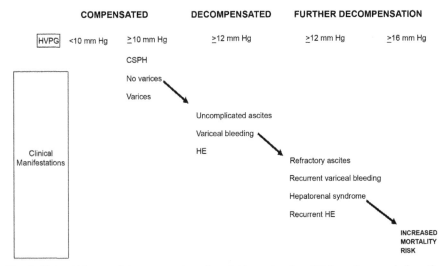

Fig. 1. Natural history of the progression of portal hypertension. HE, hepatic encephalopathy.

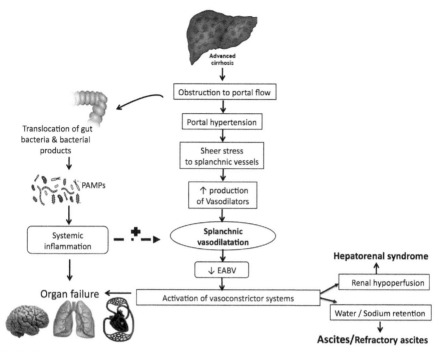

Fig. 2. The pathophysiology of refractory ascites and renal dysfunction incorporating the peripheral arterial vasodilatation and the systemic inflammation hypotheses. EABV, effective arterial blood volume; PAMP, pathogen associated molecular pattern.

a result of the portal hypertension. Thus, systemic vasodilatation also ensues[7,8] The combination of splanchnic arterial vasodilatation, leading to splanchnic pooling of the circulatory volume, and systemic arterial vasodilatation causing arterial underfilling, leads to a reduction in mean arterial pressure (MAP). At earlier stages of cirrhosis, the decrease in systemic vascular resistance (SVR) is moderate and there is a compensatory increase in cardiac output (CO) to maintain the MAP within the normal range.[9] However, as cirrhosis becomes more advanced, the degree of splanchnic arterial vasodilation becomes more severe and causes a marked reduction in SVR that cannot be compensated for by an increase in CO, thus resulting in effective arterial hypovolemia and systemic hypotension.[2,9] Of note, evidence in the literature shows that patients with advanced cirrhosis also have cirrhotic cardiomyopathy, exacerbating the reduction in CO and worsening the arterial underfilling.[10] The MAP reduction is sensed by arterial baroreceptors, triggering the activation of endogenous vasoconstrictor systems as a compensatory mechanism.[4,11] The main vasoconstrictor systems activated are the sympathetic nervous system, the renin-angiotensin-aldosterone system, as well as nonosmotic vasopressin release.[4] Activation of these vasoconstrictor systems is the body's attempt at reducing the extent of arterial vasodilatation. Furthermore, the kidneys are particularly sensitive to the vasoconstrictive effects of angiotensin and the sympathetic nervous system, resulting in renal vasoconstriction, and this stimulates renal sodium (Na) and water retention in order to expand the intravascular volume, which favors edema and ascites formation. Alteration in renal blood flow autoregulation in advanced cirrhosis, related to a rightward shift of the autoregulation curve, also contributes to renal vasoconstriction.[12]

For any given renal perfusion pressure, there is therefore less renal blood flow because of sympathetic overactivity.[12] These factors result in renal hypoperfusion and propensity toward the development of HRS.[7,12,13]

Systemic Inflammation

There is emerging evidence that systemic inflammation also plays an important role in the development of complications of portal hypertension such as HRS.[4] The main mechanism leading to systemic inflammation in advanced cirrhosis, in the absence of active bacterial infection, is bacterial translocation from the intestinal lumen into the intestinal mucosa.[4] Cirrhosis is associated with bacterial overgrowth, intestinal dysbiosis, and increased intestinal permeability.[14,15] These factors result in pathologic bacterial translocation from the intestinal lumen, through the mesenteric lymphatics, and from there into the systemic circulation, resulting in systemic endotoxemia. Recent report of increased levels of various inflammatory markers correlating with the height of HVPG supports this contention.[16] These bacterial products or pathogen-associated molecular patterns (PAMPs) interact with their corresponding pattern recognition receptors, and the downstream effect of this interaction is the generation of proinflammatory cytokines. The release of the proinflammatory cytokines and subsequent inflammatory response increase arterial nitric oxide production, thus exacerbating existing splanchnic vasodilatation and subsequent effective arterial underfilling, predisposing to the development of HRS.[4,9]

Advanced cirrhosis is now considered a proinflammatory state. Dirchwolf and colleagues[17] showed that, compared with healthy controls, patients with advanced liver disease showed significantly higher levels of proinflammatory cytokines (interleukin [IL]-6, tumor necrosis factor [TNF]-α, IL-7, IL-5, IL-12) and chemoattractants, including monocyte chemoattractant protein-1. Similar findings have been reported by other investigators.[18] These findings add credence to the systemic inflammation hypothesis.

In an animal model of cirrhosis, treatment with norfloxacin, a gut decontaminant, reduces the incidence of acute kidney injury (AKI), a syndrome that includes HRS as its most severe form.[19] This study also showed an upregulation of toll-like receptor 4 (TLR4) in the proximal renal tubules of these animals, adding weight to the evidence that an interaction with a pathogen receptor molecule, in this case TLR4, is important in mediating kidney dysfunction associated with HRS.[19] Furthermore, primary prophylaxis with norfloxacin in patients with low-protein ascites and advanced cirrhosis is associated with a significant reduction in the probability of developing HRS.[20] Selective decontamination with norfloxacin has also been shown to decrease vascular nitric oxide production and partially reverse the hyperdynamic circulatory state that predisposes to HRS in cirrhotic patients.[21] These studies provide evidence into the role of bacterial translocation and systemic inflammation in HRS development. Furthermore, a recent study by Sole and colleagues[22] showed that patients with decompensated cirrhosis and HRS had higher levels of urinary and plasma inflammatory cytokines compared with patients with decompensated cirrhosis and no AKI, or hypovolemia-induced AKI. The intensity of the inflammatory response observed in the patients with HRS-AKI correlated with lack of resolution of renal impairment and short-term mortality in these patients.[22]

Although systemic inflammation can occur in the absence of documented bacterial infection via bacterial translocation, active bacterial infection is often the main trigger for the development of HRS in patients with cirrhosis.[9] Bacterial infections occur in approximately 25% to 45% of cirrhotic patients hospitalized with an acute decompensation, with SBP and urinary tract infection (UTI) being the most common infections.[23,24] Bacterial infection–induced progressive renal failure, meeting the previous diagnostic criteria for type 1 HRS,[25] develops in about 30% of patients with SBP and 20% of patients with UTI.[24]

From the available evidence to date, it is likely that the systemic inflammatory response (in the presence or absence of active infection), exacerbates the circulatory dysfunction initiated by portal hypertension, and further contributes to a reduction in the effective arterial blood volume, predisposing to the development of RA, HRS, and other important complications of portal hypertension.

ASCITES
Diagnosis

Ascites occurs at the rate of 6% to 7% per annum in patients with cirrhosis. Therefore, in the decade after diagnosis of cirrhosis, 60% to 70% of cirrhotic patients developed ascites.[26,27] The development of ascites in cirrhosis marks a clinically significant milestone in the natural history of the disease, because it is the most common initial presentation of decompensated liver disease and therefore it indicates the start of the decompensated phase. It is associated with poor quality of life, increased morbidity, and a median survival of 2 years.[28]

The first-line treatment of patients with uncomplicated ascites is diuretics and sodium (Na) restriction. However, up to 10% per annum of patients with ascites become refractory to the standard treatment of Na restriction and diuretics.[29] Ascites is classified as refractory to diuretic therapy when there is a lack of response to maximal doses of diuretics, or diuretic intractable when the development of side effects precludes the use of maximal doses of diuretics.[30] **Box 1** shows the diagnostic criteria of RA as proposed by the International Club of Ascites (ICA).[30]

The development of RA is also associated with further complications, such as electrolyte abnormalities, especially hyponatremia, SBP, and AKI including HRS.[31] Furthermore, compared with patients with diuretic-responsive ascites, the survival of patients with RA is reduced to 50% at 6 months and 25% at 1 year.[32]

MANAGEMENT
Dietary Sodium Restriction and Sodium Balance

Cirrhotic patients who have decompensated with ascites have excess total body Na. Therefore, the mainstay of managing ascites in this patient cohort is limiting their daily Na intake.[33] A negative Na balance can be attained by reducing daily intake of Na and increasing urinary Na excretion. The ICA recommended that daily Na intake should not exceed 88 mmol (2 g).[30] Education plays a crucial role and information on where to purchase low-Na food items and recipes for low-Na meals is helpful. Patients with an abnormally high daily salt intake often notice a dramatic change with reduction in their volume of ascites by merely restricting their salt intake; this is especially true in patients whose urinary Na excretion exceeds 78 to 100 mmol/d. **Fig. 3** shows how clinicians can estimate the amount of fluid retention and therefore anticipate patients' weight gain corresponding with their Na balance. This estimation helps gauge the frequency of paracentesis required. Restricting Na intake is not necessarily equal to limiting the daily calorie intake, because there is an increasingly wide supply of low-salt food items. However, it has to be kept in mind so as to not compromise the nutritional status when implementing Na restriction. Patients with ascites should be encouraged to increase their total caloric intake while being watchful of their Na intake, because they usually are already malnourished and sarcopenic given the catabolic state of cirrhosis

---

Box 1
Diagnostic criteria of refractory ascites according to the International Club of Ascites

Diuretic-resistant ascites
- Ascites that cannot be mobilized
- Early recurrence of which cannot be prevented
  Because of lack of response to dietary sodium restriction and maximal doses of diuretics

Diuretic-intractable ascites
- Ascites that cannot be mobilized
- Early recurrence that cannot be prevented
  Because of development of diuretic-induced complications[a] that preclude the use of effective doses of diuretics.

Duration of treatment
  Greater than or equal to 1 week
  - Spironolactone 400 mg/d or amiloride 30 mg/d
  - Furosemide 160 mg/d
  - Adherence to low-sodium diet (≤90 mmol/d)

Lack of treatment response
- Mean weight loss of less than 0.8 kg over 4 days
- Urinary sodium less than sodium intake

Early recurrence of ascites
  Reappearance of grade 2 or grade 3 ascites within 4 weeks of initial mobilization

[a] Diuretic-induced complications: (1) Renal impairment; (2) Hyponatremia; (3) Hypokalemia or hyperkalemia; (4) Hepatic encephalopathy.
  Adapted from Moore KP, Wong F, Gines P, et al. The management of ascites in cirrhosis: report on the consensus conference of the International Ascites Club. Hepatology 2003;38:258-66; with permission.

---

and their burden of ascites. In one of the first real-world cross-sectional studies, Morando and colleagues[34] showed that severe Na restriction to less than 88 mmol/d can reduce mean daily calorie intake by 20% without lowering serum Na level.

Diuretic-Responsive Ascites

Apart from restricting Na intake, management of uncomplicated ascites includes initiation of diuretic therapy, which enhances renal excretion of Na.[27] Renal Na retention in

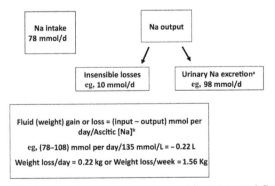

Fig. 3. Principles behind sodium balance in patients with ascites and fluid/weight loss or gain calculation. [a] Spot urine Na/K ratio greater than 1 is equivalent to 24-hour urinary Na excretion of greater than 78 mmol/d. [b] Ascitic [Na] is the same as serum [Na] 135 mmol/L

cirrhosis is predominantly secondary to increased proximal as well as distal tubular Na reabsorption rather than a decrease in filtered Na load.[27] Hyperaldosteronism is the main mechanism by which distal tubular Na reabsorption occurs; aldosterone antagonists are the diuretic of choice in the management of ascites, because they are more effective than loop diuretics alone[27] because the Na that is not being reabsorbed at the loop of Henle by loop diuretics is transported to the distal tubule and reabsorbed there because of the hyperaldosteronism, unless Na reabsorption is also blocked at that site by aldosterone antagonists. The standard of care is initiating aldosterone antagonists such as spironolactone alone at a dosage of 100 mg daily when first diagnosed with ascites; increasing in a stepwise manner weekly to a maximal dose of 400 mg/d every week.[27] In patients with recurrent or inadequately controlled ascites and those who develop hyperkalemia, loop diuretic such as furosemide can be added to the diuretic regime, starting at a dosage of 40 mg daily, increasing by 40 mg/wk to a maximal dose of 160 mg/d.[27] However, there are data to suggest that the combination of a loop and a distal diuretic is more efficacious and associated with fewer side effects than using a distal diuretic and a loop diuretic sequentially.[35] Therefore, some clinicians prefer to initiate diuretic therapy by using a combination of 100 mg of spironolactone and 40 mg of furosemide, and increasing in a stepwise fashion in increments of 100 mg of spironolactone and 40 mg of furosemide if necessary. It is important to recognize that the dose-response curve of furosemide is sigmoidal: once a maximal response is reached, increasing the dose of furosemide does not increase the diuretic response; it increases the likelihood of side effects. Patients with inadequately controlled ascites are those who lose less than 2 kg/wk. It is crucial that dose increment is accompanied by renal function monitoring to avoid diuretic-related renal dysfunction or electrolyte imbalances. The goal of treatment is water-weight loss less than or equal to 0.5 kg/d in patients without peripheral edema and 1 kg/d in those with peripheral edema.[27] Spot urine Na can also be helpful to identify patients with noncompliance to standard therapy compared with those with true RA (see **Fig. 3**), because the former have very high urinary Na concentration.

Diuretic Refractory Ascites

The standard of care in the management of RA consists of dietary Na restriction, repeated large-volume paracentesis (LVP), and insertion of transjugular intrahepatic portosystemic shunt (TIPS) in the appropriate patients. RA has a negative prognostic implication with median survival of less than a year.[36] Patients with RA who meet the minimum criteria for liver transplant (LT) should be referred to a transplant center for consideration of LT. **Fig. 4** shows the suggested clinical approach that can be adopted once patients decompensate with uncomplicated RA.

Albumin Infusions

The development of ascites in cirrhosis is related to the shift of fluid from the intravascular compartment into the abdominal cavity. In the hepatic sinusoids, portal hypertension–induced increase in hydrostatic pressure, together with low oncotic pressure caused by hypoalbuminemia, favors the egress of fluid from the circulation into the abdominal cavity.[37] Therefore, theoretically, albumin infusion can restore part of the equilibrium by correcting the hypoalbuminemia, which increases oncotic pressure, reducing ascites volume in the abdominal cavity. Furthermore, albumin also has antiinflammatory and antioxidant properties,[38] which may ameliorate the abnormal hemodynamics of advanced cirrhosis by reducing the extent of arterial vasodilatation. There has never been a dose-response study for albumin, and the recommended doses for albumin infusion were proposed by the ICA based on expert

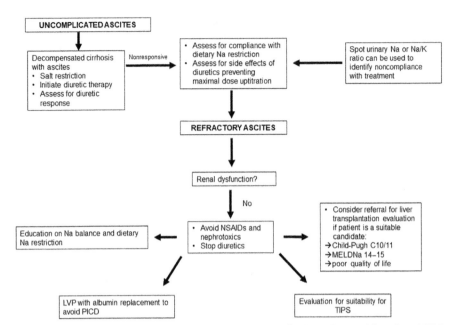

Fig. 4. Recommended stepwise approach in managing cirrhotic patients with ascites. MELD-Na, Model for End-stage Liver Disease–Sodium; NSAIDs, nonsteroidal antiinflammatory drugs; PICD, paracentesis-induced circulatory dysfunction.

opinions. Romanelli and colleagues[37] evaluated the effects of chronic albumin infusions on patient survival, recurrence of ascites, and development of other cirrhosis-related complications in 100 consecutive patients with cirrhosis and ascites. Patients who received albumin infusions had a significantly greater cumulative survival by 16 months ($P = .0078$) and lower probability of ascites recurrence (51% vs 94%, $P<.0001$) over a median follow-up period of 84 months (range, 2–120 months). The use of albumin has also been shown to prevent the development of paracentesis-induced circulatory dysfunction (PICD) (discussed later) in patients who undergo LVP,[39] likely related to its ability to maintain the intravascular volume. The prevalence of other complications of cirrhosis, such as hepatic encephalopathy (HE), variceal bleeding, and liver failure, were comparable between those two groups ($P>.05$). Albumin infusion therapy was deemed safe with no reported administration-related side effects throughout the study period. There is recent evidence from randomized clinical studies advocating the use of chronic albumin infusions in managing cirrhotic patients with ascites; this practice is widely used in some European centers, especially in Italy, where a study was conducted involving 68 liver units designed to reach a consensus among their hepatologists on the use of intravenous albumin in cirrhotic patients with ascites.[40] Expert opinion from that study is that chronic albumin infusion can help to improve the well-being and general condition of cirrhotic patients with ascites. In addition, 77% of the experts in that study agreed that the administration of albumin in the long-term can reduce the number of hospital admissions as well as length of hospital stay once admitted, which further corroborates the favorable cost/benefit ratio in the albumin-treated group as shown by Gentilini and colleagues.[41] In addition, the chronic administration of intravenous albumin in cirrhotic patients with ascites improved the rate of diuretic response, therefore lowering the rate of RA. A pilot study by Schindler and Ramadori[42] in which 12 patients with diuretic-resistant ascites were treated with intravenous albumin (mean daily dose of 22.1 g) showed that there was a significant improvement in urinary Na excretion and subsequent increase in urine volume. Albumin infusions were administered for an average of 31 days. A recent multicenter randomized controlled trial from Italy confirmed that chronic albumin infusions for 18 months in patients with diuretic-responsive ascites improved survival.[43] Whether the same survival benefits will be observed in patients with RA awaits further studies.

Transjugular Intrahepatic Portosystemic Shunt

TIPS is a radiologically inserted stent that connects a branch of the portal vein with a branch of the hepatic vein within the liver parenchyma. It functions as a side-to-side portocaval shunt and is effective at lowering portal pressure, which is central to the pathogenesis of RA and HRS.[44] TIPS is more effective than LVP at controlling ascites and can lead to ascites elimination in up to 77.6% of patients.[45–47] There is now increasing evidence that TIPS placement improves transplant-free survival rates.[46,48,49] In addition, it has a beneficial effect on nutritional status.[50] TIPS placement can be considered as a first-line treatment of carefully selected patients with RA.[48,49,51] However, placement is contraindicated in up to 60% of patients, highlighting the need for careful patient selection[31] (**Table 1**). TIPS placement before the development of RA may also be beneficial in improving survival.[48,51] Patients considered for TIPS should undergo detailed evaluation, including liver imaging, cardiac evaluation, and a full infection screen to ensure that they are no contraindications.

Complications occurring with TIPS placement include bleeding, hemoperitoneum, liver capsule rupture, and TIPS-biliary fistulae. Stent migration or kinking, stent stenosis, hemolytic anemia, and stent infection can also occur. HE is a recognized complication of portosystemic shunting after TIPS placement. The incidence of de novo or worsening HE after TIPS is estimated at 25% to 45%[52] and is significantly reduced by the use of underdilated covered stents.[53]

Large-Volume Paracentesis and Paracentesis-induced Circulatory Dysfunction

LVP remains the first-line management for RA and has been shown to be safe and effective with lower incidence of renal injury, electrolyte abnormalities, and much

Table 1 Patient selection criteria and contraindications to transjugular intrahepatic portosystemic shunt placement	
Patient Selection	
Young (<65 y)	
Normal cardiac, renal function	
No prior history of encephalopathy	
Child-Pugh score <12, MELD <18	
No sepsis, including dental sepsis	
Contraindications	
Relative	Absolute
Age >70 y	Child-Pugh ≥12 or MELD ≥18
Hepatoma	Congestive cardiac failure
Porta vein thrombosis	Severe pulmonary hypertension
Noncompliance with sodium restriction	Unrelieved biliary obstruction
	Untreated infection or uncontrolled sepsis
	Multiple hepatic cysts

Abbreviation: MELD, model for end-stage liver disease.

less systemic and hemodynamic disturbance. LVP is key in the outpatient management of patients with RA. For patients who are adherent to Na restriction, the volume of ascites removed should be no more than 6 to 8 L every 14 days. Survival rates were reportedly similar in patients who had LVP compared with patients who were on diuretics. Despite underlying coagulopathy in these patients, LVP is fairly safe, with minimal complication risks.[54] In one study, which included patients with International Normalized Ratio greater than 1.5 and platelet count less than 50×10^6/L, approximately 1% of patients experienced minimal cutaneous bleeding after LVP.[55] Bleeding risks are quoted as approximating 0.5% when patients are consented for the procedure.

Most guidelines on the management of ascites recommend the use of plasma expander after LVP of more than 5 L to prevent the development of PICD.[27,56,57] LVP of smaller volume is not associated with any renal hemodynamic perturbations.[58] The most frequently used plasma expander is human albumin solution (HAS).

PICD is a condition associated with rapid reaccumulation of ascites and a 20% risk of developing renal impairment and HRS. Immediately after LVP, venous return increases because of decrease in intra-abdominal pressure, followed by arterial vasodilatation, which peaks at day 6 following the LVP, with activation of various neurohormonal vasoconstrictor systems.[59] An alternative to HAS is saline replacement, especially when smaller-volume paracentesis is performed. Sola-Vera and colleagues[60] showed that, although albumin is more effective than saline in preventing PICD, it is a valid alternative when less than 6 L of ascites is removed. Volume replacement using colloids ameliorates some of the deleterious effects of LVP on renal and systemic hemodynamics.[60] HAS has been shown to be better than synthetic colloids in PICD prevention. There is no set rule as to whether the albumin should be given before, during, or after the paracentesis. Although the randomized controlled trial by Moreau and colleagues[61] comparing outcome and hospital-related costs in patients treated with HAS versus those given synthetic colloid (3.5% polygeline) was prematurely discontinued because of concerns about bovine-related products, HAS seemed to be more effective at preventing liver-related complications. The use of albumin is also more cost-effective, with lower median 30-day hospital costs (€1915 vs €4612).[61] The American Association for the Study of Liver Disease recommends infusion of 6 to 8 g of albumin per liter of ascites removed with paracentesis greater than 5 L.[62] This amount also seems to confer some survival advantage.[56] Not all episodes of PICD lead to the development of renal impairment.[63] Recent study from our own institution showed that routine use of HAS and limiting LVP to 8 L can prevent development of renal impairment despite PICD.[39]

Automated Low-flow Ascites Pump (alfapump)

The alfapump is an implantable battery-powered pump that transports ascites from the peritoneal cavity into the bladder (**Fig. 5**), so it can be eliminated by micturition. Emerging data show that it is effective and significantly reduces the need for LVP.[64,65] In addition, its use is associated with an improvement in nutritional status as well as health-related quality of life.[64,66] Initial trial results showed that its use was associated with a high incidence of adverse events, including infections.[64,65,67] The introduction of mandatory prophylactic antibiotic seems to have obviated this complication. Because the alfapump is equivalent to a continuous, slow, low-volume paracentesis without the use of albumin, some patients in the studies developed renal dysfunction. It has been recommended that intermittent albumin should be given as guided by renal function, because physiologic studies have shown that there are increased activities of various vasoconstrictor systems despite

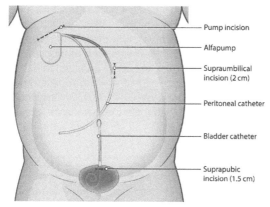

Pump incision

Alfapump

Supraumbilical
incision (2 cm)

Peritoneal catheter

Bladder catheter

Suprapubic
incision (1.5 cm)

Fig. 5. alfapump in situ. (*Courtesy of* Sequana Medical NV, Zwijnaarde, Belgium; with permission.)

low-volume paracentesis.[67] Further studies will include albumin supplementation with alfapump use. The alfapump system is commercially available in some European countries, but currently not approved in North America.

Liver Transplant

Liver transplant remains the gold standard treatment option for patients with RA and advanced liver disease who meet the minimum criteria for transplant.[68] Ascites was excluded as one of the prioritizing measures for LT when Child-Turcotte-Pugh score was replaced by the Model for End-stage Liver Disease (MELD)–based organ allocation system.[69] Ascites is a well-established predictor of mortality in patients with cirrhosis[70]; patients with RA have a 1-year mortality approaching 50%.[36,71] Persistent ascites has been shown to result in excess waiting list mortality equivalent to 4.5 MELD[72] or 3.5 Model for End-stage Liver Disease–Sodium (MELD-Na)[73] scores; this was more prominent in the group of patients with MELD score of less than 21.[73] The implication is that patients with RA are underserved by the MELD score, remaining at the lower tier of LT waiting lists unless they have coexisting issues such as hepatocellular carcinoma or hepatopulmonary syndrome that make them eligible to be awarded an exception point of 22 when listed for LT, with an increment of 3 points every 3 months. Therefore, they eventually succumb to their liver disease if not transplanted.[74] Hyponatremia has an established association with RA and is linked with high mortality in cirrhotic patients.[70,75] It is also a strong predictor of waitlist mortality,[76] with 5% to 7% increase in waiting list mortality for every 1 mmol/L decrease in serum Na level.[77] It is anticipated that the new MELD-Na score will accurately capture this group of patients, allowing them to be transplanted earlier for better posttransplant outcomes. After transplant, ascites can remain for another 3 to 4 months because it takes time for the abnormal hemodynamics and renal pathophysiology that accounts for formation of ascites in cirrhosis to fully reverse. It is important for patients to continue to adhere to their low-Na diets after transplant until ascites clearance.

HEPATORENAL SYNDROME
Introduction

Renal dysfunction is a common manifestation of advanced cirrhosis and has been estimated to occur in between 20% and 40% of patients with advanced cirrhosis admitted with decompensation.[78,79] Patients with RA are at risk for AKI, the early diagnosis of which is imperative. One of the main challenges with the diagnosis of AKI is the recognition that a normal laboratory serum creatinine (sCr) value can be falsely reassuring when managing cirrhotic patients given that most of these patients often have a lower baseline sCr levels, which are often multifactorial, one of the causes of which is sarcopenia and lower muscle mass, leading to less creatine conversion to creatinine.[80] Recommendations made by ICA[80] to aid clinicians in diagnosing AKI early during its course have helped to identify these patients, allowing early treatment and optimization of their renal function.

Diagnosis

Renal dysfunction in cirrhosis is associated with significant morbidity and mortality. It may present acutely as sudden and rapid deterioration in renal function or it may evolve slowly because of underlying chronic abnormalities, being related to hemodynamics or structural renal disease. Therefore, there is a need for early detection and management. Based on the needs for uniformity of nomenclature, and early detection of mild renal dysfunction, the Acute Dialysis Quality Initiative (ADQI) group and the ICA in 2011 proposed the following definition for kidney dysfunction in cirrhosis: AKI is defined as an increase in serum creatinine level by greater than or equal to 0.3 mg/dL in less than 48 hours, or a 50% increase from a stable baseline within the preceding 3 months.[81] The cause of AKI could be related to either rapid structural damage to the kidney or acute deterioration of renal hemodynamics. Thus, type 1 HRS is a special form of AKI. In contrast, chronic kidney disease (CKD) is defined as an estimated glomerular filtration rate (eGFR) of less than 60 mL/min for greater than or equal to 3 months.[81] In 2015, the ICA modified the definitions of AKI in patients with cirrhosis, adapting the definition of AKI from the Kidney Disease Improving Global Outcomes group.[80] The organization also described the severity of AKI by defining the 3 stages of AKI (stages 1, 2, 3). However, recent data have suggested that stage 1 AKI consists of a heterogeneous group of patients with different clinical outcomes depending on whether the final sCr level is more or less than 1.5 mg/dL.[82] For this reason, current guidelines from the European Association for the Study of the Liver recommend that clinicians should separate these two groups of patients into AKI stage 1a or 1b to describe patients whose sCr level at AKI diagnosis is less than or more than 1.5 mg/dL respectively.[83] The North American Association for the Study of the Liver has not made such a recommendation; **Table 2** highlights the new definition of AKI in cirrhosis and incorporates the modification of AKI stage 1.

Differential diagnosis of acute kidney injury in cirrhosis

AKI in cirrhosis can be caused by prerenal azotemia (PRA), HRS, or acute tubular necrosis (ATN). HRS is a unique form of AKI that occurs mainly in the setting of advanced cirrhosis because of the circulatory dysfunction mentioned earlier.[2] However, it has also been described in acute liver failure.[9] Two types of HRS were historically recognized. Type 1 HRS, now renamed HRS-AKI,[83] occurs in an acute setting and is a rapidly progressive decline in renal function associated with a high mortality.[70] The diagnostic criteria for HRS-AKI as defined by the ICA are shown in **Box 2**.[80] Type 2 HRS, renamed HRS–non-AKI (HRS-NAKI),[83] is a more chronic form of renal dysfunction that evolves over weeks to months. Despite these new terminologies, the terms type 1 and 2 HRS are still often used in clinical practice and were used in all studies on HRS therapies.[9] Distinguishing HRS-AKI from other causes of AKI is paramount because treatment varies.

Table 2
Definition of acute kidney injury in cirrhosis

- Definition of AKI: increase in sCr $\geq$0.3 mg/dL ($\geq$26.5 μmol/L) within 48 h, or a percentage increase in sCr of $\geq$50% from a known baseline[a] with the change presumed to have occurred within the prior 7 d

Stage of AKI	Definition
1	Increase in sCr $\geq$0.3 mg/dL (26.5 μmol/L) or an increase in sCr $\geq$1.5-fold to 2-fold from baseline
1a[b]	sCr <1.5 mg/dL at diagnosis
1b[b]	sCr $\geq$1.5 mg/dL at diagnosis
2	Increase in sCr >2-fold to 3-fold from baseline
3	Increase in sCr >3-fold from baseline or sCr $\geq$4.0 mg/dL (353.6 μmol/L) with an acute increase $\geq$0.3 mg/dL ($\geq$26.5 μmol/L), or renal replacement therapy initiation

[a] Baseline is a value of sCr obtained in the previous 3 months. In patients with more than 1 value obtained in the previous 3 months, the value closest to the hospital admission time should be used. In patients without a previous sCr value, the sCr on admission should be used as baseline.
[b] Only according to European Association for the Study of the Liver guidelines.
Adapted from Angeli P, Gines P, Wong F, et al. Diagnosis and management of acute kidney injury in patients with cirrhosis: revised consensus recommendations of the International Club of Ascites. Gut 2015;64:531-7; and EASL Clinical Practice Guidelines for the management of patients with decompensated cirrhosis. J Hepatol 2018;69(2):406-60; with permission.

Serum creatinine, which is routinely measured as a marker of renal dysfunction, is unable to distinguish between these various causes of AKI. Thus there is a need for other biomarkers, and these include urinary and serum neutrophil gelatinase-associated lipocalin (NGAL), urinary IL-18, urinary kidney injury molecule 1 (KIM-1), urinary liver type fatty acid binding protein 1 (L-FAP), urinary albumin, and fractional execration of Na (FENa).[84] Urinary NGAL is an iron-transporting protein rapidly accumulating in the kidney tubules and urine after nephrotoxic and ischemic insults. It is therefore a biomarker of tubular damage and is the most frequently studied biomarker in cirrhosis-related AKI.

Studies have shown that levels of urinary NGAL are significantly higher in patients with ATN, lower in patients with PRA, and intermediate in patients with HRS.[84,85]

Box 2
International Club of Ascites diagnostic criteria for hepatorenal syndrome acute kidney injury

- Cirrhosis with ascites
- Diagnosis of AKI according to IAC AKI criteria[a]
- No response after 2 consecutive days of diuretic withdrawal and plasma volume expansion with albumin 1 g per kilogram of body weight
- Absence of shock
- No current or recent treatment with nephrotoxic drugs
- Absence of parenchymal kidney disease as indicated by absence of proteinuria greater than 500 mg/d, microhematuria (>50 red blood cells per high power field), and normal renal ultrasonography

[a] As per Ref.[80]
From Garcia-Tsao G, Parikh CR, Viola A. Acute kidney injury in cirrhosis. Hepatology 2008;48:2064-77; with permission.

Although urinary NGAL has the potential to differentiate between ATN and other types of AKI, it has limitations, namely that (1) it is increased in patients with UTI because it is also produced by neutrophils, thus levels may be falsely increased in this context; (2) levels may overlap between patients with HRS and ATN and a clear threshold level differentiating between these two conditions is yet to be determined.[86] There is potential for further research into biomarkers that aid diagnosis and categorization of AKI episodes into HRS, PRA, and ATN, especially because renal biopsies are rarely performed in patients with advanced cirrhosis.

Management

The ICA recommends the algorithm indicated in **Fig. 6** in the management of patients with cirrhosis and AKI.[87]

Supportive measures

Because HRS is a diagnosis of exclusion, it is important that patients with cirrhosis who present with AKI have other diagnoses ruled out. Patients still on diuretics should have these stopped. All patients with AKI should receive a volume challenge irrespective of recent diuretic intake. The best approach is the administration of HAS, to be given at a dose of 1 g per kilogram of body weight up to 100 g/d. In patients who have PRA, the sCr level should start decreasing as the intravascular volume is being repleted. Patients who have structural renal disease have abnormal urine findings,

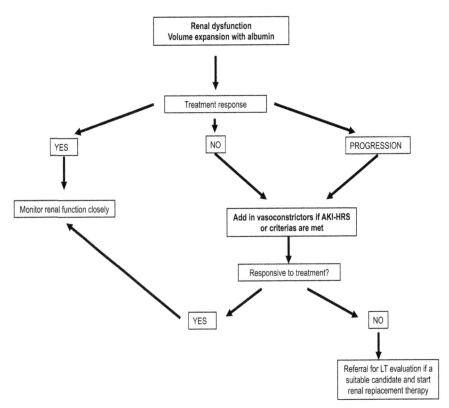

Fig. 6. Treatment algorithm for patients with cirrhosis and AKI.

including the presence of casts and sediments, and these should be treated according to the definitive diagnosis. Patients with HRS do not respond to volume challenge. Their sCr levels may continue to increase despite the volume challenge. Empiric antibiotics should be given until all cultures have been returned as negative. Patients who have proven infections should have their antibiotics modified according to sensitivity testing results.

Vasoconstrictor therapy

Vasoconstrictors combined with HAS significantly improve renal function in HRS.[88–90] Vasoconstrictors exert their beneficial effect in HRS by attenuating splanchnic arterial vasodilatation, whereas HAS infusion helps increase the effective arterial volume. HAS may also reduce the inflammatory mediator levels. The consequence of this combination treatment is an attenuation of the hemodynamic dysregulation associated with HRS, yielding better perfusion of the kidneys followed by improvement in renal function. Vasoconstrictors that have been used in clinical trials for the management of HRS include terlipressin, norepinephrine, octreotide, and midodrine. It is important to mention that all studies investigating the effects of vasoconstrictor in HRS involved patients who had been diagnosed using the classic definition of type 1 HRS.[25]

Terlipressin, a vasopressin analogue, is the most commonly used vasoconstrictor for the management of HRS worldwide. It is currently not available in North America for the treatment of HRS. A recent randomized controlled trial showed that treatment with terlipressin leads to reversal of HRS in approximately 56% of patients.[90] It also leads to an improvement in short-term survival in treated patients with HRS.[91] However, in a study performed in North America, Boyer and colleagues[92] reported that, although treatment with terlipressin was beneficial compared with placebo in type 1 HRS, this was not statistically significant for either partial or complete reversal.[92] However, in those patients who had a complete HRS reversal, their survival was significantly improved.[93] The discrepancy between this study and others previously reported may be caused by differences in patient population, short duration of terlipressin treatment, and the early use of alternative therapies that prevented an adequate follow-up of patients.[9] However, when the results of this study were pooled with those of an earlier North American study,[88] HRS reversal was significantly more frequent with terlipressin and albumin versus placebo and albumin.[93] Predictors of HRS reversal were lower baseline sCr level, lower MAP at study entry, lower total bilirubin level, and absence of known precipitating factors for HRS.[93]

Terlipressin is administered intravenously at doses ranging from 0.5 mg to 2.0 mg every 6 hours depending on the response. Treatment duration ranges from 5 to 15 days.[91] Adverse effects associated with terlipressin use include diarrhea, abdominal cramps, cardiac arrhythmias, intestinal ischemia, and hypertension.[9] Peripheral ischemia occurs in 4% to 13% of patients.[91] Terlipressin given as a continuous infusion is effective at lower doses for treating type 1 HRS and better tolerated compared with the bolus dosing regimen.[94] Terlipressin should be avoided in patients with known ischemic heart disease or peripheral vascular disease. Terlipressin is superior to the combination of midodrine and octreotide in the reversal of HRS.

Norepinephrine, or noradrenaline (NA), an α-adrenergic agonist, combined with HAS is also effective in treating type 1 HRS. In a randomized study comparing NA with terlipressin, Singh and colleagues[95] reported an HRS reversal rate of 39% in the terlipressin group compared with 43% in the NA group ($P = .76$). Similar findings have been reported by other investigators.[89] Note that although NA may be a less expensive drug to treat HRS, unlike terlipressin, which can be given via peripheral venous access, its administration requires central venous access in a monitored environment. In patients with acute-on-chronic liver failure (ACLF), terlipressin has been shown to be superior to NA in the reversal of HRS associated with ACLF.[96]

A combination therapy consisting of midodrine (α-adrenergic agonist), octreotide (somatostatin analogue), and HAS has also been used in the management of type 1 HRS. This combination is mostly used in North America, where terlipressin is not available. Although this combination has been reported to be beneficial in some patients with type 1 HRS,[97] a randomized controlled trial comparing this combination with terlipressin and HAS showed that the latter combination is significantly more effective in improving renal function in HRS (28.6% vs 70.4%; $P = .01$).[90] A meta-analysis concluded that terlipressin with HAS, and NA with HAS, are both superior to midodrine plus octreotide with HAS for reversal of HRS.[91] Following treatment, HRS may recur in up to 20% of patients, and retreatment may be required and is equally effective.

Transjugular intrahepatic portosystemic shunt

The insertion of a TIPS is associated with worsening of arterial vasodilatation for up 12 months following TIPS insertion.[98] Therefore, patients with renal dysfunction before TIPS may have worsening of their renal function after TIPS, hence there have not been any publications on the use of TIPS as a treatment of HRS for more than a decade. Patients who have their renal function normalized with vasoconstrictors may receive a TIPS as a treatment of their RA.[99] However, because most of these patients also have severe liver dysfunction, the use of TIPS is not feasible for most of these patients.

Renal replacement therapy

In patients who fail to respond to vasoconstrictor therapy and meet the indications for renal replacement therapy (RRT), it can be initiated. RRT can be intermittent hemodialysis or continuous RRT, and the latter is usually better tolerated in unstable patients. RRT should be considered as a bridge to LT in patients with HRS and not a definitive treatment option, because it is the hemodynamic changes associated with the cirrhotic liver that drive the renal dysfunction. At the eighth International Consensus Conference of the ADQI group, it was recommended that RRT should be withheld in type 1 HRS unless there is an acute reversible component or a plan for LT.[100] Treatment with RRT for patients with type I HRS who failed to respond to vasoconstrictor therapy is not associated with a survival benefit and, instead, resulted in prolonged hospital stay.[101]

Liver transplant

Patients who have RA and chronic renal dysfunction (HRS-NAKI) have a worse prognosis compared with those without HRS-NAKI, with estimated median survival of 6 months.[102] The definitive management of HRS, both AKI and non-AKI types, is LT because the diseased liver is replaced and thus the associated circulatory dysfunction predisposing to HRS is reversed. However, not all patients are eligible for LT. Patients with HRS are 1.29 times more likely to die after LT than those undergoing LT without HRS.[103] Following LT, renal recovery occurs in 76% to 80% of patients with HRS.[103,104] The 1-year survival in patients with type 1 HRS who achieve reversal after LT is significantly higher than in those who do not (97% vs 60%; $P = .0045$).[104] This study reported that the strongest predictor of HRS nonreversal was the duration of dialysis before LT and showed that patients who required dialysis for more than 14 days were 9.2 times more likely to have HRS nonreversal.[104] This finding highlights the importance of urgently listing and prioritizing patients with HRS who do not respond to vasoconstrictor for LT, because a timely LT can increase the likelihood of renal recovery after LT, improving patient survival.

Repeated episodes of AKI can also have detrimental effects on renal recovery. In our own center (Neong SF, unpublished data, 2019), patients with recurrent episodes of AKI are more likely to be treatment nonresponders compared with those who only had a single episode of AKI. It is therefore imperative that, in patients who have sustained an episode of AKI, efforts are made to optimize their renal function and remove all insults to prevent AKI recurrence.

Pretransplant impairment in renal function is a major predictor of posttransplant CKD, with a reported 5-year incidence rate of 18% to 22%.[105,106] In one of the largest studies on outcomes of cirrhotic patients transplanted for HRS-NAKI,[107] a large proportion of these patients developed stage 3 CKD as early as 3 months (53.8% vs 28.4%; _P_ = .007) after LT compared with the control group. Contrary to previous studies, patients with HRS-NAKI had comparable 1-year graft and patient survival (92.9% vs 91.6%) compared with the control group despite longer stay in intensive care units and prolonged hospitalizations. Older recipients, especially those aged 60 years and older, are at higher risk of developing stage 3 CKD after LT.[107]

Simultaneous liver and kidney transplant (SLKT) should be considered in patients with any form of AKI, including HRS with a high risk for renal nonrecovery. The definition of renal nonrecovery varies between Europe and the United Sates. **Box 3** summarizes the indication for SLKT in these two regions. Following SLKT, the 1-year survival for cirrhotic patients with AKI including HRS is approximately 91%.[108]

Prevention

The mainstay of management of HRS is to prevent its development in the first place. Therefore, measures should be undertaken in patients with advanced cirrhosis not to worsen the already present circulatory dysfunction. Therefore, it is prudent to withdraw diuretics in patients who have diuretic resistance. Patients undergoing LVP are at risk of developing renal impairment including HRS because of PICD. Therefore, these patients should receive intravenous HAS, which helps restore the effective arterial volume, because evidence suggests that its use significantly reduces the occurrence of HRS.[60]

Because patients with infections are at risk for developing HRS-AKI, patients suspected of infection should be given empiric antibiotics, which can be withdrawn if no infection is identified. Patients who have gastrointestinal bleed should receive

---

Box 3
Indications for simultaneous liver and kidney transplant in cirrhotic patients

European Association for the Study of Liver[27,99]
- AKI on RRT for $\geq$4 weeks or AKI with eGFR $\leq$35 mL/min or measured glomerular filtration rate (GFR) $\leq$25 mL/min $\geq$4 weeks
- CKD with eGFR $\leq$40 mL/min or measured GFR $\leq$30 mL/min
- CKD with proteinuria $\geq$2 g a day
- CKD with renal biopsy showing >30% global glomerulosclerosis or >30% interstitial fibrosis
- Presence of inherited metabolic disease (eg, hyperoxaluria)

United States[110]
- AKI and 6 weeks of consecutive dialysis or AKI for 6 weeks with an eGFR $\leq$25 mL/min or AKI and 6 weeks of a combination of both
- Patients with end-stage renal disease chronically administered dialysis
- CKD stage 3 for greater than 90 days with an eGFR of 30 mL/min or less
- Presence of comorbid metabolic disease (eg, hyperoxaluria)

Data from Refs.[27,99,110]

prophylactic antibiotics because their risks for bacterial infections are high. If the diagnosis of an infection is confirmed, modification of antibiotic therapy should be done according to sensitivity. In patients with SBP, there is evidence showing that, in addition to antimicrobial therapy, intravenous HAS administration significantly reduces the risk of developing HRS and also reduces mortality.[109]

Other preventive measures include avoidance of nephrotoxins such as radiographic dyes, nonsteroidal antiinflammatory agents, and aminoglycosides. Patients with RA should always receive close monitoring of renal function, electrolytes, and fluid balance status.

SUMMARY

The development of ascites is an important milestone in the natural history of cirrhosis because it heralds the start of the decompensated phase. Dietary Na restriction and diuretic therapy are the cornerstones of managing patients with uncomplicated ascites. When refractory to therapy, LVP is the current standard of care. In selected cirrhotic patients with RA, TIPS can be an effective treatment. Despite novel therapeutic options on the horizon for managing RA, the only definitive treatment that can correct underlying portal hypertension and treat RA with or without HRS is LT. It is therefore crucial that patients with RA are identified early, treated appropriately with standard of care, and referred for LT when clinically indicated to improve patient survival. Prevention of AKI is key to improving the survival of these patients.

REFERENCES

1. Ripoll C, Groszmann R, Garcia-Tsao G, et al. Hepatic venous pressure gradient predicts clinical decompensation in patients with compensated cirrhosis. Gastroenterology 2007;133:481–8.
2. Gines P, Schrier RW. Renal failure in cirrhosis. N Engl J Med 2009;361:1279–90.
3. Schrier RW, Arroyo V, Bernardi M, et al. Peripheral arterial vasodilation hypothesis: a proposal for the initiation of renal sodium and water retention in cirrhosis. Hepatology 1988;8:1151–7.
4. Bernardi M, Moreau R, Angeli P, et al. Mechanisms of decompensation and organ failure in cirrhosis: from peripheral arterial vasodilation to systemic inflammation hypothesis. J Hepatol 2015;63:1272–84.
5. Moller S, Bendtsen F. The pathophysiology of arterial vasodilatation and hyperdynamic circulation in cirrhosis. Liver Int 2018;38:570–80.
6. Fernandez M. Molecular pathophysiology of portal hypertension. Hepatology 2015;61:1406–15.
7. Adebayo D, Neong SF, Wong F. Refractory ascites in liver cirrhosis. Am J Gastroenterol 2019;114:40–7.
8. Busk TM, Bendtsen F, Moller S. Hepatorenal syndrome in cirrhosis: diagnostic, pathophysiological, and therapeutic aspects. Expert Rev Gastroenterol Hepatol 2016;16:1–9.
9. Gines P, Sola E, Angeli P, et al. Hepatorenal syndrome. Nat Rev Dis Primers 2018;4:33.
10. Krag A, Bendtsen F, Burroughs AK, et al. The cardiorenal link in advanced cirrhosis. Med Hypotheses 2012;79:53–5.
11. Schrier RW. Decreased effective blood volume in edematous disorders: what does this mean? J Am Soc Nephrol 2007;18:2028–31.

12. Stadlbauer V, Wright GA, Banaji M, et al. Relationship between activation of the sympathetic nervous system and renal blood flow autoregulation in cirrhosis. Gastroenterology 2008;134:111–9.

13. Sole C, Pose E, Sola E, et al. Hepatorenal syndrome in the era of acute kidney injury. Liver Int 2018;38:1891–901.

14. Bauer TM, Schwacha H, Steinbruckner B, et al. Small intestinal bacterial overgrowth in human cirrhosis is associated with systemic endotoxemia. Am J Gastroenterol 2002;97:2364–70.

15. Qin N, Yang F, Li A, et al. Alterations of the human gut microbiome in liver cirrhosis. Nature 2014;513:59–64.

16. Buck M, Garcia-Tsao G, Groszmann RJ, et al. Novel inflammatory biomarkers of portal pressure in compensated cirrhosis patients. Hepatology 2014;59:1052–9.

17. Dirchwolf M, Podhorzer A, Marino M, et al. Immune dysfunction in cirrhosis: distinct cytokines phenotypes according to cirrhosis severity. Cytokine 2016; 77:14–25.

18. Claria J, Stauber RE, Coenraad MJ, et al. Systemic inflammation in decompensated cirrhosis: characterization and role in acute-on-chronic liver failure. Hepatology 2016;64:1249–64.

19. Shah N, Dhar D, El Zahraa Mohammed F, et al. Prevention of acute kidney injury in a rodent model of cirrhosis following selective gut decontamination is associated with reduced renal TLR4 expression. J Hepatol 2012;56:1047–53.

20. Fernandez J, Navasa M, Planas R, et al. Primary prophylaxis of spontaneous bacterial peritonitis delays hepatorenal syndrome and improves survival in cirrhosis. Gastroenterology 2007;133:818–24.

21. Rasaratnam B, Kaye D, Jennings G, et al. The effect of selective intestinal decontamination on the hyperdynamic circulatory state in cirrhosis. A randomized trial. Ann Intern Med 2003;139:186–93.

22. Sole C, Sola E, Huelin P, et al. Characterization of inflammatory response in hepatorenal syndrome. relationship with kidney outcome and survival. Liver Int 2019;39:1246–55.

23. Fasolato S, Angeli P, Dallagnese L, et al. Renal failure and bacterial infections in patients with cirrhosis: epidemiology and clinical features. Hepatology 2007;45: 223–9.

24. Piano S, Brocca A, Mareso S, et al. Infections complicating cirrhosis. Liver Int 2018;38(Suppl 1):126–33.

25. Salerno F, Gerbes A, Gines P, et al. Diagnosis, prevention and treatment of hepatorenal syndrome in cirrhosis. Gut 2007;56:1310–8.

26. Gordon FD. Ascites. Clin Liver Dis 2012;16:285–99.

27. European Association for the Study of the Liver. EASL clinical practice guidelines on the management of ascites, spontaneous bacterial peritonitis, and hepatorenal syndrome in cirrhosis. J Hepatol 2010;53:397–417.

28. D'Amico G, Garcia-Tsao G, Pagliaro L. Natural history and prognostic indicators of survival in cirrhosis: a systematic review of 118 studies. J Hepatol 2006;44: 217–31.

29. Salerno F, Guevara M, Bernardi M, et al. Refractory ascites: pathogenesis, definition and therapy of a severe complication in patients with cirrhosis. Liver Int 2010;30:937–47.

30. Moore KP, Wong F, Gines P, et al. The management of ascites in cirrhosis: report on the consensus conference of the International Ascites Club. Hepatology 2003;38:258–66.

31. Piano S, Tonon M, Angeli P. Management of ascites and hepatorenal syndrome. Hepatol Int 2018;12(Suppl 1):122–34.

32. Cardenas A, Arroyo V. Refractory ascites. Dig Dis 2005;23:30–8.

33. Wong F. Management of ascites in cirrhosis. J Gastroenterol Hepatol 2012;27: 11–20.

34. Morando F, Rosi S, Gola E, et al. Adherence to a moderate sodium restriction diet in outpatients with cirrhosis and ascites: a real-life cross-sectional study. Liver Int 2015;35:1508–15.

35. Angeli P, Fasolato S, Mazza E, et al. Combined versus sequential diuretic treatment of ascites in non-azotaemic patients with cirrhosis: results of an open randomised clinical trial. Gut 2010;59:98–104.

36. Gines P, Cardenas A, Arroyo V, et al. Management of cirrhosis and ascites. N Engl J Med 2004;350:1646–54.

37. Romanelli RG, La Villa G, Barletta G, et al. Long-term albumin infusion improves survival in patients with cirrhosis and ascites: an unblinded randomized trial. World J Gastroenterol 2006;12:1403–7.

38. Reiberger T, Mandorfer M. Beta adrenergic blockade and decompensated cirrhosis. J Hepatol 2017;66:849–59.

39. Tan HK, James PD, Wong F. Albumin may prevent the morbidity of paracentesis-induced circulatory dysfunction in cirrhosis and refractory ascites: a pilot study. Dig Dis Sci 2016;61:3084–92.

40. Gentilini P, Bernardi M, Bolondi L, et al. The rational use of albumin in patients with cirrhosis and ascites. A Delphi study for the attainment of a consensus on prescribing standards. Dig Liver Dis 2004;36:539–46.

41. Gentilini P, Casini-Raggi V, Di Fiore G, et al. Albumin improves the response to diuretics in patients with cirrhosis and ascites: results of a randomized, controlled trial. J Hepatol 1999;30:639–45.

42. Schindler C, Ramadori G. Albumin substitution improves urinary sodium excretion and diuresis in patients with liver cirrhosis and refractory ascites. J Hepatol 1999;31:1132.

43. Caraceni P, Riggio O, Angeli P, et al. Long-term albumin administration in decompensated cirrhosis (ANSWER): an open-label randomised trial. Lancet 2018;391:2417–29.

44. Wong F, Sniderman K, Liu P, et al. Transjugular intrahepatic portosystemic stent shunt: effects on hemodynamics and sodium homeostasis in cirrhosis and refractory ascites. Ann Intern Med 1995;122:816–22.

45. Tan HK, James PD, Sniderman KW, et al. Long-term clinical outcome of patients with cirrhosis and refractory ascites treated with transjugular intrahepatic portosystemic shunt insertion. J Gastroenterol Hepatol 2015;30:389–95.

46. Salerno F, Camma C, Enea M, et al. Transjugular intrahepatic portosystemic shunt for refractory ascites: a meta-analysis of individual patient data. Gastroenterology 2007;133:825–34.

47. Saab S, Nieto JM, Lewis SK, et al. TIPS versus paracentesis for cirrhotic patients with refractory ascites. Cochrane Database Syst Rev 2006;(4):CD004889.

48. Bureau C, Thabut D, Oberti F, et al. Transjugular intrahepatic portosystemic shunts with covered stents increase transplant-free survival of patients with cirrhosis and recurrent ascites. Gastroenterology 2017;152:157–63.

49. Bucsics T, Hoffman S, Grunberger J, et al. ePTFE-TIPS vs repetitive LVP plus albumin for the treatment of refractory ascites in patients with cirrhosis. Liver Int 2018;38:1036–44.

50. Tsien C, Shah SN, McCullough AJ, et al. Reversal of sarcopenia predicts survival after a transjugular intrahepatic portosystemic stent. Eur J Gastroenterol Hepatol 2013;25:85–93.
51. Shen NT, Schneider Y, Congly SE, et al. Cost effectiveness of early insertion of transjugular intrahepatic portosystemic shunts for recurrent ascites. Clin Gastroenterol Hepatol 2018;16:1503–10.
52. Vilstrup H, Amodio P, Bajaj J, et al. Hepatic encephalopathy in chronic liver disease: 2014 practice guideline by the American Association for the Study of Liver Diseases and the European Association for the Study of the Liver. Hepatology 2014;60:715–35.
53. Schepis F, Vizzutti F, Garcia-Tsao G, et al. Under-dilated TIPS associate with efficacy and reduced encephalopathy in a prospective, non-randomized study of patients with cirrhosis. Clin Gastroenterol Hepatol 2018;16:1153–62.
54. Sharzehi K, Jain V, Naveed A, et al. Hemorrhagic complications of paracentesis: a systematic review of the literature. Gastroenterol Res Pract 2014;2014:985141.
55. Lin CH, Shih FY, Ma MH, et al. Should bleeding tendency deter abdominal paracentesis? Dig Liver Dis 2005;37:946–51.
56. Bernardi M, Caraceni P, Navickis RJ. Does the evidence support a survival benefit of albumin infusion in patients with cirrhosis undergoing large-volume paracentesis? Expert Rev Gastroenterol Hepatol 2017;11:191–2.
57. Bernardi M, Caraceni P, Navickis RJ, et al. Albumin infusion in patients undergoing large-volume paracentesis: a meta-analysis of randomized trials. Hepatology 2012;55:1172–81.
58. Peltekian KM, Wong F, Liu PP, et al. Cardiovascular, renal, and neurohumoral responses to single large-volume paracentesis in patients with cirrhosis and diuretic-resistant ascites. Am J Gastroenterol 1997;92:394–9.
59. Gines P, Tito L, Arroyo V, et al. Randomized comparative study of therapeutic paracentesis with and without intravenous albumin in cirrhosis. Gastroenterology 1988;94:1493–502.
60. Sola-Vera J, Minana J, Ricart E, et al. Randomized trial comparing albumin and saline in the prevention of paracentesis-induced circulatory dysfunction in cirrhotic patients with ascites. Hepatology 2003;37:1147–53.
61. Moreau R, Valla DC, Durand-Zaleski I, et al. Comparison of outcome in patients with cirrhosis and ascites following treatment with albumin or a synthetic colloid: a randomised controlled pilot trail. Liver Int 2006;26:46–54.
62. Runyon BA. Introduction to the revised American Association for the Study of Liver Diseases Practice Guideline management of adult patients with ascites due to cirrhosis 2012. Hepatology 2013;57:1651–3.
63. Moreau R, Asselah T, Condat B, et al. Comparison of the effect of terlipressin and albumin on arterial blood volume in patients with cirrhosis and tense ascites treated by paracentesis: a randomised pilot study. Gut 2002;50:90–4.
64. Bureau C, Adebayo D, Chalret de Rieu M, et al. Alfapump® system vs. large volume paracentesis for refractory ascites: a multicenter randomized controlled study. J Hepatol 2017;67:940–9.
65. Bellot P, Welker MW, Soriano G, et al. Automated low flow pump system for the treatment of refractory ascites: a multi-center safety and efficacy study. J Hepatol 2013;58:922–7.
66. Stepanova M, Nader F, Bureau C, et al. Patients with refractory ascites treated with alfapump® system have better health-related quality of life as compared to those treated with large volume paracentesis: the results of a multicenter randomized controlled study. Qual Life Res 2018;27:1513–20.

67. Sola E, Sanchez-Cabus S, Rodriguez E, et al. Effects of alfapump system on kidney and circulatory function in patients with cirrhosis and refractory ascites. Liver Transpl 2017;23:583–93.
68. Fortune B, Cardenas A. Ascites, refractory ascites and hyponatremia in cirrhosis. Gastroenterol Rep 2017;5:104–12.
69. Freeman RB Jr, Wiesner RH, Harper A, et al. The new liver allocation system: moving toward evidence-based transplantation policy. Liver Transpl 2002;8: 851–8.
70. Gines A, Escorsell A, Gines P, et al. Incidence, predictive factors, and prognosis of the hepatorenal syndrome in cirrhosis with ascites. Gastroenterology 1993; 105:229–36.
71. Siqueira F, Kelly T, Saab S. Refractory ascites: pathogenesis, clinical impact, and management. Gastroenterol Hepatol 2009;5:647–56.
72. Heuman DM, Abou-Assi SG, Habib A, et al. Persistent ascites and low serum sodium identify patients with cirrhosis and low MELD scores who are at high risk for early death. Hepatology 2004;40:802–10.
73. Somsouk M, Kornfield R, Vittinghoff E, et al. Moderate ascites identifies patients with low model for end-stage liver disease scores awaiting liver transplantation who have a high mortality risk. Liver Transpl 2011;17:129–36.
74. Busuttil RW, Farmer DG, Yersiz H, et al. Analysis of long-term outcomes of 3200 liver transplantations over two decades: a single-center experience. Ann Surg 2005;241:905–16.
75. Fernandez-Esparrach G, Sanchez-Fueyo A, Gines P, et al. A prognostic model for predicting survival in cirrhosis with ascites. J Hepatol 2001;34:46–52.
76. Prohic D, Mesihovic R, Vanis N, et al. Prognostic significance of ascites and serum sodium in patients with low MELD scores. Med Arch 2016;70:48–52.
77. Biggins SW, Rodriguez HJ, Bacchetti P, et al. Serum sodium predicts mortality in patients listed for liver transplantation. Hepatology 2005;41:32–9.
78. Carvalho GC, Regis Cde A, Kalil JR, et al. Causes of renal failure in patients with decompensated cirrhosis and its impact in hospital mortality. Ann Hepatol 2012; 11:90–5.
79. Garcia-Tsao G, Parikh CR, Viola A. Acute kidney injury in cirrhosis. Hepatology 2008;48:2064–77.
80. Angeli P, Gines P, Wong F, et al. Diagnosis and management of acute kidney injury in patients with cirrhosis: revised consensus recommendations of the International Club of Ascites. Gut 2015;64:531–7.
81. Wong F, Nadim MK, Kellum JA, et al. Working Party proposal for a revised classification system of renal dysfunction in patients with cirrhosis. Gut 2011;60: 702–9.
82. Piano S, Rosi S, Maresio G, et al. Evaluation of the Acute Kidney Injury Network criteria in hospitalized patients with cirrhosis and ascites. J Hepatol 2013;59: 482–9.
83. EASL clinical practice guidelines for the management of patients with decompensated cirrhosis. J Hepatol 2018;69(2):406–60.
84. Belcher JM, Sanyal AJ, Peixoto AJ, et al. Kidney biomarkers and differential diagnosis of patients with cirrhosis and acute kidney injury. Hepatology 2014; 60:622–32.
85. Ariza X, Sola E, Elia C, et al. Analysis of a urinary biomarker panel for clinical outcomes assessment in cirrhosis. PLoS One 2015;10:e0128145.
86. Piano S, Brocca A, Angeli P. Renal function in cirrhosis: a critical review of available tools. Semin Liver Dis 2018;38:230–41.

87. Wong F, Angeli P. New diagnostic criteria and management of acute kidney injury. J Hepatol 2017;66:860–1.
88. Sanyal AJ, Boyer T, Garcia-Tsao G, et al. A randomized, prospective, double-blind, placebo-controlled trial of terlipressin for type 1 hepatorenal syndrome. Gastroenterology 2008;134:1360–8.
89. Alessandria C, Ottobrelli A, Debernardi-Venon W, et al. Noradrenalin vs terlipressin in patients with hepatorenal syndrome: a prospective, randomized, unblinded, pilot study. J Hepatol 2007;47:499–505.
90. Cavallin M, Kamath PS, Merli M, et al. Terlipressin plus albumin versus midodrine and octreotide plus albumin in the treatment of hepatorenal syndrome: a randomized trial. Hepatology 2015;62:567–74.
91. Facciorusso A, Chandar AK, Murad MH, et al. Comparative efficacy of pharmacological strategies for management of type 1 hepatorenal syndrome: a systematic review and network meta-analysis. Lancet Gastroenterol Hepatol 2017;2: 94–102.
92. Boyer TD, Sanyal AJ, Wong F, et al. Terlipressin plus albumin is more effective than albumin alone in improving renal function in patients with cirrhosis and hepatorenal syndrome type 1. Gastroenterology 2016;150:1579–89.
93. Sanyal AJ, Boyer TD, Frederick RT, et al. Reversal of hepatorenal syndrome type 1 with terlipressin plus albumin vs. placebo plus albumin in a pooled analysis of the OT-0401 and REVERSE randomised clinical studies. Aliment Pharmacol Ther 2017;45:1390–402.
94. Cavallin M, Piano S, Romano A, et al. Terlipressin given by continuous intravenous infusion versus intravenous boluses in the treatment of hepatorenal syndrome: a randomized controlled study. Hepatology 2016;63:983–92.
95. Singh V, Ghosh S, Singh B, et al. Noradrenaline vs. terlipressin in the treatment of hepatorenal syndrome: a randomized study. J Hepatol 2012;56:1293–8.
96. Piano S, Schmidt HH, Ariza X, et al. Association between grade of acute on chronic liver failure and response to terlipressin and albumin in patients with hepatorenal syndrome. Clin Gastroenterol Hepatol 2018;16:1792–800.
97. Skagen C, Einstein M, Lucey MR, et al. Combination treatment with octreotide, midodrine, and albumin improves survival in patients with type 1 and type 2 hepatorenal syndrome. J Clin Gastroenterol 2009;43:680–5.
98. Azoulay D, Castaing D, Dennison A, et al. Transjugular intrahepatic portosystemic shunt worsens the hyperdynamic circulatory state of the cirrhotic patient: preliminary report of a prospective study. Hepatology 1994;19:129–32.
99. Wong F, Pantea L, Sniderman K. Midodrine, octreotide, albumin, and TIPS in selected patients with cirrhosis and type 1 hepatorenal syndrome. Hepatology 2004;40:55–64.
100. Nadim MK, Kellum JA, Davenport A, et al. Hepatorenal syndrome: the 8th international consensus conference of the Acute Dialysis Quality Initiative (ADQI) Group. Crit Care 2012;16:R23.
101. Zhang Z, Maddukuri G, Jaipaul N, et al. Role of renal replacement therapy in patients with type 1 hepatorenal syndrome receiving combination treatment of vasoconstrictor plus albumin. J Crit Care 2015;30:969–74.
102. Alessandria C, Ozdogan O, Guevara M, et al. MELD score and clinical type predict prognosis in hepatorenal syndrome: relevance to liver transplantation. Hepatology 2005;41:1282–9.
103. Utako P, Emyoo T, Anothaisintawee T, et al. Clinical outcomes after liver transplantation for hepatorenal syndrome: a systematic review and meta-analysis. Biomed Res Int 2018;2018:5362810.

104. Wong F, Leung W, Al Beshir M, et al. Outcomes of patients with cirrhosis and hepatorenal syndrome type 1 treated with liver transplantation. Liver Transpl 2015;21:300–7.
105. Ojo AO, Held PJ, Port FK, et al. Chronic renal failure after transplantation of a nonrenal organ. N Engl J Med 2003;349:931–40.
106. Pawarode A, Fine DM, Thuluvath PJ. Independent risk factors and natural history of renal dysfunction in liver transplant recipients. Liver Transpl 2003;9: 741–7.
107. Tan HK, Marquez M, Wong F, et al. Pretransplant type 2 hepatorenal syndrome is associated with persistently impaired renal function after liver transplantation. Transplantation 2015;99:1441–6.
108. Cannon RM, Jones CM, Davis EG, et al. Effect of renal diagnosis on survival in simultaneous liver-kidney transplantation. J Am Coll Surg 2019;228:536–44.e3.
109. Salerno F, Navickis RJ, Wilkes MM. Albumin infusion improves outcomes of patients with spontaneous bacterial peritonitis: a meta-analysis of randomized trials. Clin Gastroenterol Hepatol 2013;11:123–30.
110. Formica RN Jr. Simultaneous liver kidney transplantation. Curr Opin Nephrol Hypertens 2016;25:577–82.

Pulmonary Complications of Portal Hypertension

Rodrigo Cartin-Ceba, MD, MSc[a],*, Michael J. Krowka, MD[b]

KEYWORDS

- Cirrhosis • Liver transplant • Hepatopulmonary syndrome • Portal hypertension
- Portopulmonary hypertension • Hepatic hydrothorax

KEY POINTS

- Hepatic hydrothorax, an uncommon complication of portal hypertension, is the presence of a transudative pleural effusion not explained by cardiopulmonary disease.
- Portopulmonary hypertension and hepatopulmonary syndrome are serious pulmonary vascular complications of portal hypertension.
- Portopulmonary hypertension results when there is obstruction to arterial flow owing to vasoconstriction and proliferation in the pulmonary vascular bed; it is associated with significant mortality.
- Hepatopulmonary syndrome is characterized by low pulmonary vascular resistance secondary to intrapulmonary vascular dilatations and hypoxemia.
- Liver transplantation can completely resolve hepatic hydrothorax and hepatopulmonary syndrome; however, the posttransplant course in portopulmonary hypertension is less predictable.

HEPATIC HYDROTHORAX

Pleural effusion is characterized by the accumulation of fluid in the pleural cavity and is classified into transudative or exudative.[1] Hepatic hydrothorax (HH) is a transudative pleural effusion, usually greater than 500 mL, in a patient with portal hypertension without any other underlying primary cardiopulmonary source.[2,3] HH represents only 2% to 3% of all causes of pleural effusions.[4] Approximately one-half of patients with cirrhosis develop ascites; however, only 5% to 10% develop HH, which is less tolerated than ascites because it often results in dyspnea and hypoxia.[5,6] HH presents in approximately 85% of the cases on the right side, followed by the left in 13%.

Disclosures: Dr R. Cartin-Ceba has nothing to disclose. Dr M.J. Krowka was a member of the steering committee of the PORTICO Trial.
[a] Division of Pulmonary and Critical Care Medicine, Mayo Clinic Arizona, 13400 East Shea Boulevard, Scottsdale, AZ 85259, USA; [b] Division of Pulmonary and Critical Care Medicine, Mayo Clinic Rochester, 200 1st Street SW, Rochester, MN 55905, USA
* Corresponding author.
E-mail addresses: cartinceba.rodrigo@mayo.edu; cartinceceba.rodrigo@mayo.edu

Approximately 2% of cases are bilateral. In addition, HH can occur in the absence of clinical ascites owing to negative pleural pressure drawing fluid into the thorax from the abdomen.[4,7]

The most common clinical manifestations of HH include dyspnea, pleuritic chest pain, hypoxia, and nonproductive cough. Ascites and other findings of chronic liver disease are also commonly found; however, several cases of HH in the absence of ascites have been reported.

Diagnosis

HH can be typically detected on a posteroanterior chest radiograph. The diagnosis of HH is confirmed with thoracentesis to prove the presence of a transudative pleural effusion, which is similar to the ascitic fluid; thus, the protein concentration is usually low (<2.5 g/dL) and presents a serum-to-pleural fluid albumin gradient of greater than 1.1 g/dL[3] (**Box 1**). Despite similarities between the pleural and ascitic fluids, the pleural fluid tends to have slightly higher protein and albumin concentrations.[8,9] Other causes of transudative pleural effusion should be excluded such as heart or kidney failure. A thoracentesis is also done to exclude other conditions such as infection or malignancy, which are predominantly exudative effusions. The pleural fluid analysis should include the following tests: cell count and differential, Gram stain, culture, cytology, protein concentrations, albumin concentration, and lactate dehydrogenase concentration. Additional studies may be required depending on the clinical scenario including triglyceride levels to exclude chylothorax and amylase concentration to exclude pancreatitis.

In cases where the diagnosis of HH is uncertain, diagnosis clarification could be established with a radioisotope diagnostic technique where ^{99m}Tc-labeled microspheres of albumin or a sulfur colloid is injected intraperitoneally and migration into the pleural space indicates movement of fluid through diaphragmatic defects therefore confirming the diagnosis of HH,[10] this test should be ideally done shortly after a therapeutic thoracentesis. If the radioisotope fails to show up in the pleural space, an alternate etiology should be sought. Although this test has been considered the gold standard for identification of HH owing to very high specificity (≤100%), its sensitivity remains modest at approximately 71%. The sensitivity of the test can be greatly

---

Box 1
Pleural fluid characteristics of uncomplicated HH

Pleural fluid analysis

- Polymorphonuclear cell count of less than 500 cells/mm^3 and negative culture
- Total protein of concentration less than 2.5 g/dL
- Total protein pleural fluid to serum total protein ratio of less than 0.5
- Lactate dehydrogenase pleural fluid to serum ratio of less than 0.6
- Serum to pleural fluid albumin gradient of greater than 1.1 g/dL
- Pleural pH of 7.4 to 7.55
- Pleural fluid amylase concentration less than the serum amylase concentration
- Pleural glucose level similar to serum level

(*Data from* Moore KP, Wong F, Gines P, et al. The management of ascites in cirrhosis: report on the consensus conference of the International Ascites Club. Hepatology 2003;38:258–66.)

improved ($\leq$100%) by performing a thoracentesis before the administration of radio-isotopes to decrease pleural pressure.

Spontaneous bacterial empyema

Similar to spontaneous bacterial peritonitis in patients with ascites, patients with HH may develop spontaneous bacterial empyema (SBEM), which is a spontaneous infection of a preexisting HH. The name empyema is somewhat misleading, because there is usually no purulent material in the pleural cavity and the condition is treated differently as compared with empyema complicating pneumonia. The pathogenesis is unclear, movement of infected ascitic fluid to the pleural space is considered one of the main mechanisms; however, 2 studies have shown that 40% to 50% of episodes of SBEM are not associated with concomitant spontaneous bacterial peritonitis .[11,12] The most common bacteria causing SBEM are *Escherichia coli, Streptococcus* species, *Enterococcus* species, *Klebsiella pneumoniae*, and *Pseudomonas aeruginosa*.[13] The diagnostic criteria for SBEM include[11]:

- Positive pleural fluid culture and neutrophil cell count of greater than 250 cells/mm^3, or
- Negative pleural fluid culture and a neutrophil cell count of greater than 500 cells/mm^3, and
- No evidence of pneumonia on chest imaging.

Treatment of SBEM includes prompt initiation of a third generation cephalosporin for 7 to 10 days,[12] and there is no need for placement of a chest tube unless there is presence of frank purulence in the pleural space.

Pathophysiology and Pathogenesis

Multiple potential mechanisms have been described in the literature for the development of HH, including azygous vein hypertension with leakage of plasma, passage of peritoneal fluid via lymphatics, thoracic duct lymphatic leakage, and hypoalbuminemia causing decreased oncotic pressure[14]; however, the most accepted mechanism is the migration of ascitic fluid from the peritoneal cavity to the pleural space through small diaphragmatic defects generally located in the tendinous portion of the diaphragm and facilitated by the negative intrathoracic pressure.[15]

Management and Treatment

The medical treatment of HH is very similar to the treatment of ascites, including dietary sodium restriction and diuresis.[16] Patients with confirmed HH should also be referred for liver transplantation (LT) evaluation if they are suitable candidates. Patients should be advised to consume no more than 88 mEq (2000 mg) of sodium per day.

A combination of a loop diuretic (furosemide) and an aldosterone receptor antagonist (spironolactone) is often effective and uptitration may be necessary based on the response and symptomatology. If, despite sodium restriction and diuresis, the response is inadequate or if the patient develops complications associated with the diuresis, the HH is considered refractory and escalation of therapy may include repeated therapeutic thoracenteses, transjugular intrahepatic portosystemic shunting (TIPS), pleurodesis, surgical repair of diaphragmatic defects, and LT. Refractory HH has been described in 20% to 25% of cases.[17]

Thoracentesis

A therapeutic thoracentesis is often successful in decreasing the size of the pleural effusion and in alleviating respiratory symptoms. For the most part, repeated therapeutic thoracenteses are well-tolerated, although there are potential complications such as pain, pneumothorax, hemothorax, and reexpansion pulmonary edema. In general, it is recommended to consider other therapeutic alternatives when the thoracentesis is required every 2 to 3 weeks.[18,19]

Transjugular intrahepatic portosystemic shunt

Given its benefit in decompressing the increased portal pressures, most studies of TIPS for treatment of HH found in the contemporary literature have shown response rates in the 70% to 80% range.[20–24] It is important to consider the potential complications of TIPS, including worsening encephalopathy, renal failure, and bleeding related to the procedure. A pre-TIPS Model for End-stage Liver Disease (MELD) score of greater than 15 or a Child-Pugh score of greater than 10 portend a worse prognosis and an increased risk of complications.[20]

Indwelling pleural catheters

Traditionally, the placement of chest tubes for HH has been considered a relative contraindication owing to concerns of infection and leakage of excessive fluids, proteins, and electrolytes.[25–27] Once the chest tube is placed, it may be difficult to remove it owing to continuous reaccumulation of the fluid.[25] A study of 1981 patients with HH showed that patients who underwent chest tube placement had an increased risk of mortality as compared with patients that underwent only thoracentesis (odds ratio, 2.1; 95% confidence interval [CI], 1.4–3.1).[28] Despite these concerns, newer studies evaluating the use of indwelling pleural catheters in HH and in benign pleural effusions have reported less frequent and less ominous complications.[29–32] The results of a recent meta-analysis evaluating the use of indwelling pleural catheters in patients with nonmalignant effusions reported an infection rate of 2.3% (95% CI, 0%–4.7%), and a rate of spontaneous pleurodesis of 163 of 325 patients (51.3%).[31] Most recent studies do not report significant volume and electrolyte losses with the use of indwelling pleural catheters.[29–32] A recent retrospective multicenter study of patients with HH showed that, in 79 patients where an indwelling pleural catheter was placed for either palliation or as a bridge to LT, 10% developed pleural space infection, 2.5% died secondary to catheter-related sepsis, and 28% achieved spontaneous pleurodesis with a median time from catheter insertion to pleurodesis of 55 days.[33] Given new evidence, indwelling pleural catheters may be considered with caution in a selected group of patients with refractory HH if there is contraindication for TIPS as a palliative treatment or as a bridge to LT. Potential risks including a high risk of infection should be discussed with the patient.

Other surgical procedures

Pleurodesis (chemical or mechanical) has been used in refractory HH with variable success and significant risk of complications, including fever, renal failure, worsening encephalopathy, and pneumothorax. The results of a recent meta-analysis of 13 studies, including 180 patients who underwent pleurodesis by chemical and/or mechanical technique using either conventional thoracoscopy or video-assisted thoracic surgery, reported the pooled rate of complete response of 72% (95% CI, 65%–79%).[34] However, complications related to chemical pleurodesis were reported in 6 studies including 63 patients, and the pooled incidence of adverse events was very high at 82% (95% CI, 66%–94%).[34]

Surgical repair of diaphragmatic defects may be considered via a thoracoscopic approach and using surgical mesh reinforcement. A retrospective analysis of 63 patients with refractory HH who underwent thoracoscopic mesh onlay reinforcement to repair diaphragmatic defects found that, after a median 20.5 months, only 4 patients experienced recurrence, and patients with higher MELD scores and impaired renal function at baseline had higher mortality.[35]

A rare complication of hydrothorax that needs surgical correction is a trapped lung, which occurs owing to fibrous visceral pleural thickening from a chronic inflammatory process that prevents lung reexpansion. Surgical removal of the fibrosed visceral pleura to allow for the expansion of the underlying lung is often required; however, such s procedure carries significant risk of complications both before and after LT. A recent case series from a single center showed that surgery in LT recipients with pleural space complications is associated with significant 30-day mortality and morbidity.[36]

Liver transplantation
Transplantation is the definitive treatment for HH and these patients should be referred for LT evaluation provided there are no contraindications to transplantation. Outcomes of HH patients who undergo LT are similar to those patients who undergo LT for other reasons.[37]

PORTOPULMONARY HYPERTENSION

Portopulmonary hypertension (POPH) is a well-known serious pulmonary vascular complication of portal hypertension that is associated with significant mortality and is related to neither the etiology of liver disease nor the severity of portal hypertension. POPH is defined as pulmonary arterial hypertension (PAH) that occurs as a consequence of portal hypertension with or without cirrhosis.[38] During the most recent Sixth World Symposium on Pulmonary Hypertension, POPH continued to be part of group 1 of the classification of pulmonary hypertension because of its pathologic and hemodynamic similarities with other causes of precapillary pulmonary hypertension. The criteria following hemodynamic data obtained during a right heart catheterization (RHC) for the definition of POPH are summarized in **Box 2**.[39]

Box 2
Diagnostic criteria for POPH and HPS

POPH

- Portal hypertension

- MPAP of greater than 25 mm Hg

- PVR of greater than 3 wood units (240 dyn.s.cm^{-5})

- PAWP of less than 15 mm Hg

HPS

- Liver disease (usually cirrhosis with portal hypertension)

- Positive CE-TTE

- Abnormal arterial oxygenation
  - Alveolar-arterial oxygen gradient of 15 mm Hg or greater (>20 mm Hg if age >64 years)

Abbreviations: CE-TTE, contrast-enhanced transthoracic echocardiography; HPS, hepatopulmonary syndrome; MPAP, mean pulmonary artery pressure; PAWP, pulmonary artery wedge pressure; PVR, pulmonary vascular resistance.
From Krowka MJ, Fallon MB, Kawut SM, Fuhrmann V, Heimbach JK, Ramsay MA, et al. International Liver Transplant Society Practice Guidelines: Diagnosis and Management of Hepatopulmonary Syndrome and Portopulmonary Hypertension. Transplantation. 2016;100(7):1440-52; with permission.

Approximately 20% of patients with cirrhosis have a moderate increase in pulmonary arterial pressures as assessed by echocardiography; however, only a fraction of these patients truly have POPH.[40] This observation is likely related to other pulmonary hemodynamic patterns encountered in advanced liver disease such as excess volume owing to fluid retention (with increased left-sided filling pressures) or a hyperdynamic state with increased cardiac output (CO), which is often present in patients with end-stage liver disease.[41,42] Distinguishing these patterns by RHC is important to provide correct management[43] (**Fig. 1**). An increase in both pulmonary vascular resistance (PVR) and pulmonary artery wedge pressure (PAWP) can confuse the interpretation of pulmonary hemodynamics,[42] a phenomenon that is seen in up to 25% patients with POPH.[44] In these cases, true precapillary pulmonary hypertension (POPH) is manifest by an increased transpulmonary gradient (mean pulmonary artery pressure [MPAP]-PAWP of >12 mm Hg). These patients should not be excluded from the diagnosis of POPH owing to an elevated PAWP alone.

POPH should be distinguished from hepatopulmonary syndrome (HPS; **Table 1**).[41,45] In HPS, arterial hypoxemia (which may be severe) is caused by intrapulmonary vascular dilatations (IPVD), as opposed to vascular obstructions of POPH. HPS presents with normal PVR and a high flow state characterized by an increased CO. This distinction is important if LT is being considered owing to differences in risk, treatment options, and outcomes.[45]

Epidemiology of Portopulmonary Hypertension

POPH affects predominantly adults and is remarkably rare in the pediatric age group.[46] Autoimmune liver disorders and female gender are more frequently associated with POPH.[47] Poor correlation exists between the severity of POPH and the degree of liver dysfunction as characterized by the Child-Turcotte-Pugh or MELD

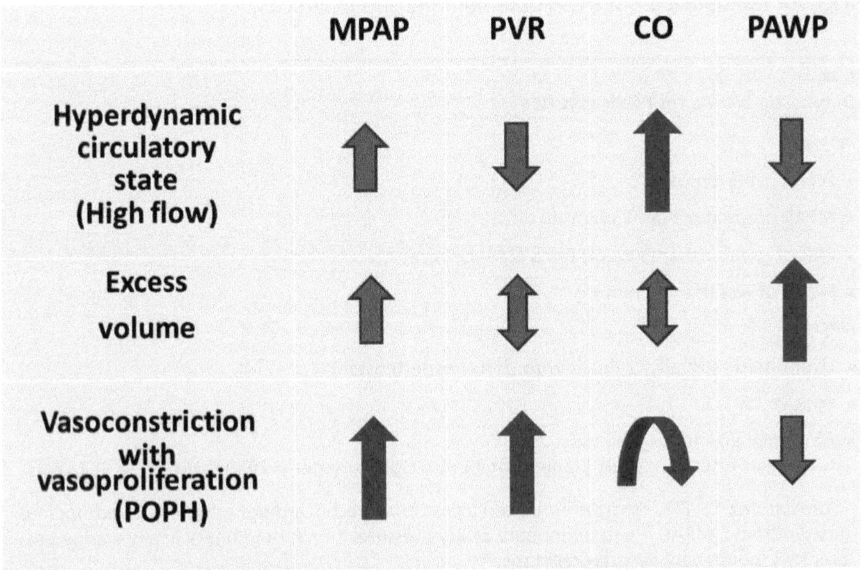

	MPAP	PVR	CO	PAWP
Hyperdynamic circulatory state (High flow)	↑	↓	↑	↓
Excess volume	↑	↕	↕	↑
Vasoconstriction with vasoproliferation (POPH)	↑	↑	↷	↓

Fig. 1. Pulmonary hemodynamic patterns documented by RHC in advanced liver disease. CO, cardiac output; MPAP, mean pulmonary artery pressure (normal <25 mm Hg); PAWP, pulmonary artery wedge pressure; PVR, pulmonary vascular resistance (normal less than 240 dyne.s.cm-5 [or 3 Wood units]).

Table 1
Differences between POPH and Hepatopulmonary syndrome (HPS)

	POPH	HPS
Primary pathophysiology	PAH	Intrapulmonary vascular dilatations
Genetic predisposition	Documented	Documented
Pathology	PAH owing to plexiform lesions, thrombosis, obliterative pulmonary arteriopathy	Intrapulmonary vascular dilatations causing intrapulmonary shunting and consequent hypoxemia
Severity of hypoxemia	+ (Typically mild)	+++ (Mild to very severe depending on degree of shunting)
Right ventricular function	Significantly elevated RVSP with RV dilatation/systolic dysfunction and low cardiac output	Normal or mildly elevated RVSP (owing to high flow state) with normal RV size and function
Clinical findings	Loud second heart sound, systolic murmur, RV heave, lower extremity edema along with features of portal hypertension (varices, splenomegaly, ascites, etc)	Clubbing, cyanosis, systolic flow murmur, platypnea, orthodeoxia along with signs of end stage liver disease
Screening advised	Yes, transthoracic echocardiography	Yes, contrast-enhanced TTE
Treatment	Pulmonary artery-specific therapy	Supportive care and management of underlying liver disease until LT (which is curative for HPS)
LT recommended/feasible?	Only in patients where the PAH is adequately controlled before transplantation.	Recommended/feasible in all patients (even in severe hypoxemia).
MELD exception points available	Yes	Yes

Abbreviations: RV, right ventricular; RVSP, right ventricular systolic pressure.

(*Adapted from* Angeli P, Gines P, Wong F, et al. Diagnosis and management of acute kidney injury in patients with cirrhosis: revised consensus recommendations of the International Club of Ascites. Gut 2015;64:531–7; and EASL Clinical Practice Guidelines for the management of patients with decompensated cirrhosis. J Hepatol 2018;69(2):406–60.)

scores.[44,48] When comparing POPH with idiopathic PAH hemodynamics, POPH is characterized by a higher CO and less severity as measured by MPAP and PVR.[39]

An unselected series of 17,901 autopsies revealed that PAH was 5 times more likely in patients with cirrhosis than those without liver disease.[49] Hadengue and associates[48] reported the largest prospective study of patients with portal hypertension (n = 507) in which portopulmonary hemodynamic measurements and concluded that 2% had POPH. Contemporary observational studies have demonstrated that POPH is a relatively common condition among LT candidates and in pulmonary hypertension registries. In the French pulmonary hypertension registry experience over a

12-month period (2002–2003), Humbert and coworkers[50] reported a 10.4% frequency of POPH (70/674) from 17 university hospitals. In the United States, the REVEAL (Registry to Evaluate Early And Long-term PAH disease management) registry documented a 5.3% POPH frequency (174/3525), in which there were 68% prevalent and 32% incident cases, satisfying the criteria of an MPAP of 25 mm Hg or greater, a PVR of 240 dyn.s.cm^{-5} or greater, and a PAWP of 15 mm Hg or greater.[44,46] Following slightly different PVR diagnostic criteria as a part of outpatient RHC diagnostic assessments, the largest POPH-LT center experiences reported to date are as follows: 8.5% (Baylor Dallas, 102/1205; PVR of >120 dyn.s.cm^{-5}), 6.1% (Clichy, France 10/165; PVR of >120 dyn.s.cm^{-5}), and 5.3% (Mayo Clinic 66/1235; PVR of >240 dyns.s.cm^{-5}).[42,51,52]

Pathophysiology and Pathogenesis

Genetic predisposition may play a role because not all patients with portal hypertension owing to cirrhosis develop POPH.[53] Furthermore, the histopathologic changes from POPH are indistinguishable from the changes observed in other phenotypes of pulmonary artery hypertension.[43,54] POPH is characterized by a spectrum of obstructive and remodeling changes in the pulmonary arterial bed, as observed in autopsy and lung explant studies. Initially, medial hypertrophy with smooth muscle proliferation and a transition to myofibroblasts has been documented. As this proliferative pathologic process advances, plexogenic arteriopathy eventually develops.[43,54]

Multiple circulating growth factors, neurohormone levels, and cytokine levels are present in portal hypertension, with many potential candidate mediators in the development of POPH. The pulmonary vascular pathology occurs within the context of a hyperdynamic state caused by extrahepatic (splanchnic) vasodilation.[46] It is unknown if this persistent high-flow state initiates (by shear stress) or exacerbates (in combination with circulating mediators) the pulmonary vascular proliferative process. A case control study of 31 POPH cases and 104 controls evaluating single nucleotide polymorphisms showed associations with estrogen receptor 1, aromatase, phosphodiesterase 5, angiopoietin 1, and calcium-binding protein A4.[53] The mechanistic link between estrogen signaling, serum estradiol levels, circulating endothelial progenitor cells, and the development of POPH is a current research hypothesis of interest.[55,56] Pulmonary endothelial cells lack prostacyclin synthase in patients with POPH (hence a lack of prostacyclin vasodilation).[57] The pulmonary vascular bed is exposed to increased levels of circulating endothlin-1 in the setting of cirrhosis (a potent vasoconstrictor and facilitator of smooth muscle proliferation)[58,59] and may be deficient in local nitric oxide effect (for vasodilation).[60] The role of other circulating and receptor factors that may affect the pulmonary endothelium owing to the existence of portal hypertension is speculative. These factors include vasoconstrictive/proliferative mediators such as serotonin, thromboxane, vasoactive intestinal peptide, and vascular endothelial growth factor, as well as the possible imbalance of endothelin A receptor-mediating vasoconstriction, and endothelin B receptors (mediating vasodilation) in the pulmonary arterial bed.[60]

Clinical Manifestations

Dyspnea at rest or with exertion is by far the most common presenting symptom of POPH. Other causes of dyspnea that are common in patients with portal hypertension need to be excluded, namely, ascites, anemia, fluid retention, and muscle wasting. Symptoms such as chest pain or syncope are usually markers of severe POPH.[46] Physical findings in POPH may be absent or subtle and nonspecific; however, the presence of a hyperdynamic precordium, an accentuated second heart sound (best heard at the apex), and a systolic murmur owing to tricuspid valve regurgitation may be noted. With severe POPH, findings of right heart failure such as marked distension of the jugular veins, peripheral edema, ascites and a right ventricular third heart sound (S3) could be seen. The lung examination is usually normal and it is uncommon to have clubbing or cyanosis as seen in HPS. Mild hypoxemia is common and often associated with abnormal overnight pulse oximetry. The chest roentgenogram usually demonstrates cardiomegaly and enlargement of the central pulmonary arteries as the duration and severity of POPH progresses.[46] The electrocardiogram may show a rightward electrical axis, a right bundle branch block pattern, and when POPH is severe the presence of inverted T waves in the precordial V1 to V4 leads can be seen, which suggests a severe effect on the right ventricle. Pulmonary function tests are usually not helpful in the diagnosis or management of POPH because reduced single breath diffusing capacity (a common abnormality seen in PAH) is frequently seen in most patients with advanced liver disease.

Screening for Portopulmonary Hypertension

Transthoracic echocardiography (TTE) has been the most practical method to screen for POPH.[61–63] By assessing the tricuspid regurgitant peak velocity, estimating the right atrial pressure by inferior vena cava changes with inspiration and using the modified Bernoulli equation, an estimate of the right ventricle systolic pressure (RVSP) can be determined in approximately 80% of patients with portal hypertension.[61] This quantitative approach allows one to decide which patients should proceed to RHC for the definitive characterization of pulmonary hemodynamics. An RVSP of greater than 50 mm Hg has been the cutoff criteria used to proceed to RHC at our institution[64]; rarely, immeasurable tricuspid regurgitant peak velocity with abnormal qualitative right ventricular size or function results in RHC. TTE was noted to have a 97% sensitivity and 77% specificity to detect moderate to severe PAH before LT.[61] Based on different RVSP cutoffs, other investigators have recommended that LT candidates with an RVSP of greater than 38 mm Hg should be referred for RHC.[65] Specific screening recommendations by the International Liver Transplant Society include screening with TTE in all patients with portal hypertension who are candidates for TIPS or LT, and to repeat the screening with TTE while awaiting LT, although the optimal interval is unclear.[39]

Management and Treatment

The most important decisions in the management of POPH are deciding who needs pulmonary artery PAH-specific therapy and determining the risks for potential LT (**Fig. 2**). Patients with POPH with a MPAP of greater than 35 mm Hg are particularly vulnerable to poor outcomes with attempted LT, especially if there is no effort to treat the POPH with current PAH-specific medications. The immediate goal in the treatment of POPH is to improve pulmonary hemodynamics by reducing the obstruction to pulmonary arterial flow (decreased MPAP, decreased PVR, and increased CO), ultimately improving and/or normalizing right ventricular function. This goal can be accomplished by medications that result in vasodilation and antiplatelet aggregation, and that have antiproliferative effects.[46] Drug therapy may augment the lack of pulmonary endothelial prostacyclin synthase deficiency (prostacyclin infusion), block circulating endothelin-1 (ET-1) effects (endothelin receptor antagonists) and enhance local nitric oxide vasodilatation effects (phosphodiesterase inhibitors and soluble guanylate cyclase stimulator).[46,66]

Although the treatment of POPH typically follows the same algorithm as for other forms of PAH, aside from 1 study evaluating the effect of riociguat (a soluble

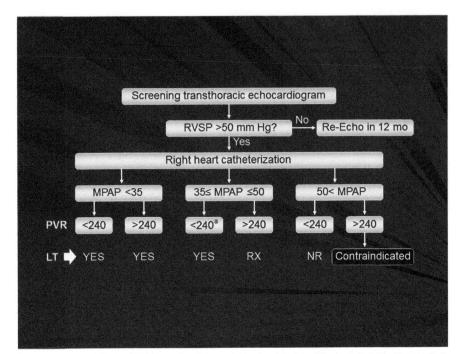

Fig. 2. Current POPH screening evaluation and treatment algorithm used at the Mayo Clinic. MPAP, mean pulmonary artery pressure (normal, <25 mm Hg); PVR, pulmonary vascular resistance [normal, <240 dyne.s.cm^{-5} (or 3 Wood units)]; NR, never reported; RVSP, right ventricular systolic pressure estimated by TTE; RX, pulmonary artery hypertension-specific therapy advised before LT; Contraindicated: high risk of intraoperative event at graft reperfusion. [a] Provided right ventricular function size and function are adequate.

guanylate cyclase stimulator) in PAH,[66] and a recently finalized clinical trial performed only in patients with POPH,[67] all the randomized controlled trials evaluating PAH-specific therapies have excluded patients with POPH. Uncontrolled studies, small series, and case reports have suggested that PAH-targeted therapies used for other types of PAH could be beneficial for patients with POPH[68–85]; for example, PAH therapies may sometimes be given preoperatively as a bridge to LT. A summary of the evidence regarding therapy in POPH is presented in **Table 2**. By improving hemodynamic and clinical parameters, PAH therapy can lead to a response that meets LT eligibility criteria; however, careful patient selection is required and this approach is not currently generally established. Specific guidelines for the management and treatment of patients with POPH have been published recently.[39]

Prostacyclin analogues
In a summary of 48 patients treated with intravenous epoprostenol from 5 studies, MPAP decreased by 25% (from 48 to 36 mm Hg), PVR decreased by 52% (from 550 to 262 dyn.s.cm^{-5}), and CO increased by 38% (from 6.3 to 8.7 L/min; all $P<.01$).[70–73,86] Other prostanoids (intravenous treprostinil and inhaled iloprost) have resulted in significant pulmonary hemodynamic improvements in POPH.[77,81,83] An ongoing observational, open-label, multicenter trial is evaluating the efficacy and safety of treprostinil in patients with POPH (ClinicalTrials.gov/NCT01028651).

Table 2
Pulmonary arterial-specific therapy use in POPH

PAH-Specific Therapy Group	Drug	Study's First Author	Number of Subjects Included	Study Main Outcomes
Endothelin receptor antagonist	Bosentan	Hoeper et al,[76] 2007	18	1- and 3-y survivals of 94% and 89%, respectively
	Bosentan	Savale et al,[87] 2013	34	Event-free survival estimates were 82%, 63% and 47% at 1, 2, and 3 y respectively
	Ambrisentan	Cartin-Ceba et al,[69] 2011	13	At 1 y, MPAP and PVR improved in 8/8; PVR normalized in 5
	Ambrisentan	Halank et al,[73] 2011	14	Improve in 6-min walk distance, no adverse effects
	Macitentan	Sitbon et al,[67] 2018	85	PVR reduction by 35%, and significantly improved mPAP and cardiac index compared with placebo
Phosphodiesterase inhibitors	Sildenafil	Reichenberger et al,[82] 2006	12	Improvement at 3 mo; not sustained at 1 y
	Sildenafil	Gough et al,[72] 2009	11	PVR decreased in all at first RHC follow-up
	Sildenafil	Hemnes et al,[74] 2009	10	At 1 y, MPAP and PVR decreased in 3/5 patients
	Sildenafil	Fisher et al,[88] 2015	20	Hemodynamics and functional class improved
Soluble guanylate cyclase stimulator	Riociguat	Ghofrani et al,[66] 2013; Cartin-Ceba et al,[92] 2018	13	Improvements in 6-min walking distance, PVR, and several other secondary efficacy parameters over 12 wk

(continued on next page)

Table 2
(continued)

PAH-Specific Therapy Group	Drug	Study's First Author	Number of Subjects Included	Study Main Outcomes
Prostanoids	Epoprostenol	Kuo et al,[80] 1997	4	MPAP and PVR improved
	Epoprostenol	Krowka et al,[177] 1999	15	15 MPAP and PVR improved
	Epoprostenol	Ashfaq et al,[68] 2007	16	Successful LT in 11 patients; 5-y survival 67%
	Epoprostenol	Fix et al,[71] 2007	19	PVR improved in 14/14; MPAP improved in 11/14
	Epoprostenol	Sussman et al,[84] 2006	8	MPAP and PVR improved in 7/8
	Treprostinil	Sakai et al,[83] 2009	3	Successful LT in 2 patients (moderate POPH)
	Inhaled iloprost	Hoeper et al,[76] 2007	13	1- and 3-y survivals of 77% and 46%, respectively
	Inhaled iloprost	Melgosa et al,[81] 2010	21	Acute, but no long-term hemodynamic improvement
	Epoprostenol	Awdish & Cajigas,[178] 2013	21	Clearance for transplant in 52% of patients within 1 y
Combination therapy	Sildenafil alone or combined with prostanoid in 9 patients	Hollatz et al,[77] 2012	11	MPAP and PVR improved in all patients, all underwent LT and 7/11 are off PAH-specific therapy
	Sildenafil and Bosentan combined in 6 patients, 1 patient only on prostanoids	Raevens et al,[65] 2013	7	MPAP and PVR improved in the 5/6 patients treated with combination of sildenafil and bosentan, 2 underwent LT

Abbreviations: IV, intravenous; MPAP, mean pulmonary artery pressure.

(From Salerno F, Gerbes A, Gines P, Wong F, Arroyo V. Diagnosis, prevention and treatment of the hepatorenal syndrome in cirrhosis: a consensus work-shop of the international ascites club. Gut 2007;56:1310–18; with permission.)

Endothelin receptor antagonists

Both bosentan and ambrisentan have been found to be well-tolerated in patients with POPH. Hoeper and colleagues[76] documented 1- and 3-year survival rates of 94% and 89%, respectively, in 18 patients with POPH and Child class A severity liver disease using the nonselective endothelin antagonist bosentan. No liver toxicity was noted. Cartin-Ceba and colleagues[69] reported 13 patients with POPH using the endothelin receptor antagonist ambrisentan (10 mg/d) and documented the 1-year improvement in each of 8 patients with POPH (MPAP decreased from 58 to 41 mm Hg and PVR decreased from 445 to 174 dyn.s.cm^{-5}; $P = .004$). Of note, 5 of the 8 patients normalized their PVR. In further support of ambrisentan in POPH, Halank and colleagues[73] described significant improvements in both exercise capacity and symptoms in 14 patients with POPH. Importantly, neither of the uncontrolled ambrisentan studies was associated with significant hepatic toxicity. More recently, Savale and colleagues[87] described 34 patients with POPH (Child class A or B severity of liver disease) treated with bosentan documenting significant hemodynamic improvement (more so in the Child class B subgroup) and event-free survival estimates were 82%, 63%, and 47% at 1, 2, and 3 years, respectively.

The first randomized, placebo-controlled, clinical study in patients with POPH, called PORTICO, which evaluated the safety and effectiveness of macitentan, showed that treatment with macitentan significantly reduced the patients' PVR by 35%, and significantly improved MPAP and cardiac index, compared with patients receiving the placebo; however, no significant differences in disease severity or in the 6-minute walk distance test were found between the 2 groups.[67] Macitentan was well-tolerated, and its safety profile was consistent with that reported in previous clinical trials, with swelling of the legs or arms and headache being the most common adverse events reported. Overall, these findings favor the use of macitentan as a potential therapeutic strategy for patients with POPH.[67] An ongoing observational, open-label, multicenter trial is evaluating the efficacy and safety of ambrisentan in patients with POPH (ClinicalTrials.gov/NCT01224210).

Phosphodiesterase-5 inhibitors

The use of phosphodiesterase inhibition (sildenafil) to enhance nitric oxide vasodilating effect, either alone or in combination with other PAH-specific therapies, has successfully improved POPH pulmonary hemodynamics and facilitated successful LT. Most of the published experiences have been in patients with less severe forms of POPH.[72,74,82] A recent study on 20 patients using sildenafil showed improvements in hemodynamics and in functional class.[88]

Soluble guanylate cyclase stimulator

Riociguat is the first-in-class soluble guanylate cyclase stimulator[66] and the first drug to be approved in 2 separate pulmonary hypertension indications: PAH (PATENT-1 study) and inoperable or persistent/recurrent chronic thromboembolic pulmonary hypertension.[66,89] Riociguat has a dual mode of action, acting in synergy with endogenous nitric oxide and also directly stimulating soluble guanylate cyclase, independent of nitric oxide availability.[90,91] In a post hoc analysis of the first randomized, controlled trial in PAH to include patients with POPH (PATENT-1), a total of 13 patients with POPH were included. Eleven patients received riociguat and 2 patients received placebo; riociguat treatment was associated with improvements in important primary and secondary efficacy parameters over 12 weeks in patients with POPH, and was generally well-tolerated, with a similar safety profile to that seen in the overall PATENT-1 population.[92]

Other conventional therapies

Right ventricular function may be impaired by the use of beta-blockers, which are usually used to prevent gastrointestinal bleeding by reducing the degree of portal hypertension. In moderate to severe POPH (n = 10; mean MPAP = 52 mm Hg), withdrawal of beta-blockade increased CO by 28% and decreased PVR by 19%, with no change in MPAP and increased the 6-minute walk distance by 79 m.[93] TIPS, as a treatment for gastrointestinal bleeding or refractory ascites, can temporarily increase MPAP, CO, and PVR. In a study of 16 patients with cirrhosis without pulmonary hypertension, the increase in MPAP was greater than that noted in CO, suggesting an increase in the PVR after TIPS.[94] Current guidelines recommend against TIPS in patients with severe POPH (mPAP of >45 mm Hg).[39] Other recommendations from the guidelines include the avoidance of anticoagulation and also avoidance of calcium channel blockers as treatment for POPH.[39]

Liver transplantation

Although LT is a potentially curative intervention for these patients (at least from a hemodynamic perspective in a highly selected group of patients), POPH is not per se an indication for LT. The outcome of POPH after LT remains unpredictable despite screening, careful patient selection, higher allocation priority, and advances in single and combination PAH-specific therapies.[95–104] Effective PAH-specific therapy has resulted in successful LT and subsequent liberation from pre-LT PAH-specific therapy in some individuals. Since 2006, LT waitlist candidates with POPH have been eligible to receive waitlist priority upgrades (MELD exceptions) based on formalized criteria set forth by the Organ Procurement and Transplantation Network,[105] and these criteria are summarized in **Box 3**. Despite the introduction of MELD score exception, a study evaluated data on 155 patients with POPH with a MELD score exception approved from the Organ Procurement and Transplantation Network database from 2006 to 2012 and demonstrated that, since the implementation of a formalized MELD

Box 3
MELD exception criteria for POPH and HPS

POPH

1. Moderate to severe POPH diagnosis confirmed by RHC
   a. MPAP of 35 mm Hg or greater
   b. PVR of 3 Wood units or greater (240 dyn.s.cm^{-5})
   c. PAWP of 15 mm Hg or less

2. PAH-specific therapy initiated; improvement documented
   a. MPAP of less than 35 mm Hg
   b. PVR of less than 5 Wood units (400 dyn.s.cm^{-5})[a]
   c. Satisfactory right ventricular function by TTE

3. MELD exception updated every 3 months
   a. Give additional MELD exception if RHC data satisfies criteria 2

HPS

1. Pao$_2$ of less than 60 mm Hg while breathing room air in the sitting position and not explained by a primary pulmonary disease

2. MELD points updated every 3 months

Abbreviations: MELD, Model end-stage liver disease; Pao$_2$, partial pressure of arterial oxygen.
    [a] If PVR is normal, a higher MPAP may be allowed and reconsidered owing to physiology that is now high flow rather than obstruction to flow owing to the therapy.

exception policy for POPH, the majority of patients awarded such points have not met Organ Procurement and Transplantation Network criteria for such exception points owing to missing or incomplete data, with nearly one-third not having hemodynamic data consistent with POPH.[106] In addition, the authors of that study found that this subset of patients with POPH MELD exceptions presented a significant risk of waitlist mortality, particularly in those with hemodynamic criteria consistent with POPH, with several early post-LT deaths in both groups attributable to right heart failure/persistent pulmonary hypertension.[106] The results of a recent study that evaluated the predictors of waitlist mortality in patients with POPH found that the severity of liver disease and POPH (as assessed by MELD and PVR, respectively) were significantly associated with waitlist, but not posttransplant, mortality in patients with approved MELD exceptions for POPH.[107] Another recent study in 300 patients undergoing LT showed that at the time of LT, 10% of patients had a MPAP of 35 mm Hg or greater, the majority of whom had volume overload or a hyperdynamic state.[108] In addition, among patients with an intraoperative MPAP of 35 mm Hg or greater and those with previously diagnosed POPH, there were no intraoperative deaths or mortalities during transplant hospitalization, suggesting that LT in selected patients with increased MPAP (normal PVR and satisfactory right ventricular function by TTE), even above 35 mm Hg, is safe and should not be a reason to exclude these patients from LT if aggressively managed.[108]

Prognosis

The overall prognosis of POPH has been confounded by small series from eras in which none of the current PAH-specific medications were available compared with the present, when there is increasing experience in PAH-specific therapies and LT. Robalino and Moodie[109] reported a 5-year survival of 4% (n = 78) in an era before the availability of continuous intravenous prostacyclin infusion. Swanson and associates[110] reported a 5-year survival rate of 14% in patients with POPH (n = 19) denied LT and not treated with any of the current pulmonary vascular therapies. From the French National Center for PAH (n = 154 over a 20-year span until 2004), Le Pavec and coworkers[111] described 1-, 3-, and 5-year survival rates of 88%, 75%, and 68%, respectively for patients with POPH (mainly Child classification A and alcohol as the etiology of cirrhosis). Causes of death in all series mentioned herein were equally distributed between right heart failure owing to POPH and direct complications of liver disease (bleeding, sepsis, and hepatocellular carcinoma). More recently, the REVEAL registry reported 2 important POPH observations.[44] First, the use of any PAH-specific therapy for POPH was delayed compared with patients diagnosed with idiopathic PAH. Specifically, at the time of entry into the registry only 25% were on PAH-specific therapy; by the end of 12 months of follow-up, 74% of those alive were on treatment. Second, although baseline hemodynamics in POPH (MPAP and PVR) were significantly better than those with idiopathic PAH, the 1- and 3-year survivals were worse and the 5-year survival for all patients with POPH was 40% versus 64% for idiopathic PAH. Liver disease etiologies and causes of death were not determined and survival was not analyzed by the type of PAH-specific therapy. A recent report by Khaderi and colleagues[112] described excellent long-term outcomes of 7 patients with POPH who underwent LT, with all patients able to come off intravenous epoprostenol after LT and a survival of 85% after 7.8 years of follow-up.

HEPATOPULMONARY SYNDROME

A clinical triad characterizes the HPS: (1) the presence of portal hypertension, chronic liver disease, or congenital portosystemic shunts, (2) abnormal arterial oxygenation defined by an elevated alveolar-arterial gradient ($\geq$15 mm Hg or $\geq$20 mm Hg if age is >64 years), and (3) the presence of IPVD as detected by contrast-enhanced bubble TTE (CE-TTE, delayed appearance of bubbles >3 cardiac cycles).[39,41,113] HPS is seen in roughly 5% to 32% of patients with advanced liver disease presenting for LT evaluation and its varying prevalence reflects varying hypoxemia criteria used in different HPS studies in the literature.[45] The classic description of the condition dates back to 1884, where the occurrence of cyanosis and clubbing in cirrhosis was first described by Flückiger.[114] The term "hepatopulmonary syndrome" was first suggested in 1977 by Kennedy and Knudson,[115] who described the association of severe hypoxemia with IPVD in patients with liver disease. HPS is an independent risk factor for mortality and morbidity in patients with advanced liver disease, resulting in a doubling of the risk of death in patients with advanced liver failure.[116] There is no relationship between the presence of HPS and the etiology or the severity of the underlying liver disease and HPS may be seen in patients with mild liver disease. HPS has also been diagnosed in patients with presinusoidal portal hypertension with otherwise normal liver function.

Pathogenesis and Pathophysiology

A rat common bile duct ligation model of HPS has immensely helped in the understanding of this syndrome.[117,118] In this model, proliferating cholangiocytes in the liver produce and secrete ET-1.[117,118] Sheer stress results in the upregulation of the endothelin B receptor in the pulmonary vasculature that subsequently binds the increased circulating ET-1 and augments pulmonary nitrous oxide (NO) production via endothelial NO synthase.[118–122] In this model, there is also increased pulmonary intravascular monocytes caused by increased pulmonary NO levels and bacterial translocation resulting in increased blood levels of tumor necrosis factor alpha.[123,124] The increased pulmonary monocytes then contribute to the formation of IPVD by increasing levels of NO via inducible nitric oxide synthase[125,126] and carbon monoxide via heme oxygenase-1.[127,128] In addition, levels of vascular endothelial growth factor are also increased.[126,129] In addition IPVD, pulmonary angiogenesis is enhanced by the complimentary effects of ET-1, pulmonary monocytes, and vascular endothelial growth factor on the pulmonary vasculature; the role of angiogenesis in HPS is also supported by the presence of neovascularization in the lungs of common bile duct ligation rats with HPS, and the improvement in oxygenation with anti-angiogenesis therapy with sorafenib.[126–131] In humans, NO has been considered a mediator of IPVD in patients with cirrhosis with HPS because they have higher exhaled levels of NO compared with patients without HPS, and exhaled NO levels normalize after LT.[132–134] Pulmonary angiogenesis has also been implicated in humans because single nucleotide polymorphisms that regulate angiogenesis are associated with the presence of HPS in patients with cirrhosis.[135] ET-1 may also play a role in human disease, as it was shown in a single study in which blood levels of ET-1 in the hepatic vein were higher in patients with cirrhosis with IPVD and HPS compared with those without IPVD, and blood ET-1 levels correlated with the degree of bile duct proliferation in the corresponding liver biopsy specimens.[136]

The pulmonary vasculature in patients with cirrhosis has been demonstrated to have decreased pulmonary vascular tone with a poor or absent hypoxemic vasoconstrictor response.[137–139] The capillary network is the choke point in the pulmonary circulation, with a normal diameter of between 8 and 15 µm. The capillary network in patients with HPS is characterized by the presence of abnormally dilated precapillary and capillary vessels ($\geq$15 µm) that result in diffusion abnormalities and shunting of blood across the pulmonary vasculature.[114,140] These dilated vessels are called IPVDs and can be detected noninvasively by the passage of microbubbles (CE-TTE) or 99m technetium macroaggregated albumin. IPVDs are typically too small to be seen on regular pulmonary angiography.[141,142] The pulmonary angiogram can appear to be busy or spongy owing to these diffuse capillary dilatations. Pulmonary and pleural based true arteriovenous malformations may also be seen occasionally.[114]

Hypoxemia in HPS is thus thought to relate to a number of factors, including (1) shortening of the pulmonary transit time across IPVDs resulting in reduced exposure of the capillary blood to the alveolus, (2) impaired diffusion across IPVDs owing to increased alveolar-capillary distance and decreased diffusion efficiency, and (3) true intrapulmonary shunting across IPVDs and across pulmonary and pleural based arteriovenous malformations.

Clinical Manifestations

Patients typically present with dyspnea and hypoxemia in the setting of chronic liver disease. The presence of chronic liver disease stigmata along with clubbing and cyanosis is classic for the diagnosis of HPS. The degree of hypoxemia can vary from mild to severe and in some cases be quite refractory to standard oxygen supplementation. Hypoxemia can be evaluated noninvasively with a finger pulse oximeter with the patient in different positions (sitting, supine, and standing). This maneuver may uncover evidence for platypnea (worsening dyspnea on assuming an upright or sitting/standing position) or orthodeoxia (worsening hypoxemia on assuming an upright or sitting/standing position). Most patients with HPS experience a gradual worsening in the degree of hypoxemia over time, but this process is quite variable and does not always correlate with the status of the underlying liver disease. All potential causes of hypoxemia need to be considered before a diagnosis of HPS is made. For example, in patients with coexisting lung disease (chronic obstructive pulmonary disease, lung fibrosis, etc) it is very important to determine the extent of hypoxemia related to HPS versus the underlying lung disease. A 99m technetium macroaggregated albumin perfusion lung scan can provide a quantitative estimation of the degree of intrapulmonary shunting and is very helpful in this situation. A high brain shunt index fraction (normal, $\leq 6\%$) would argue for HPS being the dominant cause of the patient's hypoxemia, because other intrinsic lung disorders causing hypoxemia have normal brain uptake.

Screening and Initial Testing for Hepatopulmonary Syndrome

To avoid unnecessary arterial blood gases in all patients with advanced liver disease, patients can be screened for HPS via pulse oximetry (SpO_2). With a threshold value of less than 96%, pulse oximetry had a sensitivity and specificity of 100% and 88%, respectively, for detecting patients with a partial pressure of oxygen less than 60 mm Hg[143] and seems to be a cost-effective screening test for detecting HPS in suitable LT candidates.[144] Current guidelines recommend such a screening approach.[39] However, a recent multicenter prospective cohort study has questioned the screening role of SpO_2 for the diagnosis of HPS after finding that an SpO_2 less than 96% had low sensitivity (28%; 95% CI, 18%–28%) for finding significant hypoxemia, an SpO_2 above any proposed cutoff did not rule out HPS, did not substantially change the pretest probability of HPS, and would miss detecting most patients with HPS in an LT evaluation clinic.[145] Arterial blood gases are necessary to establish the presence of hypoxemia and its severity. Patients with a sitting room air PaO_2 of less than 80 mm Hg can be then evaluated further with a CE-TTE study to confirm HPS.[39] In patients with a low SpO_2 or PaO_2 values, a CE-TTE will confirm the presence of IPVDs as well as exclude structural heart disease, intracardiac shunts, and coexistent pulmonary hypertension (**Fig. 3**). Room air and 100% oxygen blood gases in the supine and sitting position help to quantify the degree of hypoxemia and estimate the shunt fraction.[45] A chest radiograph will identify the presence of obvious pulmonary parenchymal disease. A computed tomography scan of the chest is very helpful in clarifying and quantifying abnormalities seen on the chest radiograph and is crucial in patients with coexistent pulmonary parenchymal disease (such as emphysema or interstitial lung disease). Pulmonary function tests typically show a decreased diffusing capacity that is decreased in proportion to the severity of the hypoxemia. Nonspecific spirometry abnormalities including restriction may also be noted.

Detecting Intrapulmonary Vascular Dilatations

The most sensitive method of detecting IPVDs in HPS is the CE-TTE (bubble study). The most commonly used method involves injection of agitated saline via either a central or peripheral intravenous catheter. The saline bubbles are typically 10 to 90 μm in diameter and considerably larger than the diameter of normal pulmonary capillaries (8–15 μm), which do not allow passage into the left heart.[45] However IPVDs (typically ≥15 μm) allow free passage of these bubbles into the left heart, resulting in the detection of an intrapulmonary shunt.[45] In patients with an intracardiac shunt, bubbles typically appear in the left cardiac chambers within 1 to 2 cycles of their appearance in the right atrium. In a positive bubble study for intrapulmonary shunting, bubbles will appear in the left atrium 3 to 6 cardiac cycles after their first appearance in right ventricle. The degree of shunting can be visually (semiquantitatively) estimated as being trivial, mild, moderate, or severe based on the quantity of bubbles passing

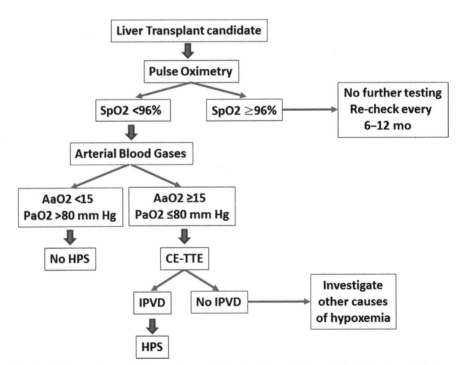

Fig. 3. HPS screening and diagnostic work flow in LT candidates. AaO₂, Alveolar-arterial oxygen gradient; CE-TTE, contrast-enhanced TTE.

through to the left heart. Although very sensitive for detecting IPVDs, the bubble study is not specific for the diagnosis of HPS and many patients with cirrhosis may have some degree of intrapulmonary shunting and not otherwise qualify for a diagnosis of HPS owing to a lack of hypoxemia.[146] A more specific test for seems to be the 99m technetium macroaggregated albumin perfusion lung scan.[146] A significantly abnormal shunt fraction (normal, ≤6%) is almost always associated with a clinical diagnosis of moderate to severe HPS.[146]

Management and Treatment

Medical therapies in hepatopulmonary syndrome

The management of HPS is supportive with supplemental oxygen because there are no medical options that have been proven beneficial or provide a sustained response. Supplemental oxygen has never been shown to reliably help dyspnea or improve quality of life in patients with HPS. Uncontrolled studies have included several agents that work through different mechanisms: methylene blue(inhibits the effect of nitric oxide on guanylate cyclase),[147–149] N(G)-nitro-L-arginine methyl ester (L-NAME, decreases nitric oxide production),[150,151] somatostatin,[152] cyclooxygenase inhibitors,[153,154] almitrine (pulmonary vasoconstrictor),[138,155] propranolol (ameliorates portal hypertension),[156,157] antibiotics (selective gut decontamination),[158,159] pentoxifylline (a tumor necrosis factor alpha inhibitor),[160] and garlic.[161,162] In a recent randomized, double-blind ,placebo-controlled trial using sorafenib, a tyrosine kinase inhibitor used as a blocker of angiogenesis, sorafenib failed to improve the alveolar–arterial oxygen gradient at 3 months in patients with HPS.[163] Finally, there has been no good evidence to support the use of TIPS in HPS.[39,133] Overall, medical therapies other than LT have not achieved consistent results in large cohorts of patients and these therapies should only be resorted to when other options do not exist for critically ill patients with refractory hypoxemia.

Liver transplantation

LT is the only intervention that improves the oxygenation and survival of patients with HPS. A series of case reports in the 1990s documented essentially complete reversal of IPVDs and clubbing in a number of patients with severe HPS.[164–166] These initial reports led to a wave of subsequent studies that looked at outcomes after LT and the resolution of HPS in these patients.[100,167–172] Recent reports have shown favorable outcomes in patients with HPS who undergo LT, even in those with severe hypoxemia.[168–170] MELD exception points for HPS were formalized in 2006 and allowed for the granting of additional MELD points to patients with HPS with a room air sitting PaO$_2$ of less than 60 mm Hg (see **Box 3**).[173] Our group has published on LT outcomes in the MELD exception era and has shown excellent outcomes in these patients.[169] Other investigators have found no association between pretransplant oxygenation and waitlist survival in patients with HPS MELD exception points; however, a pretransplant room air PaO$_2$ of 44 mm Hg or less was associated with increased posttransplant mortality.[106] The same study showed that HPS MELD exception patients had a lower overall mortality compared with others awaiting LT, suggesting that the appropriateness of the HPS exception policy should be reassessed.[106] Recent guidelines recommend that severe hypoxemia owing to HPS (PaO$_2$ of <60 mm Hg) should be considered an indication for LT and those individuals should be given standard MELD exception scores.[39] A recent European report regarding LT outcomes in patients with HPS showed that waitlist mortality and posttransplant survival in patients with severe HPS were fairly balanced under current standard exception policy, without disadvantaging the general transplant population.[174]

Combined Portopulmonary Hypertension and Hepatopulmonary Syndrome

A few cases of combined POPH and HPS have been reported in the literature.[175] A recent case report documented the development of HPS as a consequence of the use of pulmonary vasodilators in a patient with POPH.[176]

SUMMARY

HH, HPS, and POPH are the most common pulmonary complications of portal hypertension. HH presents in 5% to 10% of patients with cirrhosis and is defined as a transudative pleural effusion not explained by cardiopulmonary disease, most commonly seen on the right side. POPH and HPS are serious pulmonary vascular complications of portal hypertension with prevalence among LT candidates of approximately 6% and 5% to 32%, respectively. POPH develops when there is obstruction to arterial flow owing to vasoconstriction and proliferation in the pulmonary vascular bed; it is associated with significant mortality and is related to neither the etiology of liver disease nor the severity of portal hypertension. On the other hand, low PVR, IPVD and hypoxemia characterize HPS. LT can completely resolve HH and HPS; however, the posttransplant course in POPH is less predictable and LT in patients with POPH is indicated only in a selected group of patients.

REFERENCES

1. Light RW. The light criteria: the beginning and why they are useful 40 years later. Clin Chest Med 2013;34(1):21–6.
2. Kinasewitz GT, Keddissi JI. Hepatic hydrothorax. Curr Opin Pulm Med 2003; 9(4):261–5.
3. Badillo R, Rockey DC. Hepatic hydrothorax: clinical features, management, and outcomes in 77 patients and review of the literature. Medicine (Baltimore) 2014; 93(3):135–42.
4. Garbuzenko DV, Arefyev NO. Hepatic hydrothorax: an update and review of the literature. World J Hepatol 2017;9(31):1197–204.
5. Krok KL, Cardenas A. Hepatic hydrothorax. Semin Respir Crit Care Med 2012; 33(1):3–10.
6. Singh A, Bajwa A, Shujaat A. Evidence-based review of the management of hepatic hydrothorax. Respiration 2013;86(2):155–73.
7. Strauss RM, Boyer TD. Hepatic hydrothorax. Semin Liver Dis 1997;17(3): 227–32.
8. Chen A, Ho YS, Tu YC, et al. Diaphragmatic defect as a cause of massive hydrothorax in cirrhosis of liver. J Clin Gastroenterol 1988;10(6):663–6.
9. Lazaridis KN, Frank JW, Krowka MJ, et al. Hepatic hydrothorax: pathogenesis, diagnosis, and management. Am J Med 1999;107(3):262–7.
10. Hewett LJ, Bradshaw ML, Gordon LL, et al. Diagnosis of isolated hepatic hydrothorax using peritoneal scintigraphy. Hepatology 2016;64(4):1364–6.
11. Xiol X, Castellote J, Baliellas C, et al. Spontaneous bacterial empyema in cirrhotic patients: analysis of eleven cases. Hepatology 1990;11(3):365–70.
12. Xiol X, Castellvi JM, Guardiola J, et al. Spontaneous bacterial empyema in cirrhotic patients: a prospective study. Hepatology 1996;23(4):719–23.
13. Chen CH, Shih CM, Chou JW, et al. Outcome predictors of cirrhotic patients with spontaneous bacterial empyema. Liver Int 2011;31(3):417–24.
14. Kiafar C, Gilani N. Hepatic hydrothorax: current concepts of pathophysiology and treatment options. Ann Hepatol 2008;7(4):313–20.

15. Lieberman FL, Hidemura R, Peters RL, et al. Pathogenesis and treatment of hydrothorax complicating cirrhosis with ascites. Ann Intern Med 1966;64(2): 341–51.
16. Norvell JP, Spivey JR. Hepatic hydrothorax. Clin Liver Dis 2014;18(2):439–49.
17. Sese E, Xiol X, Castellote J, et al. Low complement levels and opsonic activity in hepatic hydrothorax: its relationship with spontaneous bacterial empyema. J Clin Gastroenterol 2003;36(1):75–7.
18. Baikati K, Le DL, Jabbour II, et al. Hepatic hydrothorax. Am J Ther 2014;21(1): 43–51.
19. Cardenas A, Kelleher T, Chopra S. Review article: hepatic hydrothorax. Aliment Pharmacol Ther 2004;20(3):271–9.
20. Dhanasekaran R, West JK, Gonzales PC, et al. Transjugular intrahepatic portosystemic shunt for symptomatic refractory hepatic hydrothorax in patients with cirrhosis. Am J Gastroenterol 2010;105(3):635–41.
21. Gordon FD, Anastopoulos HT, Crenshaw W, et al. The successful treatment of symptomatic, refractory hepatic hydrothorax with transjugular intrahepatic portosystemic shunt. Hepatology 1997;25(6):1366–9.
22. Jeffries MA, Kazanjian S, Wilson M, et al. Transjugular intrahepatic portosystemic shunts and liver transplantation in patients with refractory hepatic hydrothorax. Liver Transpl Surg 1998;4(5):416–23.
23. Spencer EB, Cohen DT, Darcy MD. Safety and efficacy of transjugular intrahepatic portosystemic shunt creation for the treatment of hepatic hydrothorax. J Vasc Interv Radiol 2002;13(4):385–90.
24. Strauss RM, Martin LG, Kaufman SL, et al. Transjugular intrahepatic portal systemic shunt for the management of symptomatic cirrhotic hydrothorax. Am J Gastroenterol 1994;89(9):1520–2.
25. Liu LU, Haddadin HA, Bodian CA, et al. Outcome analysis of cirrhotic patients undergoing chest tube placement. Chest 2004;126(1):142–8.
26. Orman ES, Lok AS. Outcomes of patients with chest tube insertion for hepatic hydrothorax. Hepatol Int 2009;3(4):582–6.
27. Runyon BA, Greenblatt M, Ming RH. Hepatic hydrothorax is a relative contraindication to chest tube insertion. Am J Gastroenterol 1986;81(7):566–7.
28. Ridha A, Al-Abboodi Y, Fasullo M. The outcome of thoracentesis versus chest tube placement for hepatic hydrothorax in patients with cirrhosis: a nationwide analysis of the national inpatient sample. Gastroenterol Res Pract 2017;2017: 5872068.
29. Chalhoub M, Harris K, Castellano M, et al. The use of the PleurX catheter in the management of non-malignant pleural effusions. Chron Respir Dis 2011;8(3): 185–91.
30. Chen A, Massoni J, Jung D, et al. Indwelling tunneled pleural catheters for the management of hepatic hydrothorax. A pilot study. Ann Am Thorac Soc 2016; 13(6):862–6.
31. Patil M, Dhillon SS, Attwood K, et al. Management of benign pleural effusions using indwelling pleural catheters: a systematic review and meta-analysis. Chest 2017;151(3):626–35.
32. Sharaf-Eldin M, Bediwy AS, Kobtan A, et al. Pigtail catheter: a less invasive option for pleural drainage in Egyptian patients with recurrent hepatic hydrothorax. Gastroenterol Res Pract 2016;2016:4013052.
33. Shojaee S, Rahman N, Haas K, et al. Indwelling tunneled pleural catheters for refractory hepatic hydrothorax in patients with cirrhosis: a multicenter study. Chest 2019;155(3):546–53.

34. Hou F, Qi X, Guo X. Effectiveness and safety of pleurodesis for hepatic hydrothorax: a systematic review and meta-analysis. Dig Dis Sci 2016;61(11):3321–34.
35. Huang PM, Kuo SW, Chen JS, et al. Thoracoscopic mesh repair of diaphragmatic defects in hepatic hydrothorax: a 10-year experience. Ann Thorac Surg 2016;101(5):1921–7.
36. Shirali AS, Grotts J, Elashoff D, et al. Predictors of outcomes after thoracic surgery in orthotopic liver transplant recipients with pleural disease. Semin Thorac Cardiovasc Surg 2019 [pii:S1043-0679(19)30028-0] [Epub ahead of print].
37. Xiol X, Tremosa G, Castellote J, et al. Liver transplantation in patients with hepatic hydrothorax. Transpl Int 2005;18(6):672–5.
38. Simonneau G, Montani D, Celermajer DS, et al. Haemodynamic definitions and updated clinical classification of pulmonary hypertension. Eur Respir J 2019;53(1) [pii:1801913].
39. Krowka MJ, Fallon MB, Kawut SM, et al. International liver transplant society practice guidelines: diagnosis and management of hepatopulmonary syndrome and portopulmonary hypertension. Transplantation 2016;100(7):1440–52.
40. Castro M, Krowka MJ. Hepatopulmonary syndrome. A pulmonary vascular complication of liver disease. Clin Chest Med 1996;17(1):35–48.
41. Rodriguez-Roisin R, Krowka MJ, Herve P, et al. Pulmonary-hepatic vascular disorders (PHD). Eur Respir J 2004;24(5):861–80.
42. Krowka MJ. Evolving dilemmas and management of portopulmonary hypertension. Semin Liver Dis 2006;26(3):265–72.
43. Krowka MJ. Pulmonary hypertension: diagnostics and therapeutics. Mayo Clin Proc 2000;75(6):625–30.
44. Krowka MJ, Miller DP, Barst RJ, et al. Portopulmonary hypertension: a report from the US-based REVEAL registry. Chest 2012;141(4):906–15.
45. Rodriguez-Roisin R, Krowka MJ. Hepatopulmonary syndrome–a liver-induced lung vascular disorder. N Engl J Med 2008;358(22):2378–87.
46. Krowka MJ. Portopulmonary hypertension. Semin Respir Crit Care Med 2012;33(1):17–25.
47. Kawut SM, Krowka MJ, Trotter JF, et al. Clinical risk factors for portopulmonary hypertension. Hepatology 2008;48(1):196–203.
48. Hadengue A, Benhayoun MK, Lebrec D, et al. Pulmonary hypertension complicating portal hypertension: prevalence and relation to splanchnic hemodynamics. Gastroenterology 1991;100(2):520–8.
49. McDonnell PJ, Toye PA, Hutchins GM. Primary pulmonary hypertension and cirrhosis: are they related? Am Rev Respir Dis 1983;127(4):437–41.
50. Humbert M, Sitbon O, Chaouat A, et al. Pulmonary arterial hypertension in France: results from a national registry. Am J Respir Crit Care Med 2006;173(9):1023–30.
51. Colle IO, Moreau R, Godinho E, et al. Diagnosis of portopulmonary hypertension in candidates for liver transplantation: a prospective study. Hepatology 2003;37(2):401–9.
52. Ramsay MA, Simpson BR, Nguyen AT, et al. Severe pulmonary hypertension in liver transplant candidates. Liver Transpl Surg 1997;3(5):494–500.
53. Roberts KE, Fallon MB, Krowka MJ, et al. Genetic risk factors for portopulmonary hypertension in patients with advanced liver disease. Am J Respir Crit Care Med 2009;179(9):835–42.

54. Edwards BS, Weir EK, Edwards WD, et al. Coexistent pulmonary and portal hypertension: morphologic and clinical features. J Am Coll Cardiol 1987;10(6): 1233–8.

55. Yeager ME, Frid MG, Stenmark KR. Progenitor cells in pulmonary vascular remodeling. Pulm Circ 2011;1(1):3–16.

56. Arnal JF, Fontaine C, Billon-Gales A, et al. Estrogen receptors and endothelium. Arterioscler Thromb Vasc Biol 2010;30(8):1506–12.

57. Tuder RM, Cool CD, Geraci MW, et al. Prostacyclin synthase expression is decreased in lungs from patients with severe pulmonary hypertension. Am J Respir Crit Care Med 1999;159(6):1925–32.

58. Kamath PS, Carpenter HA, Lloyd RV, et al. Hepatic localization of endothelin-1 in patients with idiopathic portal hypertension and cirrhosis of the liver. Liver Transpl 2000;6(5):596–602.

59. Benjaminov FS, Prentice M, Sniderman KW, et al. Portopulmonary hypertension in decompensated cirrhosis with refractory ascites. Gut 2003;52(9):1355–62.

60. Pellicelli AM, Barbaro G, Puoti C, et al. Plasma cytokines and portopulmonary hypertension in patients with cirrhosis waiting for orthotopic liver transplantation. Angiology 2010;61(8):802–6.

61. Kim WR, Krowka MJ, Plevak DJ, et al. Accuracy of Doppler echocardiography in the assessment of pulmonary hypertension in liver transplant candidates. Liver Transpl 2000;6(4):453–8.

62. Donovan CL, Marcovitz PA, Punch JD, et al. Two-dimensional and dobutamine stress echocardiography in the preoperative assessment of patients with end-stage liver disease prior to orthotopic liver transplantation. Transplantation 1996;61(8):1180–8.

63. Cotton CL, Gandhi S, Vaitkus PT, et al. Role of echocardiography in detecting portopulmonary hypertension in liver transplant candidates. Liver Transpl 2002;8(11):1051–4.

64. Krowka MJ, Swanson KL, Frantz RP, et al. Portopulmonary hypertension: results from a 10-year screening algorithm. Hepatology 2006;44(6):1502–10.

65. Raevens S, Colle I, Reyntjens K, et al. Echocardiography for the detection of portopulmonary hypertension in liver transplant candidates: an analysis of cutoff values. Liver Transpl 2013;19(6):602–10.

66. Ghofrani HA, Galie N, Grimminger F, et al. Riociguat for the treatment of pulmonary arterial hypertension. N Engl J Med 2013;369(4):330–40.

67. Sitbon O, Bosch J, Cottreel E, et al. Late Breaking Abstract - efficacy and safety of macitentan in portopulmonary hypertension: the PORTICO trial. Eur Respir J 2018;52(suppl 62):OA267.

68. Ashfaq M, Chinnakotla S, Rogers L, et al. The impact of treatment of portopulmonary hypertension on survival following liver transplantation. Am J Transplant 2007;7(5):1258–64.

69. Cartin-Ceba R, Swanson K, Iyer V, et al. Safety and efficacy of ambrisentan for the treatment of portopulmonary hypertension. Chest 2011;139(1):109–14.

70. Eriksson C, Gustavsson A, Kronvall T, et al. Hepatotoxity by bosentan in a patient with portopulmonary hypertension: a case-report and review of the literature. J Gastrointest Liver Dis 2011;20(1):77–80.

71. Fix OK, Bass NM, De Marco T, et al. Long-term follow-up of portopulmonary hypertension: effect of treatment with epoprostenol. Liver Transpl 2007;13(6): 875–85.

72. Gough MS, White RJ. Sildenafil therapy is associated with improved hemodynamics in liver transplantation candidates with pulmonary arterial hypertension. Liver Transpl 2009;15(1):30–6.

73. Halank M, Knudsen L, Seyfarth HJ, et al. Ambrisentan improves exercise capacity and symptoms in patients with portopulmonary hypertension. Z Gastroenterol 2011;49(9):1258–62.

74. Hemnes AR, Robbins IM. Sildenafil monotherapy in portopulmonary hypertension can facilitate liver transplantation. Liver Transpl 2009;15(1):15–9.

75. Hoeper MM. Liver toxicity: the Achilles' heel of endothelin receptor antagonist therapy? Eur Respir J 2009;34(3):529–30.

76. Hoeper MM, Seyfarth HJ, Hoeffken G, et al. Experience with inhaled iloprost and bosentan in portopulmonary hypertension. Eur Respir J 2007;30(6):1096–102.

77. Hollatz TJ, Musat A, Westphal S, et al. Treatment with sildenafil and treprostinil allows successful liver transplantation of patients with moderate to severe portopulmonary hypertension. Liver Transpl 2012;18(6):686–95.

78. Kahler CM, Graziadei I, Vogelsinger H, et al. Successful treatment of portopulmonary hypertension with the selective endothelin receptor antagonist Sitaxentan. Wien Klin Wochenschr 2011;123(7–8):248–52.

79. Findlay JY, Harrison BA, Plevak DJ, et al. Inhaled nitric oxide reduces pulmonary artery pressures in portopulmonary hypertension. Liver Transpl Surg 1999;5(5):381–7.

80. Kuo PC, Johnson LB, Plotkin JS, et al. Continuous intravenous infusion of epoprostenol for the treatment of portopulmonary hypertension. Transplantation 1997;63(4):604–6.

81. Melgosa MT, Ricci GL, Garcia-Pagan JC, et al. Acute and long-term effects of inhaled iloprost in portopulmonary hypertension. Liver Transpl 2010;16(3):348–56.

82. Reichenberger F, Voswinckel R, Steveling E, et al. Sildenafil treatment for portopulmonary hypertension. Eur Respir J 2006;28(3):563–7.

83. Sakai T, Planinsic RM, Mathier MA, et al. Initial experience using continuous intravenous treprostinil to manage pulmonary arterial hypertension in patients with end-stage liver disease. Transpl Int 2009;22(5):554–61.

84. Sussman N, Kaza V, Barshes N, et al. Successful liver transplantation following medical management of portopulmonary hypertension: a single-center series. Am J Transplant 2006;6(9):2177–82.

85. Raevens S, De Pauw M, Reyntjens K, et al. Oral vasodilator therapy in patients with moderate to severe portopulmonary hypertension as a bridge to liver transplantation. Eur J Gastroenterol Hepatol 2013;25(4):495–502.

86. Matsubara O, Nakamura T, Uehara T, et al. Histometrical investigation of the pulmonary artery in severe hepatic disease. J Pathol 1984;143(1):31–7.

87. Savale L, Magnier R, Le Pavec J, et al. Efficacy, safety, and pharmacokinetics of bosentan in portopulmonary hypertension. Eur Respir J 2013;41(1):96–103.

88. Fisher JH, Johnson SR, Chau C, et al. Effectiveness of phosphodiesterase-5 inhibitor therapy for portopulmonary hypertension. Can Respir J 2015;22(1):42–6.

89. Ghofrani HA, D'Armini AM, Grimminger F, et al. Riociguat for the treatment of chronic thromboembolic pulmonary hypertension. N Engl J Med 2013;369(4):319–29.

90. Grimminger F, Weimann G, Frey R, et al. First acute haemodynamic study of soluble guanylate cyclase stimulator riociguat in pulmonary hypertension. Eur Respir J 2009;33(4):785–92.

91. Stasch JP, Pacher P, Evgenov OV. Soluble guanylate cyclase as an emerging therapeutic target in cardiopulmonary disease. Circulation 2011;123(20): 2263–73.

92. Cartin-Ceba R, Halank M, Ghofrani HA, et al. Riociguat treatment for portopulmonary hypertension: a subgroup analysis from the PATENT-1/-2 studies. Pulm Circ 2018;8(2). 2045894018769305.

93. Provencher S, Herve P, Jais X, et al. Deleterious effects of beta-blockers on exercise capacity and hemodynamics in patients with portopulmonary hypertension. Gastroenterology 2006;130(1):120–6.

94. Van der Linden P, Le Moine O, Ghysels M, et al. Pulmonary hypertension after transjugular intrahepatic portosystemic shunt: effects on right ventricular function. Hepatology 1996;23(5):982–7.

95. Austin MJ, McDougall NI, Wendon JA, et al. Safety and efficacy of combined use of sildenafil, bosentan, and iloprost before and after liver transplantation in severe portopulmonary hypertension. Liver Transpl 2008;14(3):287–91.

96. Bandara M, Gordon FD, Sarwar A, et al. Successful outcomes following living donor liver transplantation for portopulmonary hypertension. Liver Transpl 2010;16(8):983–9.

97. Castro M, Krowka MJ, Schroeder DR, et al. Frequency and clinical implications of increased pulmonary artery pressures in liver transplant patients. Mayo Clin Proc 1996;71(6):543–51.

98. Fukazawa K, Pretto EA Jr. Poor outcome following aborted orthotopic liver transplantation due to severe porto-pulmonary hypertension. J Hepatobiliary Pancreat Sci 2010;17(4):505–8.

99. Kawut SM, Taichman DB, Ahya VN, et al. Hemodynamics and survival of patients with portopulmonary hypertension. Liver Transpl 2005;11(9):1107–11.

100. Krowka MJ, Mandell MS, Ramsay MA, et al. Hepatopulmonary syndrome and portopulmonary hypertension: a report of the multicenter liver transplant database. Liver Transpl 2004;10(2):174–82.

101. Saner FH, Nadalin S, Pavlakovic G, et al. Portopulmonary hypertension in the early phase following liver transplantation. Transplantation 2006;82(7):887–91.

102. Scouras NE, Matsusaki T, Boucek CD, et al. Portopulmonary hypertension as an indication for combined heart, lung, and liver or lung and liver transplantation: literature review and case presentation. Liver Transpl 2011;17(2):137–43.

103. Starkel P, Vera A, Gunson B, et al. Outcome of liver transplantation for patients with pulmonary hypertension. Liver Transpl 2002;8(4):382–8.

104. Taura P, Garcia-Valdecasas JC, Beltran J, et al. Moderate primary pulmonary hypertension in patients undergoing liver transplantation. Anesth Analg 1996; 83(4):675–80.

105. Krowka MJ, Fallon MB, Mulligan DC, et al. Model for end-stage liver disease (MELD) exception for portopulmonary hypertension. Liver Transpl 2006;12(12 Suppl 3):S114–6.

106. Goldberg DS, Krok K, Batra S, et al. Impact of the hepatopulmonary syndrome MELD exception policy on outcomes of patients after liver transplantation: an analysis of the UNOS database. Gastroenterology 2014;146(5):1256–65.e1.

107. DuBrock HM, Goldberg DS, Sussman NL, et al. Predictors of waitlist mortality in portopulmonary hypertension. Transplantation 2017;101(7):1609–15.

108. DeMartino ES, Cartin-Ceba R, Findlay JY, et al. Frequency and outcomes of patients with increased mean pulmonary artery pressure at the time of liver transplantation. Transplantation 2017;101(1):101–6.

109. Robalino BD, Moodie DS. Association between primary pulmonary hypertension and portal hypertension: analysis of its pathophysiology and clinical, laboratory and hemodynamic manifestations. J Am Coll Cardiol 1991;17(2):492–8.

110. Swanson KL, Wiesner RH, Nyberg SL, et al. Survival in portopulmonary hypertension: Mayo Clinic experience categorized by treatment subgroups. Am J Transplant 2008;8(11):2445–53.

111. Le Pavec J, Souza R, Herve P, et al. Portopulmonary hypertension: survival and prognostic factors. Am J Respir Crit Care Med 2008;178(6):637–43.

112. Khaderi S, Khan R, Safdar Z, et al. Long-term follow-up of portopulmonary hypertension patients after liver transplantation. Liver Transpl 2014;20(6):724–7.

113. Rodriquez-Roisin R, Krowka MJ, Herve P, et al. Highlights of the ERS Task Force on pulmonary-hepatic vascular disorders (PHD). J Hepatol 2005;42(6):924–7.

114. Krowka MJ, Cortese DA. Hepatopulmonary syndrome. Current concepts in diagnostic and therapeutic considerations. Chest 1994;105(5):1528–37.

115. Kennedy TC, Knudson RJ. Exercise-aggravated hypoxemia and orthodeoxia in cirrhosis. Chest 1977;72(3):305–9.

116. Fallon MB, Krowka MJ, Brown RS, et al. Impact of hepatopulmonary syndrome on quality of life and survival in liver transplant candidates. Gastroenterology 2008;135(4):1168–75.

117. Fallon MB, Abrams GA, Luo B, et al. The role of endothelial nitric oxide synthase in the pathogenesis of a rat model of hepatopulmonary syndrome. Gastroenterology 1997;113(2):606–14.

118. Fallon MB, Abrams GA, McGrath JW, et al. Common bile duct ligation in the rat: a model of intrapulmonary vasodilatation and hepatopulmonary syndrome. Am J Physiol 1997;272(4 Pt 1):G779–84.

119. Ling Y, Zhang J, Luo B, et al. The role of endothelin-1 and the endothelin B receptor in the pathogenesis of hepatopulmonary syndrome in the rat. Hepatology 2004;39(6):1593–602.

120. Liu M, Tian D, Wang T, et al. Correlation between pulmonary endothelin receptors and alveolar-arterial oxygen gradient in rats with hepatopulmonary syndrome. J Huazhong Univ Sci Technol Med Sci 2005;25(5):494–6.

121. Luo B, Tang L, Wang Z, et al. Cholangiocyte endothelin 1 and transforming growth factor beta1 production in rat experimental hepatopulmonary syndrome. Gastroenterology 2005;129(2):682–95.

122. Zhang M, Luo B, Chen SJ, et al. Endothelin-1 stimulation of endothelial nitric oxide synthase in the pathogenesis of hepatopulmonary syndrome. Am J Physiol 1999;277(5):G944–52.

123. Luo B, Liu L, Tang L, et al. ET-1 and TNF-alpha in HPS: analysis in prehepatic portal hypertension and biliary and nonbiliary cirrhosis in rats. Am J Physiol Gastrointest Liver Physiol 2004;286(2):G294–303.

124. Sztrymf B, Libert JM, Mougeot C, et al. Cirrhotic rats with bacterial translocation have higher incidence and severity of hepatopulmonary syndrome. J Gastroenterol Hepatol 2005;20(10):1538–44.

125. Thenappan T, Goel A, Marsboom G, et al. A central role for CD68(+) macrophages in hepatopulmonary syndrome. Reversal by macrophage depletion. Am J Respir Crit Care Med 2011;183(8):1080–91.

126. Zhang J, Yang W, Luo B, et al. The role of CX(3)CL1/CX(3)CR1 in pulmonary angiogenesis and intravascular monocyte accumulation in rat experimental hepatopulmonary syndrome. J Hepatol 2012;57(4):752–8.

127. Carter EP, Hartsfield CL, Miyazono M, et al. Regulation of heme oxygenase-1 by nitric oxide during hepatopulmonary syndrome. Am J Physiol Lung Cell Mol Physiol 2002;283(2):L346–53.
128. Zhang J, Ling Y, Luo B, et al. Analysis of pulmonary heme oxygenase-1 and nitric oxide synthase alterations in experimental hepatopulmonary syndrome. Gastroenterology 2003;125(5):1441–51.
129. Zhang J, Luo B, Tang L, et al. Pulmonary angiogenesis in a rat model of hepatopulmonary syndrome. Gastroenterology 2009;136(3):1070–80.
130. Mejias M, Garcia-Pras E, Tiani C, et al. Beneficial effects of sorafenib on splanchnic, intrahepatic, and portocollateral circulations in portal hypertensive and cirrhotic rats. Hepatology 2009;49(4):1245–56.
131. Chang CC, Chuang CL, Lee FY, et al. Sorafenib treatment improves hepatopulmonary syndrome in rats with biliary cirrhosis. Clin Sci (Lond) 2013;124(7): 457–66.
132. Cremona G, Higenbottam TW, Mayoral V, et al. Elevated exhaled nitric oxide in patients with hepatopulmonary syndrome. Eur Respir J 1995;8(11):1883–5.
133. Koch DG, Fallon MB. Hepatopulmonary syndrome. Clin Liver Dis 2014;18(2): 407–20.
134. Rolla G, Brussino L, Colagrande P, et al. Exhaled nitric oxide and impaired oxygenation in cirrhotic patients before and after liver transplantation. Ann Intern Med 1998;129(5):375–8.
135. Roberts KE, Kawut SM, Krowka MJ, et al. Genetic risk factors for hepatopulmonary syndrome in patients with advanced liver disease. Gastroenterology 2010; 139(1):130–9.e24.
136. Koch DG, Bogatkevich G, Ramshesh V, et al. Elevated levels of endothelin-1 in hepatic venous blood are associated with intrapulmonary vasodilatation in humans. Dig Dis Sci 2012;57(2):516–23.
137. Andrivet P, Cadranel J, Housset B, et al. Mechanisms of impaired arterial oxygenation in patients with liver cirrhosis and severe respiratory insufficiency. Effects of indomethacin. Chest 1993;103(2):500–7.
138. Nakos G, Evrenoglou D, Vassilakis N, et al. Haemodynamics and gas exchange in liver cirrhosis: the effect of orally administered almitrine bismesylate. Respir Med 1993;87(2):93–8.
139. Agusti AG, Roca J, Rodriguez-Roisin R. Mechanisms of gas exchange impairment in patients with liver cirrhosis. Clin Chest Med 1996;17(1):49–66.
140. Schraufnagel DE, Kay JM. Structural and pathologic changes in the lung vasculature in chronic liver disease. Clin Chest Med 1996;17(1):1–15.
141. Keal EE, Harington M. Cirrhosis and hypoxia. Proc R Soc Med 1970;63(6): 621–2.
142. Wolfe JD, Tashkin DP, Holly FE, et al. Hypoxemia of cirrhosis: detection of abnormal small pulmonary vascular channels by a quantitative radionuclide method. Am J Med 1977;63(5):746–54.
143. Arguedas MR, Singh H, Faulk DK, et al. Utility of pulse oximetry screening for hepatopulmonary syndrome. Clin Gastroenterol Hepatol 2007;5(6):749–54.
144. Roberts DN, Arguedas MR, Fallon MB. Cost-effectiveness of screening for hepatopulmonary syndrome in liver transplant candidates. Liver Transpl 2007;13(2): 206–14.
145. Forde KA, Fallon MB, Krowka MJ, et al. Pulse oximetry is insensitive for detection of hepatopulmonary syndrome in patients evaluated for liver transplantation. Hepatology 2019;69(1):270–81.

146. Abrams GA, Nanda NC, Dubovsky EV, et al. Use of macroaggregated albumin lung perfusion scan to diagnose hepatopulmonary syndrome: a new approach. Gastroenterology 1998;114(2):305–10.

147. Groneberg DA, Fischer A. Methylene blue improves the hepatopulmonary syndrome. Ann Intern Med 2001;135(5):380–1.

148. Rolla G, Bucca C, Brussino L. Methylene blue in the hepatopulmonary syndrome. N Engl J Med 1994;331(16):1098.

149. Schenk P, Madl C, Rezaie-Majd S, et al. Methylene blue improves the hepatopulmonary syndrome. Ann Intern Med 2000;133(9):701–6.

150. Brussino L, Bucca C, Morello M, et al. Effect on dyspnoea and hypoxaemia of inhaled N(G)-nitro-L-arginine methyl ester in hepatopulmonary syndrome. Lancet 2003;362(9377):43–4.

151. Gomez FP, Barbera JA, Roca J, et al. Effects of nebulized N(G)-nitro-L-arginine methyl ester in patients with hepatopulmonary syndrome. Hepatology 2006; 43(5):1084–91.

152. Krowka MJ, Dickson ER, Cortese DA. Hepatopulmonary syndrome. Clinical observations and lack of therapeutic response to somatostatin analogue. Chest 1993;104(2):515–21.

153. Shijo H, Sasaki H, Yuh K, et al. Effects of indomethacin on hepatogenic pulmonary angiodysplasia. Chest 1991;99(4):1027–9.

154. Song JY, Choi JY, Ko JT, et al. Long-term aspirin therapy for hepatopulmonary syndrome. Pediatrics 1996;97(6 Pt 1):917–20.

155. Krowka MJ, Cortese DA. Severe hypoxemia associated with liver disease: Mayo Clinic experience and the experimental use of almitrine bismesylate. Mayo Clin Proc 1987;62(3):164–73.

156. Agusti AG, Roca J, Bosch J, et al. Effects of propranolol on arterial oxygenation and oxygen transport to tissues in patients with cirrhosis. Am Rev Respir Dis 1990;142(2):306–10.

157. Lambrecht GL, Malbrain ML, Coremans P, et al. Orthodeoxia and platypnea in liver cirrhosis: effects of propranolol. Acta Clin Belg 1994;49(1):26–30.

158. Anel RM, Sheagren JN. Novel presentation and approach to management of hepatopulmonary syndrome with use of antimicrobial agents. Clin Infect Dis 2001;32(10):E131–6.

159. Gupta S, Faughnan ME, Lilly L, et al. Norfloxacin therapy for hepatopulmonary syndrome: a pilot randomized controlled trial. Clin Gastroenterol Hepatol 2010; 8(12):1095–8.

160. Tanikella R, Philips GM, Faulk DK, et al. Pilot study of pentoxifylline in hepatopulmonary syndrome. Liver Transpl 2008;14(8):1199–203.

161. Abrams GA, Fallon MB. Treatment of hepatopulmonary syndrome with Allium sativum L. (garlic): a pilot trial. J Clin Gastroenterol 1998;27(3):232–5.

162. De BK, Dutta D, Pal SK, et al. The role of garlic in hepatopulmonary syndrome: a randomized controlled trial. Can J Gastroenterol 2010;24(3):183–8.

163. Kawut SM, Ellenberg SS, Krowka MJ, et al. Sorafenib in Hepatopulmonary Syndrome: A Randomized, Double-Blind, Placebo-Controlled Trial. Liver Transpl 2019;25(8):1155–64.

164. Laberge JM, Brandt ML, Lebecque P, et al. Reversal of cirrhosis-related pulmonary shunting in two children by orthotopic liver transplantation. Transplantation 1992;53(5):1135–8.

165. Schwarzenberg SJ, Freese DK, Regelmann WE, et al. Resolution of severe intrapulmonary shunting after liver transplantation. Chest 1993;103(4):1271–3.

166. Stoller JK, Moodie D, Schiavone WA, et al. Reduction of intrapulmonary shunt and resolution of digital clubbing associated with primary biliary cirrhosis after liver transplantation. Hepatology 1990;11(1):54–8.
167. Arguedas MR, Abrams GA, Krowka MJ, et al. Prospective evaluation of outcomes and predictors of mortality in patients with hepatopulmonary syndrome undergoing liver transplantation. Hepatology 2003;37(1):192–7.
168. Gupta S, Castel H, Rao RV, et al. Improved survival after liver transplantation in patients with hepatopulmonary syndrome. Am J Transplant 2010;10(2):354–63.
169. Iyer VN, Swanson KL, Cartin-Ceba R, et al. Hepatopulmonary syndrome: favorable outcomes in the MELD exception era. Hepatology 2013;57(6):2427–35.
170. Iyer VN, Swanson KL, Krowka MJ. Survival benefits of liver transplant in severe hepatopulmonary syndrome. Am J Respir Crit Care Med 2013;188(4):514.
171. Lange PA, Stoller JK. The hepatopulmonary syndrome. Effect of liver transplantation. Clin Chest Med 1996;17(1):115–23.
172. Taille C, Cadranel J, Bellocq A, et al. Liver transplantation for hepatopulmonary syndrome: a ten-year experience in Paris, France. Transplantation 2003;75(9): 1482–9 [discussion: 46–7].
173. Fallon MB, Mulligan DC, Gish RG, et al. Model for end-stage liver disease (MELD) exception for hepatopulmonary syndrome. Liver Transpl 2006;12(12 Suppl 3):S105–7.
174. Raevens S, Rogiers X, Geerts A, et al. Outcome of liver transplantation for hepatopulmonary syndrome: a Eurotransplant experience. Eur Respir J 2019;53(2) [pii:1801096].
175. Pham DM, Subramanian R, Parekh S. Coexisting hepatopulmonary syndrome and portopulmonary hypertension: implications for liver transplantation. J Clin Gastroenterol 2010;44(7):e136–40.
176. Olsson KM, Meyer K, Berliner D, et al. Development of hepatopulmonary syndrome during combination therapy for portopulmonary hypertension. Eur Respir J 2019;53(1) [pii:1801880].
177. Krowka MJ, Frantz RP, McGoon MD, et al. Improvement in pulmonary hemodynamics during intravenous epoprostenol (prostacyclin): a study of 15 patients with moderate to severe portopulmonary hypertension. Hepatology 1999; 30(3):641–8.
178. Awdish RL, Cajigas HR. Early initiation of prostacyclin in portopulmonary hypertension: 10 years of a transplant center's experience. Lung 2013;191(6): 593–600.

Pharmacologic Management of Portal Hypertension

Chalermrat Bunchorntavakul, MD[a,b], K. Rajender Reddy, MD[b,*]

KEYWORDS

- Portal hypertension • Variceal hemorrhage • Terlipressin • Somatostatin
- Propranolol • Carvedilol

KEY POINTS

- Terlipressin, somatostatin, or octreotide, in combination with early endoscopic therapy, are recommended for the treatment of acute variceal hemorrhage.
- Nonselective β-blockers decrease the risk of variceal hemorrhage and hepatic decompensation, particularly in those 30% to 40% of patients with good hemodynamic response.
- Carvedilol, statins, and anticoagulants have shown promising results in the management of portal hypertension.
- Recent advances in the pharmacologic treatment of portal hypertension have focused on modifying an increased intrahepatic resistance by increasing availability of nitric oxide and/or modulating vasoactive substances.
- Novel pharmacologic agents are being developed for portal hypertension.

INTRODUCTION

Portal hypertension (PHT) is the major driver for most complications of cirrhosis leading to death or liver transplantation, for example, variceal hemorrhage (VH), ascites, and the hepatorenal syndrome (HRS). The best practical method to assess portal pressure (PP) is the measurement of the hepatic venous pressure gradient (HVPG) through catheterization of the hepatic vein (normal HVPG is 3–5 mm Hg), and most complications of PHT develop when the HVPG is greater than 10 mm Hg (defined as clinically significant PHT).[1–3] Pharmacologic management of PHT is aimed at reducing PP (by decreasing the HVPG to <10–12 mm Hg or a ≥10%–20% decrease in the HVPG) without causing systemic hypotension. For several decades, somatostatin (SMT), octreotide, or terlipressin have been used, together with urgent endoscopic therapy, to treat acute VH. Over the long term, however, nonselective

Conflict of interest: None.
[a] Division of Gastroenterology and Hepatology, Department of Medicine, Rajavithi Hospital, College of Medicine, Rangsit University, Rajavithi Road, Ratchathewi, Bangkok 10400, Thailand; [b] Division of Gastroenterology and Hepatology, Department of Medicine, University of Pennsylvania, 2 Dulles, 3400 Spruce Street, Philadelphia, PA 19104, USA
* Corresponding author.
E-mail address: rajender.reddy@uphs.upenn.edu

Clin Liver Dis 23 (2019) 713–736
https://doi.org/10.1016/j.cld.2019.06.004
1089-3261/19/© 2019 Elsevier Inc. All rights reserved.

liver.theclinics.com

β-blockers (NSBBs) have been a mainstay strategy for the prevention of VH and also decreasing the risk of hepatic decompensation.[1-3] However, current pharmacologic treatments for PHT are still far from ideal; for example, the optimal hemodynamic target can only be achieved in 30% to 40% of patients receiving NSBBs.[1-4] Owing to the advances in the knowledge of the pathophysiology of PHT and in drug development, several pharmacologic agents, such as carvedilol, statins, and anticoagulants, have been evaluated and seem to exert benefits in patients with PHT.[5-7] Further, several potential agents with various targets are under investigation for the management of PHT and some of them have initially shown promising results. The key aims of pharmacologic management of PHT nowadays are not only to prevent major complications of PHT, but also to improve or even favorably modify the natural history of cirrhosis and PHT, such as prevention of clinical decompensation and mortality, as well as the reversal of cirrhosis and PHT.

RATIONAL BASIS OF PHARMACOLOGIC THERAPY FOR PORTAL HYPERTENSION

According to Ohm's law, the pressure gradient across the portal system is determined by portal blood flow and vascular resistance opposing the flow. Therefore, drugs or procedures that decrease the hepatic vascular resistance and/or portal blood flow will decrease PP.[3] In patients with advanced chronic liver disease, PP increases initially as a consequence of an increased intrahepatic resistance to portal flow attributed to structural changes toward cirrhosis (eg, progressive fibrosis, vascular distortion from regenerative nodules, sinusoidal remodeling and microvascular thrombi).[2,3] This "structural" component explains approximately 70% of the increased intrahepatic resistance and could be targeted pharmacologically by treating the etiology of liver disease, and using antifibrotic agents and anticoagulants.[2] However, approximately 30% of the increased intrahepatic resistance is attributed to an increased intrahepatic vascular tone, which is attributed to endothelial dysfunction resulting from disequilibrium between increased production/response to vasoconstrictors and reduced production/response to vasodilators, mainly nitric oxide (NO).[2,3,8] This "functional" component may be responsive to drugs that improve endothelial functions (eg, statins) and vasodilators (eg, nitrates, α-adrenergic antagonists, and angiotensin-II receptor blockers [ARBs]; Fig. 1).[2]

As the liver disease progresses and HVPG increases to 10 mm Hg or greater (defined as clinically significant PHT), portosystemic collaterals begin to develop and blood flow increases owing to splanchnic arteriolar vasodilatation, which then worsens PHT despite the formation of widespread portosystemic collaterals that divert most portal flow to systemic circulation.[2,3] NSBBs (β-2 adrenergic blocking effect), SMT, and vasopressin act by causing splanchnic vasoconstriction, thereby decreasing the portal venous inflow.[2] The formation of collaterals is a consequence not only of dilatation of preexisting vascular channels owing to increased PP, but also neoangiogenesis through multiple signaling pathways (eg, vascular endothelial growth factor derived, platelet-derived growth factor receptor derived, and stem cell growth factor derived; see Fig. 1).[3,9] Apart from the development of esophageal varices (EV), patients with clinically significant PHT have an increased risk of developing overt clinical decompensation (eg, ascites, VH, and encephalopathy).[10] In those without EV, pharmacologic treatment to achieve a small decrease in the HVPG (<10% of baseline value) has led to a decrease in the rate of EV formation and, theoretically, as such would be able to prevent the development of clinical decompensation.[11]

Increased splanchnic NO production is the key factor that leads to vasodilatation and increased splanchnic blood flow.[2,3] Vasodilation occurs not only in the splanchnic, but

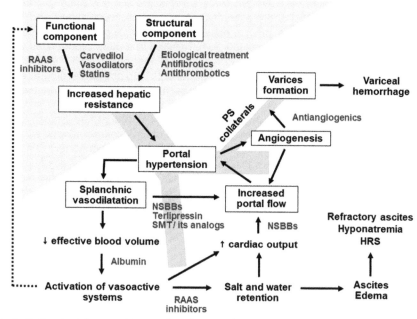

Fig. 1. Pathophysiology and targets for pharmacologic treatment of PHT. PS, portosystemic; RAAS, renin–angiotensin–aldosterone system. (*Adapted from* Garcia-Tsao G, Abraldes JG, Berzigotti A, et al. Portal hypertensive bleeding in cirrhosis: Risk stratification, diagnosis, and management: 2016 practice guidance by the American Association for the study of liver diseases. Hepatology (Baltimore, Md) 2017;65(1):310-335; with permission.)

also in the systemic circulation, leading to activation of neurohumoral and vasoconstrictive systems (eg, adrenergic and renin–angiotensin–aldosterone system), sodium and water retention, increased blood volume, and increased cardiac output (hyperdynamic circulatory state) that in turn further increase portal venous inflow and PP.[2,3] As liver disease further progresses, circulatory dysfunction and ascites evolve. In patients with symptomatic PHT, pharmacologic therapy should be more aggressive, targeted at decreasing the PP to less than 12 mm Hg or a 20% or greater decrease in the HVPG from baseline, because this mark decreases the risk of EV bleeding and rebleeding, clinical decompensation, and mortality.[1,12]

PHARMACOLOGIC AGENTS USED FOR PORTAL HYPERTENSION IN CURRENT CLINICAL PRACTICE
Acute Variceal Hemorrhage and the Hepatorenal Syndrome

Somatostatin and its analogs (eg, octreotide)
SMT is a 14 amino acid peptide secreted by neural, endocrine, and enteroendocrine cells that inhibits gastrointestinal and pancreatic secretion. It has a very short biologic half-life (1.2–4.8 minutes), which necessitates a continuous intravenous (IV) infusion to maintain an adequate serum concentration.[1,13–15] SMT induces splanchnic vasoconstriction (through the inhibition of vasodilatory peptides, mainly glucagon, and also by a direct vasoconstrictive effect) and consequently reduces PP.[1,14] In patients with cirrhosis, wedged hepatic venous pressure decreased rapidly by approximately 30% after a 250-μg bolus injection, and both wedged hepatic venous pressure and portal blood flow decreased approximately 17% during continuous infusion of

250 μg/h.[16] During acute VH, SMT produces a significant and sustained decrease in HVPG (approximately 15%) and prevents secondary increases by meals and blood transfusion (which may be a main mechanism in preventing early rebleeding).[17] Notably, higher dose SMT infusion (500 μg/h) resulted in a more pronounced effect on the HVPG and azygos blood flow than the classical dose of 250 μg/h.[18] Thus, a randomized controlled trial (RCT) suggested that patients with active bleeding at emergency endoscopy (high risk for hemostasis failure) may benefit from higher doses of SMT (250 μg ×3 boluses followed by a 500 μg/h IV infusion; **Table 1**).[19]

Octreotide is an 8 amino acid synthetic analogue of SMT that has a much longer duration of action and possesses somewhat similar pharmacologic effects, although its affinity for SMT receptors is different from that of the natural hormone.[1,13,14] Apart from IV administration, octreotide can also be given subcutaneously (peak serum concentration within 30 minutes and elimination half-life is 1.5 h); however, this route of administration is not recommended for acute VH (see **Table 1**). Additionally, octreotide prevents postprandial splanchnic hyperemia and enhances the hemodynamic effects of propranolol in patients with PHT.[20–22] Apart from octreotide, other long-acting synthetic analogs of SMT, such as lanreotide, vapreotide, and seglitide, have very limited evidence for the management of PHT.[1,15]

SMT and its analogs, in combination with early endoscopic variceal ligation (EVL), are recommended for the treatment of acute VH.[2,23] In a Cochrane meta-analysis of 21 RCT (n = 2588) on acute VH comparing SMT and its analogs with all other therapies, the drugs significantly increased the rate of hemostasis (risk ratio, 0.68; 95% confidence interval, 0.54–0.87), but without significant effects on mortality.[24] These vasoactive agents have improved the efficacy of endoscopic therapy to achieve initial control of bleeding.[25] Octreotide is currently the only vasoactive drug available in the United States, and in a meta-analysis of 13 RCT, it was shown to significantly improve hemostasis after acute VH but without effects on mortality.[26] SMT and its analogs are safe and severe side effects are rare (vomiting and hyperglycemia occur in approximately 20% of patients, and are usually mild and manageable).[1,15]

Vasopressin and its analogs (eg, terlipressin)

Vasopressin, an endogenous peptide hormone, decreases the portal venous inflow by causing splanchnic vasoconstriction, which then results in reduced PP. However, it is

Table 1
Vasoactive agents for acute VH: characteristics and dosing

	SMT	Octreotide	Terlipressin
Characteristics	Natural SMT	Synthetic analogue of SMT	Long-acting synthetic analogue of vasopressin
Main mechanisms	Inhibits the release of vasodilatory peptides (mainly glucagon)	Inhibits the release of vasodilatory peptides (mainly glucagon)	Splanchnic vasoconstrictors
Recommended dose	Initial IV bolus 250 μg (can be repeated in 1st h if ongoing bleeding) Continue infusion 250–500 μg/h Duration: 2–5 d	Initial IV bolus 50 μg (can be repeated in 1st h if ongoing bleeding) Continue infusion 50 μg/h Duration: 2–5 d	Initial 48 h: 2 mg IV q 4 h until control of bleeding Maintenance: 1 mg q 4 h Duration: 2–5 d

Adapted from Garcia-Tsao G, Abraldes JG, Berzigotti A, et al. Portal hypertensive bleeding in cirrhosis: Risk stratification, diagnosis, and management: 2016 practice guidance by the American Association for the study of liver diseases. Hepatology (Baltimore, Md) 2017;65(1):310-335; with permission.

not routinely used for acute VH owing to its substantial systemic side effects, such as reduced cardiac output, bradycardia, and systemic vasoconstriction.[2] To decrease its systemic side effects, vasopressin IV infusion should ideally be accompanied by IV nitroglycerin and should not be used for more than 1 day.[2] Terlipressin (triglycyl lysine vasopressin) is a synthetic analogue of vasopressin with longer biologic activity and better cardiovascular safety profile.[1] Like vasopressin, it decreases cardiac output, increases systemic vascular resistance, and causes splanchnic vasoconstriction, resulting in a rapid decrease in PP (approximately 20% in 15 to 30 minutes after a single IV injection, which lasts for approximately 4 hours) while it may also increase systemic arterial blood pressure (BP).[1,27,28] As compared with SMT, terlipressin has more sustained hemodynamic effects in reducing PP[29] and also significantly reducing PP in patients who did not respond to standard dose SMT.[30]

Terlipressin is currently indicated for the treatment of acute VH (see **Table 1**) and type 1 HRS.[2,23] In a meta-analysis of 20 RCT (n = 1609) comparing terlipressin with placebo or other treatments for acute VH, terlipressin significantly improved hemostasis (odds ratio [OR], 2.94; P = .0008) and decreased the in-hospital mortality (O,R 0.31; P = .008), compared with no vasoactive drugs.[31] Terlipressin had a significantly higher rate of complications (O,R 2.44; P = .04) compared with SMT, and had a significantly lower hemostasis rate (OR, 0.37; P = .007) compared with octreotide.[31] Additionally, in a meta-analysis evaluating several vasoactive drugs (30 RCT; 4 RCT used terlipressin),[32] and a large RCT (n = 780) comparing terlipressin, SMT, and octreotide (followed by endoscopic therapy) for acute VH, there were no differences in mortality and hemostasis rates among the vasoactive agents. To date, terlipressin is the only pharmacologic agent shown to decrease mortality in acute VH, although this is finding mainly due to the observations from RCTs conducted before 1990 comparing terlipressin with no vasoactive drug.[31,33,34]

For HRS, terlipressin is recommended as the first-line pharmacologic treatment because it counteracts the main pathogenesis, which included marked splanchnic vasodilation in patients with cirrhosis and ascites, which subsequently results in decreased effective circulatory volume and severe renal vasoconstriction.[23,35] Further, it has been shown to have beneficial effects in increasing arterial BP, renal blood flow, and urinary sodium excretion.[35] Telipressin can be used as IV boluses at the initial dose of 0.5 to 1.0 mg every 4 to 6 hours, in combination with IV albumin 20 to 40 g/d, to further improve effective circulatory volume.[23] Administration of terlipressin by continuous IV infusion at initial dose of 2 mg/d is also suggested because it decreases the total daily required dose of the drug and, also its side effects.[23,36] In case of nonresponse (a decrease in serum creatinine to <25% from the peak value), after 2 days, the dose of terlipressin should be increased in a stepwise manner to a maximum of 12 mg/d (2 mg every 4–6 hours).[23] In 2 well-performed meta-analyses, terlipressin plus albumin was shown to improve renal function and also short-term survival in patients with HRS.[37,38] The most common side effects of terlipressin are diarrhea, abdominal pain, circulatory overload, and cardiovascular ischemic complications, which have been reported in up to 30% to 50% of patients; the rate of discontinuation owing to side effects (mainly ischemic complications) has been 4% to 22%.[23,38,39] Therefore, terlipressin should not be used in patients with who are older than 70 years of age, or have a history of coronary artery disease, cardiomyopathies, cardiac arrhythmias, cerebrovascular disease, peripheral arterial disease, uncontrolled hypertension, severe asthma, and chronic obstructive pulmonary disease.[40]

Other vasoactive agents including α-adrenergic drugs, such as noradrenaline and oral midodrine plus subcutaneous octreotide, administered with albumin have also been evaluated for the treatment of HRS. Based on hemodynamic studies, noradrenaline has strong effects in decreasing splanchnic vasodilatation and increasing arterial BP, but without (or mild) significant effects on PP, renal blood flow, and urinary sodium excretion.[35] Octreotide has moderate effects in reducing splanchnic vasodilatation and PP, mild effects in increasing arterial BP, but without significant effects on renal blood flow, and urinary sodium excretion.[35] Midodrine, an α1-adreanergic agonist, has mild to moderate effects in increasing arterial BP, but without (or mild) significant effects on renal blood flow and urinary sodium excretion (there are no available data regarding the effects on PP and splanchnic circulation).[35] Several RCT suggested that noradrenaline (continuous IV infusion 0.5–3 mg/h) can be an alternative to terlipressin, because it has shown to be as effective as terlipressin regarding the increase in mean arterial BP, the reversal of HRS, and survival, although it may be associated with fewer side effects.[41,42] However, there have been a limited number of patients evaluated with noradrenaline as a treatment for HRS and its use often requires close monitoring in an intensive care unit.[41,42] Of note, terlipressin with albumin is superior to midodrine plus octreotide with albumin for reversal of HRS.[43]

Long-Term Strategy: Prevention of Variceal Hemorrhage, Delaying Progression of Portal Hypertension and Its Complications

Nonselective β-blockers and carvedilol

NSBBs (eg, propranolol, nadolol, and timolol) act by blocking both β-1 cardiac receptors leading to decreased cardiac output, and β-2 vascular receptors, allowing unopposed α-1 adrenergic activity that results in splanchnic vasoconstriction, which then lead to a decrease in PP and portal–collateral blood flow.[1] Other beneficial effects of NSBBs include the decrease of azygos blood flow and variceal pressure, as well as shortening the intestinal transit time and decreasing intestinal permeability, which have been associated with decreased bacterial overgrowth and thereby a decreased risk of bacterial translocation and spontaneous bacterial peritonitis.[1,44–46]

In 1980, an RCT by Lebrec and colleagues[47,48] demonstrated that propranolol (at doses that decreased the heart rate by approximately 25%) significantly reduced the risk of rebleeding from EV. Since then, more than 800 articles have been published regarding the use of propranolol or nadolol in cirrhosis, and in fact NSBBs have become one of the most effective preventative therapies, against VH, in patients with cirrhosis, both for primary and secondary prophylaxis (combined with EVL).[2,23,49] A meta-analysis of 19 RCTs comparing NSBBs with EVL showed that EVL was associated with lower rates of VH, but without differences in mortality.[50] The beneficial effect of EVL on bleeding was not confirmed in subgroup analyses limited to 7 RCTs with adequate randomization or full paper articles.[50] Therefore, it has been recommended by the American and the European Guidelines that either NSBBs or EVL are reasonable considerations for the prevention of first VH in patients with medium or large EV and the choice of treatment should be based on local expertise, patient preference, and patient characteristics.[2,23] However, NSBBs may be more preferable because, unlike EVL, which has only a local effect on EV obliteration, they also exert other potential beneficial effects by decreasing the PP, including decreasing the incidence of hepatic decompensation and death.[2,23,51,52]

NSBBs are relatively safe, inexpensive, and easy to use, although careful monitoring of heart rate and BP together with dose titration is required to achieve the best hemodynamic outcomes (**Table 2**). It should be noted that only 30% to 40% of the patients under long-term therapy with NSBBs have a good hemodynamic response (a decrease of the HVPG to <12 mm Hg or ≥10%–20% of the pretreatment value), which is a robust indicator of protection from VH and liver decompensation.[4,51] In a

Table 2
NSBBs for PHT: characteristics, dosing and therapy goal

	Propranolol	Nadolol	Carvedilol
Characteristics	β-1 and β-2 adrenergic receptor antagonist (NSBB)	β-1 and β-2 adrenergic receptor antagonist (long-acting NSBB)	β-1 and β-2 adrenergic receptor antagonist, with intrinsic anti-α1 adrenergic activity
Mechanisms	Decreases portal flow through a decrease in cardiac output (β-1 blockade) and splanchnic vasoconstriction by unopposed α1 activity (β-2 blockade)	Decreases portal flow through a decrease in cardiac output (β-1 blockade) and splanchnic vasoconstriction by unopposed α1 activity (β-2 blockade)	Decreases portal flow (as NSBB), but also acts as a vasodilator of intrahepatic circulation (α1 blockade)
Recommended dose	20–40 mg BID Adjust every 2–3 d until treatment goal is achieved Maximal dose: 320 mg/d in patients without ascites; 160 mg/d in patients with ascites	20–40 mg OD Adjust every 2–3 d until treatment goal is achieved Maximal dose: 160 mg/d in patients without ascites; 80 mg/d in patients with ascites	Start with 6.25 mg OD After 3 d increase to 6.25 mg BID Maximal dose: 12.5 mg/d (except in patients with persistent arterial HT)
Therapy goal	Resting HR 55–60 bpm SBP should not decrease <90 mm Hg	Resting HR 55–60 bpm SBP should not decrease <90 mm Hg	SBP should not decrease <90 mm Hg

Abbreviations: BID, 2 times per day; HR, heart rate; HT, hypertension; OD, once daily.
Adapted from Garcia-Tsao G, Abraldes JG, Berzigotti A, et al. Portal hypertensive bleeding in cirrhosis: Risk stratification, diagnosis, and management: 2016 practice guidance by the American Association for the study of liver diseases. Hepatology (Baltimore, Md) 2017;65(1):310-335; with permission.

prospective study of 83 patients with compensated cirrhosis and large EV treated with nadolol, an HVPG decrease of 10% or more significantly deceased the risk of hepatic decompensation (eg, ascites and HRS) as compared with those without HVPG response.[51] Recently, this beneficial effect has been confirmed in a large RCT (PREDESCI study) of 201 patients with compensated cirrhosis and clinically significant PHT treated with either NSBBs (propranolol or carvedilol as guided by the HVPG response) or placebo. In this study, HVPG responders had a significant decrease in the incidence of first clinical decompensation as compared with the placebo group (hazard ratio, 0.51; 95% confidence interval, 0.26–0.97; $P = .0412$).[52] Of note, patients with subclinical PHT have a lesser degree of a hyperdynamic circulation and thus a significantly lesser degree of PP decrease is noted after acute β-blockade, than in those with clinically significant PHT, suggesting that NSBBs are more suitable to prevent decompensation of cirrhosis in patients with clinically significant PHT.[53]

There are a few limitations to the use of NSBBs in cirrhosis; approximately 15% of patients may have absolute or relative contraindications to therapy (eg, refractory asthma, respiratory failure, advanced atrioventricular block, and severe arterial hypotension), and another 15% require dose reduction or discontinuation attributed to common side effects (eg, fatigue, weakness, and shortness of breath).[2] In addition, there have been concerns regarding the use of NSBBs in patients with refractory ascites because these patients are characterized by both splanchnic and systemic vasodilatation, low systemic BP, and decreased renal perfusion, and NSBBs can cause hypotension and impair cardiac output, which may precipitate HRS and mortality.[49] Since the first study, which raised the possible deleterious effects of NSBBs on survival in patients with advanced cirrhosis,[54] several relevant studies have been published and yielded somewhat conflicting results. In a meta-analysis of 3 RCTs and 8 observational studies (n = 3145), NSBB use was not associated with increased all-cause mortality in patients with ascites or in those with refractory ascites.[55] Taken together, refractory ascites and SBP are not absolute contraindications for treatment with NSBBs; however, in these patients, high doses of NSBBs (>160 mg/d of propranolol or >80 mg/d of nadolol) should be avoided.[2] In patients with refractory ascites and severe circulatory dysfunction (BP of <90 mm Hg, serum sodium of <130 mEq/L, or HRS), the dose of NSBBs should be decreased or the drug temporarily held and NSBBs may be reintroduced if circulatory dysfunction improves.[2]

Carvedilol is an NSBB with mild intrinsic anti-α1-adrenergic activity (one-tenth of its β-blocker activity) and has the capability of enhancing the release of NO, which in turn causes vasodilation.[7] It was developed for the treatment of arterial hypertension and heart failure. By blocking the α1-adrenergic receptor, carvedilol decreases the hepatic vascular tone and hepatic resistance, resulting in a further decrease in PP, but can also enhance arterial hypotension and aggravate sodium retention.[7] It is advised that carvedilol be started at low doses and titrated up slowly, particularly in patients older than 65 years of age and those with advanced liver disease because of decreased hepatic metabolism of the drug. Thus, the drug should be taken with food to slow the speed of absorption and decrease the likelihood of side effects.[7,56] There have been several studies evaluating the effects of carvedilol on HVPG.[57] Two meta-analyses demonstrated that carvedilol was associated with a significantly greater decrease in HVPG than those induced by propranolol or nadolol (mean difference of 7%–9% of reduction in the HVPG), and there were no major differences in side effects apart from slightly greater decrease in the arterial BP by carvedilol.[57,58] In addition, carvedilol achieves a good hemodynamic response in more than 50% of nonresponders to standard NSBBs.[1,56] Further, the sequential use of propranolol followed by carvedilol in nonresponders to propranolol achieved a good hemodynamic response in more than 70% of cases.[52,56] In terms of clinical outcomes, carvedilol was as effective as EVL for the primary prevention of VH[59,60] and was as effective as EVL or nadolol plus isosorbide-5-mononitrate (ISMN) for the secondary prevention of VH, although there have only been a limited number of patients evaluated where it was used for secondary prophylaxis.[61,62] In summary, carvedilol may be an alternative to NSBB for the prevention of VH (particularly as primary prophylaxis) and is the first choice for patients who did not respond to propranolol, are not hypotensive, and are without refractory ascites.

Vasodilators (eg, nitrates and α-adrenergic antagonists)

Several vasodilators may decrease hepatic vascular resistance and may potentiate the hemodynamic effects of NSBBs in reducing PP. The effect of ISMN, an exogenous NO donor, is typically used to prevent or relieve angina chest pain in patients with ischemic heart disease by dilating blood vessels to facilitate blood flow to the coronary artery. In patients with cirrhosis, ISMN has shown to decrease PP without decreasing hepatic blood flow (at low doses 10–20 mg).[1,63,64] However, in meta-analysis of 10 RCTs on primary and 17 RCTs on the secondary prevention of VH, the combination of NSBBs and ISMN was not significantly better than NSBBs alone regarding overall bleeding or mortality rates, and had a higher rate of side effects (eg, headache and lightheadedness).[65] Notably, a small prospective study reported that the addition of ISMN can improve hemodynamic response in about one-third of patients who did not respond to propranolol (á la carte treatment) with a corresponding decrease in VH.[66]

Prazosin, an α-adrenergic antagonist, decreased the HVPG while increasing hepatic blood flow and, thus, may enhance the hemodynamic effects of NSBBs even more than ISMN.[67,68] However, the clinical outcome of the combination of NSBBs and prazosin for VH has not been evaluated in a well-performed RCT, partly because more recent attention has been toward carvedilol (the hemodynamic effects of carvedilol are theoretically similar to those of the combination of NSBBs and prazosin). It should be emphasized that vasodilators decrease intrahepatic vascular resistance, but also cause systemic vasodilatation, which decreases the arterial BP and potentially activates endogenous vasoactive systems (may worsen ascites); therefore, these drugs should not be used as monotherapy for PHT.

Renin–angiotensin–aldosterone inhibitors

Renin–angiotensin–aldosterone inhibitors, for example, ARBs, angiotensin-converting enzyme inhibitors and aldosterone antagonists may have some role in the management of PHT because angiotensin II is associated with dynamic and static increases in intrahepatic resistance attributable to the contraction of smooth muscle cells, the contraction and proliferation of hepatic stellate cells, and the deposition of fibrous tissue.[69–71] In addition, these drugs also alleviate an increase in portal venous inflow via sodium and water retention through the renin–angiotensin–aldosterone system.[71] Although a well-performed clinical study is lacking, several hemodynamic studies (with relatively small sample sizes) performed to evaluate the effects of ARBs on HVPG yielded conflicting results.[71–73] A meta-analysis in 2010 (19 RCT; 9 ARBs, 3 angiotensin-converting enzyme inhibitors, 7 aldosterone antagonists) demonstrated that ARBs/angiotensin-converting enzyme inhibitors decreased the HVPG in patients with Child-Pugh class A cirrhosis and without adverse events.[71] However, in a more recent meta-analysis of 11 RCT evaluating only ARBs (n = 394), there was no overall significant decrease in the HVPG as compared with controls and, further, there was an increased risk of symptomatic hypotension.[73] The addition of candesartan to propranolol conferred no benefit relative to propranolol monotherapy.[72]

Statins

Statins are a heterogeneous group of molecules that inhibit the activity of hydroxymethylglutarylcoenzyme A reductase, a key enzyme in the synthesis of cholesterol, and which have been used extensively for the management of dyslipidemia to reduce cardiovascular morbidity and mortality.[74] Besides their lipid-lowering properties, statins also exhibit multiple pleiotropic effects, such as antioxidative, antiproliferative and antiinflammatory properties, as well as their capability to improve endothelial dysfunction and stimulate neoangiogenesis.[74–76] These pleiotropic effects may be beneficial for some chronic conditions, including chronic liver disease and PHT. The dynamic component of increased intrahepatic resistance is an imbalance in the vascular tone-regulating pathways (eg, Ras homolog gene family member A/Rho-kinase and NO) and with a shift toward vasoconstriction. In experimental models, statins have improved endothelial function and lowered intrahepatic resistance through inhibition of hepatic Ras homolog gene family member A/Rho-kinase signaling and activation of endothelial NO synthase pathway.[77–79] Thus, statins can prevent further microvascular dysfunction, as well as the splanchnic vasodilatation and hepatic inflammation induced by lipopolysaccharides (endotoxemia).[80] Apart from the dynamic component, statins may also decrease the structural component of increased intrahepatic resistance through their antifibrotic properties by modulating Rho-kinase activity and Kruppel-like factor 2 expression.[74,77]

There have been 3 RCTs that evaluated the effects of statins on HVPG in a small number of patients with cirrhosis and PHT (most were Child-Pugh class A).[81–83] Statin therapy was associated with a decrease in HVPG, whereas no significant changes were observed in patients treated with placebo. Notably, in 32% and 60% of patients treated with simvastatin and in 91% of patients treated with atorvastatin in the 3 studies, a clinically significant decrease in the HVPG (>20%) was observed.[74,81–83] Further, 4 retrospective cohort studies that included a large number of patients with cirrhosis from various etiologies have reported that statins significantly decreased the risk of hepatic decompensation and death.[84–87] In a meta-analysis of 13 studies (3 RCTs and 10 cohort studies), statin use in patients with cirrhosis was associated with a 46% lower risk of hepatic decompensation, a 27% lower risk of variceal bleeding or progression of PHT, and a 46% lower mortality.[5] In a large RCT of 158 patients with cirrhosis and PHT, the addition of simvastatin (40 mg/d) to standard therapy (EVL + NSBB) alone did not decrease the rebleeding rate at 2 years of follow-up (25% vs 28%; P = .583, respectively), but was associated with a decrease in overall mortality (9% vs 22%; P = .030, respectively), which mainly was liver related.[88] It should be noted that the survival benefit was only seen among patients with Child-Pugh class A or B cirrhosis (not class C) and survival was not the primary end point of the study.[88] Taken together, statins have a beneficial effect on the evolution of cirrhosis by decreasing PP (which may be also by decreasing systemic and hepatic inflammation), decreasing the risk of decompensation and possibly improving survival.[74]

Statins are generally well-tolerated and significant side effects, mainly muscular toxicity and hepatotoxicity, are rare. The spectrum of statin-associated muscle toxicity include several manifestations and range from myalgia (8%–20% of cases) to the most severe and less frequent form, rhabdomyolysis (<1 cases per 1,000,000 patient-years).[74,89] The risk of muscle adverse events caused by statins seems to be related to statin systemic exposure, so the risk of statin-related muscle toxicity is increased in patients treated with higher doses of statins.[74] Although mild, transient elevation of liver enzymes are not uncommon, significant hepatotoxicity (alanine aminotransferase of >5× the upper limit of normal) related to statins is very rare (<2 cases per 1,000,000 patient-years) and likely idiosyncratic in nature.[74,90,91] Because statins undergo first-pass hepatic metabolism, generally through the cytochrome P450 system, patients with chronic liver disease are at risk of decreased hepatic clearance and may possibly be at greater risk for complications from statin therapy.[92] Based on available retrospective cohort studies and RCTs in patients with cirrhosis (Child-Pugh class A to C, but the number of patients with Child-Pugh class C was low), statins seem to be well-tolerated and similar to the control group and no treatment-related serious adverse events have been reported,[74,92] except in the largest RCT performed to date, where rhabdomyolysis developed in 3% of patients receiving simvastatin 40 mg/d (all had advanced cirrhosis).[88]

Despite the data on the possible benefit of statins in decreasing PP and adverse outcomes of decompensation and death, their use exclusively in patients with cirrhosis to prevent these events has not been advocated by guidelines, and rightly so, for reasons of needing a large randomized trial to confirm the benefits.[74] Yet, if patients with cirrhosis have a nonhepatic indication for the use of a statin, it should be readily used and data from large cohorts suggest that they are underused for a variety of reasons, including safety concerns.[91,93]

Anticoagulants (eg, warfarin and direct-acting anticoagulants)
Patients with cirrhosis have an increased risk of venous thrombotic events, mainly portal vein thrombosis (PVT), whereas bleeding seems to be related to the severity of PHT rather than to a hemostatic imbalance.[94] PVT occurs in approximately 20% of patients with cirrhosis, and particularly in those with advanced cirrhosis, and is associated with poor outcomes.[95] In a meta-analysis of 8 studies (n = 353), patients with cirrhosis and PVT who receive anticoagulant therapy have increased recanalization and decreased progression of thrombosis, compared with patients who do not receive anticoagulants, with no excess risk of major and minor bleedings and a lesser incidence of VH.[95] Therefore, anticoagulants are often the first-line therapy for patients with cirrhosis and PVT (recanalization rates of ≤40%–90%) if there are no contraindications.[94,95] Although PVT should be avoided, studies on the prevention of PVT in cirrhosis by anticoagulants are lacking, mainly owing to concerns that anticoagulants may tip the unsteady hemostatic balance of patients with advanced cirrhosis toward bleeding.[94]

In an RCT evaluating enoxaparin (4000 IU/d, subcutaneously) versus no treatment in preventing PVT in patients with advanced cirrhosis (n = 70), a 12-month course of enoxaparin was relatively safe and effective in preventing PVT in patients with cirrhosis (incidence of PVT: 0% vs 16.6%; P = .025, respectively).[6] Moreover, enoxaparin delayed the occurrence of hepatic decompensation (38.2% vs 83%; $P<.0001$, respectively) and improved survival (23.5% vs 26.1%; P = .02, respectively) as compared with no treatment.[6] The mechanisms of the beneficial effects of low-molecular weight heparin on liver disease progression, which seem to be more than just the mere prevention of PVT, is unclear, although it is possible that anticoagulation also improves intrahepatic microcirculation (decreasing intrahepatic resistance and PP) and intestinal microcirculation (decreasing bacterial translocation and the risk of bacterial infections).[2,6,94]

Direct-acting anticoagulants (DOACs; eg, rivaroxaban and apixaban) have significant pharmacologic advantages over vitamin K antagonists (eg, warfarin), which include a rapid onset of action, rapid resolution of the anticoagulation effect on discontinuation, fewer drug–drug interactions, predictable pharmacokinetics, and also, importantly, eliminating the requirement for regular monitoring of prothrombin time.[96] Although DOACs are metabolized by the liver to varying degrees, and their pharmacokinetics are potentially altered in patients with advanced liver disease, the overall incidence of hepatotoxicity attributed to these agents has been considered to be low (<4%).[96,97] Although the large trials that led to the approval of DOACs excluded patients with cirrhosis, based on limited studies and pharmacokinetics, DOACs seem to be as safe and efficacious as traditional anticoagulants in patients with compensated cirrhosis; however, more studies are needed in patients with decompensated cirrhosis to determine the optimal drug and dose in this patient population.[97] Notably, the recent guideline from the European Heart Rhythm Association for the use of DOACs in patients with atrial fibrillation indicates that DOACs are contraindicated in Child-Pugh class C cirrhosis and suggests that apixaban, dabigatran, and edoxaban may be used cautiously in patients with Child-Pugh class B cirrhosis.[98]

Currently, there are at least 2 ongoing RCTs evaluating the effects of prophylactic anticoagulation in patients with cirrhosis (without PVT): Childbenox (NCT02271295: from France) evaluating enoxaparin 4000 IU/d subcutaneously versus no treatment and Cirroxaban (NCT02643212: from Spain) evaluating rivaroxaban 10 mg/d versus placebo. The primary outcomes of both RCTs are survival and liver disease progression at 24 months, whereas the development of PVT is the secondary outcome.

Table 3
Selected potentially novel pharmacologic therapeutics in PHT

Agents	Main Effects	Data from Animal and Human Studies
Agents that reduce intrahepatic resistance by increasing NO availability		
Obeticholic acid (FXR agonist)[102,103]	Increases availability of NO through actions on AMDA-mediated regulation of eNOS activity; Reduces inflammation and oxidative stress in the liver; Antifibrotic effects	Obeticholic acid is associated with a trend toward drop in HVPG in patients with cirrhosis
Sapropterin (BH4 analog)[104]	Increases availability of NO (BH4 is an essential cofactor for the synthesis of NO by eNOS)	Sapropterin did not reduce PP and endothelial dysfunction in patients with cirrhosis
PDE-5 inhibitors for example, sildenafil,[105] udenafil[106]	Potentiates the vasodilatory effects of cGMP by preventing its degradation by PDE-5; Enhances the vasodilatory effects of NO	Sildenafil reduced MAP without reducing PP in patients with cirrhosis; Udenafil reduces PP approximately 20% in patients with cirrhosis
Serelaxin (recombinant human relaxin-2)[107]	Vasoprotective effects in the renal and systemic circulation via RXFP1; Enhances the vasodilatory effects of NO; Possible antifibrotic effects	Serelaxin reduced PP and increases RBF in patients with cirrhosis
Flavonoids in dark chocolate[108]	Increases NO availability and possibly reduces liver injury via antioxidative effects	Dark chocolate attenuated the postprandial increase in HVPG in patients with cirrhosis
Ascorbic acid[109]	Increases NO availability via antioxidative effects	Ascorbic acid (3 g IV) improved endothelial dysfunction and attenuated the postprandial increase in HVPG in patients with cirrhosis
SOD modulators for example, SOD analogs,[110] recombinant human SOD,[111] and gene transfer[112]	Enhances NO availability by enhancing the activity of SOD (an important antioxidant enzymes); Possible antifibrotic effects	Tempol (SOD analog) increased intrasinusoidal NO and reduced PP in cirrhotic rats; Recombinant human manganese SOD reduced PP (without changing MAP) and liver fibrogenesis in cirrhotic rats; SOD gene transfer improved endothelial dysfunction and reduced PP in cirrhotic rats

Agent	Mechanism	Evidence
Resveratrol (polyphenol flavonoid)[113]	Increases NO availability by upregulation of eNOS and antioxidative effects	Resveratrol improved endothelial dysfunction, reduced PP and activation of HSCs in cirrhotic rats
Agents that reduce intrahepatic resistance by modulating vasoactive substances		
TXA2/PGE-receptor antagonists for example, terutroban,[114] MS-PPOH[115]	Improves vasoconstriction and endothelial dysfunction through inhibition of TXA2/PGE pathway. Possible antifibrotic effects	Terutroban reduced PP in cirrhotic rats. MS-PPOH reduced PP (without increasing MAP) and increased urine sodium excretion in cirrhotic rats. RCT of ifetroban (NCT01436500) is ongoing
Montelukast (leukotriene inhibitor)[116]	Improves vasoconstriction and endothelial dysfunction through inhibition of TXA2/PGE pathway	Montelukast reduced PP in cirrhotic rats
ET antagonists for example, bosentan (nonselective),[117] tezaosentan (nonselective),[118,119] ambrisentan (ET$_A$ antagonist)[117] and macitentan (ET$_{A>B}$ antagonist)	Enhances vasodilatation by blocking ET receptors on endothelial and HSCs. Possible antifibrotic effects. Possible antiangiogenic effects	Bosentan (but not ambrisentan) reduced PP in cirrhotic rats. Bosentan and ambrisentan reduced neovascularization and PS collaterals in cirrhotic rats. Tezaosentan did not reduce PP in patients with cirrhosis. RCTs of ambrisentan (EudraCT 2011–001139–22) and macitentan (NCT01136692) are ongoing
Palosuran (urotensin II receptor antagonist)[120,121]	Enhances vasodilatation by blocking urotensin (a vasoconstrictor that is upregulated in cirrhosis)	Palosuran reduced PP and increased RBF, urine sodium and water excretion in cirrhotic rats
Droxidopa (synthetic precursor of norepinephrine)[122]	Vasoprotective effects on the hemodynamic and renal alterations	Droxidopa reduced portal blood flow (without changing in PP), increased MAP and diuresis in rats with PHT
Antiangiogenic agents		
TKIs for example, sorafenib,[123–125] sunitinib,[126] brivanib[127]	Antiangiogenesis (with or without antitumor) effects through the suppression of the Raf/MEK/ERK signaling pathway and blockade of signaling from the receptors of VEGF, PDGF, and SCGF	Sorafenib decreased PP and portal blood flow in patients with cirrhosis. Sorafenib potentiated the effects of propranolol on the reduction of PP, PS shunting, and neovascularization in cirrhotic rats. Sunitinib and brivanib decreased PP, fibrotic markers, and neovascularization in cirrhotic rats

(continued on next page)

Table 3
(continued)

Agents	Main Effects	Data from Animal and Human Studies
Agents that target gut microflora and bacterial translocation		
Antibiotics for example, rifaximin,[128-130] norfloxacin	Reduces bacterial translocation and endotoxemia (endotoxins exacerbate hyperdynamic circulation, promote intrahepatic release of ET and COX)	Intestinal decontamination with rifaximin reduced HVPG and endotoxin levels in patients with alcoholic cirrhosis Long-term rifaximin reduced mortality and PHT-related complications (eg, VH, HE, SBP, HRS) in patients with cirrhosis RCT of norfloxacin (vs VSL#3) is ongoing (NCT01134692)
Probiotics for example, VSL#3,[131,132] Bifidobacterium spp.	Improves intestinal dysbiosis; which reduces circulatory dysfunction, proinflammatory markers and endotoxemia	VSL#3 reduced HVPG, improved the hepatic and systemic hemodynamics and serum sodium levels in patients with cirrhosis VSL#3 improved liver functions and decreased HE and hospitalization in patients with cirrhosis
Agents that modulate metabolic hormones		
Metformin[133]	Reduces HSC activation, hepatic inflammation, superoxide and NO scavenging Possible antifibrotic effects	Metformin decreased intrahepatic resistance, PP, and fibrosis in cirrhotic rats
Liraglutide (GLP-1 analog)[134]	Reduced HSC activation and cell proliferation Antifibrotic effects	Liraglutide reduced intrahepatic resistance, PP and fibrosis in cirrhotic rats
Fenofibrate (PPAR-α agonist)[135]	Increases NO availability by upregulation of eNOS Improved vasodilatory response to ACh Possible antifibrotic effects	Fenofibrate reduced PP approximately 30% and fibrosis in cirrhotic rats
Leptin inhibitors[136]	Increases NO availability via antioxidative effects	Leptin receptor antibody reduced PP (without changing MAP) in cirrhotic rats
Antiapoptotic agents		
Emricasan (pan-caspase inhibitor)[137,138]	Reduces apoptosis and hepatic inflammation Improves intrahepatic vasoconstriction and splanchnic vasodilation Possible antifibrotic effects	Emricasan reduced PP in patients with cirrhosis and severe PHT

Dietary approaches		
Taurine (amino-sulfonic acid)[139]	Reduces oxidative endoplasmic reticulum stress and inhibits HSCs	Taurine 6 g/d reduced HVPG approximately 12% in patients with cirrhosis
Caffeine[140]	Various vasoactive effects through different mechanisms Antifibrotic effects Possible antiangiogenic effects	Caffeine decreased PP, hyperdynamic circulation, neovascularization and fibrosis in cirrhotic rats
Curcumin[141]	Induces splanchnic vasoconstriction through inhibition of eNOS activation Antiangiogenic effects via VEGF pathway	Curcumin decreased PP, hyperdynamic circulation and neovascularization in cirrhotic rats

Abbreviations: ACh, acetylcholine; AMDA, asymmetric-dimethylarginine; BH4, tetrahydrobiopterin; cGMP, cyclic guanosine monophosphate; COX, cyclooxygenase; eNOS, endothelial NO synthase; ET, endothelin; FXR, farnesoid X receptor; GLP-1, glucagon-like peptide-1; HE, hepatic encephalopathy; HSC, hepatic stellate cells; MAP, mean arterial BP; MS-PPOH, N-(methylsulfonyl)-2-(2-propynyloxy)-benzenehexanamide; PDE-5, phosphodiesterase; PDGF, platelet-derived growth factor receptor; PPAR-α, peroxisome proliferator-activated receptor α; PS, portosystemic; RBF, renal blood flow; RXFP1, relaxin family peptide receptor-1; SBP, spontaneous bacterial peritonitis; SCGF, stem cell growth factor; SOD, superoxide dismutase; TKI, tyrosine kinase inhibitors; TXA2/PGE, thromboxane-A2/prostaglandin-endoperoxide; VEGF, vascular endothelial growth factor.

POTENTIAL NOVEL PHARMACOLOGIC AGENTS FOR PORTAL HYPERTENSION

Recent advances in the pharmacologic treatment of PHT have been mainly focused on the pathway of increased intrahepatic resistance. The first proposed approach is by modulating the hepatic vascular tone and improving endothelial dysfunction, mostly by treatments targeting at increasing the availability of NO in the intrahepatic circulation (eg, statins, obeticholic acid, tetrahydrobiopterin, antioxidants, and serelaxin) and/or antagonizing increased endogenous vasoconstrictors (eg, terutroban, endothelin antagonists, and ARBs).[99–101] Other strategies, to decrease intrahepatic resistance, have included targeting fibrogenesis (eg, simtuzumab, obeticholic acid, and specific treatment of the etiology of the liver disease), microvascular occlusion (eg, anticoagulants), and neoangiogenesis (eg, antiangiogenic agents).[9,99,100] In addition, there is a miscellaneous group of drugs that may decrease PP through distinct mechanisms, such as emricasan, fibrates, rifaximin, probiotics, or taurine (**Table 3**).[99,100] There is an interplay between structural and hemodynamic components that leads to PHT and thus it is important to consider evaluating therapies that target several potential pathways. Drugs that improve endothelial function may also suppress fibrogenesis, and angiogenesis, thus serving to decrease fibrogenesis while improving vascular tone.

SUMMARY

PHT is a common complication of advanced liver disease. Pharmacologic management to reduce PP has played an important role in the prevention and treatment of most complications of cirrhosis, especially VH; however, the impact on survival has been limited with the current therapeutic options. Recent advances have mainly focused on modifying the existent increased intrahepatic resistance through NO and/or modulating vasoactive substances and inflammatory and neurohormonal stimuli outside the liver. These approaches, in combination with etiology-specific therapy, are likely to lead to increasing benefit on survival and quality of life while awaiting liver transplantation, the ultimate rescue strategy.

REFERENCES

1. Berzigotti A, Bosch J. Pharmacologic management of portal hypertension. Clin Liver Dis 2014;18(2):303–17.
2. Garcia-Tsao G, Abraldes JG, Berzigotti A, et al. Portal hypertensive bleeding in cirrhosis: risk stratification, diagnosis, and management: 2016 practice guidance by the American Association for the study of liver diseases. Hepatology 2017;65(1):310–35.
3. Baiges A, Hernandez-Gea V, Bosch J. Pharmacologic prevention of variceal bleeding and rebleeding. Hepatol Int 2018;12(Suppl 1):68–80.
4. Bosch J, Garcia-Pagan JC. Prevention of variceal rebleeding. Lancet 2003; 361(9361):952–4.
5. Kim RG, Loomba R, Prokop LJ, et al. Statin use and risk of cirrhosis and related complications in patients with chronic liver diseases: a systematic review and meta-analysis. Clin Gastroenterol Hepatol 2017;15(10):1521–30.e8.
6. Villa E, Camma C, Marietta M, et al. Enoxaparin prevents portal vein thrombosis and liver decompensation in patients with advanced cirrhosis. Gastroenterology 2012;143(5):1253–60.e4.
7. Bosch J. Carvedilol for portal hypertension in patients with cirrhosis. Hepatology 2010;51(6):2214–8.

8. Iwakiri Y, Groszmann RJ. Vascular endothelial dysfunction in cirrhosis. J Hepatol 2007;46(5):927–34.

9. Garbuzenko DV, Arefyev NO, Kazachkov EL. Antiangiogenic therapy for portal hypertension in liver cirrhosis: current progress and perspectives. World J Gastroenterol 2018;24(33):3738–48.

10. Ripoll C, Groszmann R, Garcia-Tsao G, et al. Hepatic venous pressure gradient predicts clinical decompensation in patients with compensated cirrhosis. Gastroenterology 2007;133(2):481–8.

11. Groszmann RJ, Garcia-Tsao G, Bosch J, et al. Beta-blockers to prevent gastroesophageal varices in patients with cirrhosis. N Engl J Med 2005;353(21):2254–61.

12. D'Amico G, Garcia-Pagan JC, Luca A, et al. Hepatic vein pressure gradient reduction and prevention of variceal bleeding in cirrhosis: a systematic review. Gastroenterology 2006;131(5):1611–24.

13. Harris AG. Somatostatin and somatostatin analogues: pharmacokinetics and pharmacodynamic effects. Gut 1994;35(3 Suppl):S1–4.

14. Reynaert H, Geerts A. Pharmacological rationale for the use of somatostatin and analogues in portal hypertension. Aliment Pharmacol Ther 2003;18(4):375–86.

15. Abraldes JG, Bosch J. Somatostatin and analogues in portal hypertension. Hepatology 2002;35(6):1305–12.

16. Bosch J, Kravetz D, Rodes J. Effects of somatostatin on hepatic and systemic hemodynamics in patients with cirrhosis of the liver: comparison with vasopressin. Gastroenterology 1981;80(3):518–25.

17. Villanueva C, Ortiz J, Minana J, et al. Somatostatin treatment and risk stratification by continuous portal pressure monitoring during acute variceal bleeding. Gastroenterology 2001;121(1):110–7.

18. Cirera I, Feu F, Luca A, et al. Effects of bolus injections and continuous infusions of somatostatin and placebo in patients with cirrhosis: a double-blind hemodynamic investigation. Hepatology 1995;22(1):106–11.

19. Moitinho E, Planas R, Banares R, et al. Multicenter randomized controlled trial comparing different schedules of somatostatin in the treatment of acute variceal bleeding. J Hepatol 2001;35(6):712–8.

20. Albillos A, Rossi I, Iborra J, et al. Octreotide prevents postprandial splanchnic hyperemia in patients with portal hypertension. J Hepatol 1994;21(1):88–94.

21. Vorobioff JD, Gamen M, Kravetz D, et al. Effects of long-term propranolol and octreotide on postprandial hemodynamics in cirrhosis: a randomized, controlled trial. Gastroenterology 2002;122(4):916–22.

22. Vorobioff JD, Ferretti SE, Zangroniz P, et al. Octreotide enhances portal pressure reduction induced by propranolol in cirrhosis: a randomized, controlled trial. Am J Gastroenterol 2007;102(10):2206–13.

23. European Association for the Study of the Liver. Electronic address: easloffice@easloffice.eu, European Association for the Study of the Liver. EASL clinical practice guidelines for the management of patients with decompensated cirrhosis. J Hepatol 2018;69(2):406–60.

24. Gotzsche PC, Hrobjartsson A. Somatostatin analogues for acute bleeding oesophageal varices. Cochrane Database Syst Rev 2008;(3):CD000193.

25. Banares R, Albillos A, Rincon D, et al. Endoscopic treatment versus endoscopic plus pharmacologic treatment for acute variceal bleeding: a meta-analysis. Hepatology 2002;35(3):609–15.

26. Corley DA, Cello JP, Adkisson W, et al. Octreotide for acute esophageal variceal bleeding: a meta-analysis. Gastroenterology 2001;120(4):946–54.

27. Moller S, Hansen EF, Becker U, et al. Central and systemic haemodynamic effects of terlipressin in portal hypertensive patients. Liver 2000;20(1):51–9.

28. Narahara Y, Kanazawa H, Taki Y, et al. Effects of terlipressin on systemic, hepatic and renal hemodynamics in patients with cirrhosis. J Gastroenterol Hepatol 2009;24(11):1791–7.

29. Baik SK, Jeong PH, Ji SW, et al. Acute hemodynamic effects of octreotide and terlipressin in patients with cirrhosis: a randomized comparison. Am J Gastroenterol 2005;100(3):631–5.

30. Villanueva C, Planella M, Aracil C, et al. Hemodynamic effects of terlipressin and high somatostatin dose during acute variceal bleeding in nonresponders to the usual somatostatin dose. Am J Gastroenterol 2005;100(3):624–30.

31. Zhou X, Tripathi D, Song T, et al. Terlipressin for the treatment of acute variceal bleeding: a systematic review and meta-analysis of randomized controlled trials. Medicine 2018;97(48):e13437.

32. Wells M, Chande N, Adams P, et al. Meta-analysis: vasoactive medications for the management of acute variceal bleeds. Aliment Pharmacol Ther 2012; 35(11):1267–78.

33. Ioannou GN, Doust J, Rockey DC. Systematic review: terlipressin in acute oesophageal variceal haemorrhage. Aliment Pharmacol Ther 2003;17(1):53–64.

34. Soderlund C, Magnusson I, Torngren S, et al. Terlipressin (triglycyl-lysine vasopressin) controls acute bleeding oesophageal varices. A double-blind, randomized, placebo-controlled trial. Scand J Gastroenterol 1990;25(6):622–30.

35. Cavallin M, Fasolato S, Marenco S, et al. The treatment of hepatorenal syndrome. Dig Dis 2015;33(4):548–54.

36. Cavallin M, Piano S, Romano A, et al. Terlipressin given by continuous intravenous infusion versus intravenous boluses in the treatment of hepatorenal syndrome: a randomized controlled study. Hepatology 2016;63(3):983–92.

37. Allegretti AS, Israelsen M, Krag A, et al. Terlipressin versus placebo or no intervention for people with cirrhosis and hepatorenal syndrome. Cochrane Database Syst Rev 2017;(6):CD005162.

38. Facciorusso A, Chandar AK, Murad MH, et al. Comparative efficacy of pharmacological strategies for management of type 1 hepatorenal syndrome: a systematic review and network meta-analysis. Lancet Gastroenterol Hepatol 2017;2(2): 94–102.

39. Boyer TD, Sanyal AJ, Wong F, et al. Terlipressin plus albumin is more effective than albumin alone in improving renal function in patients with cirrhosis and hepatorenal syndrome type 1. Gastroenterology 2016;150(7):1579–89.e2.

40. Moreau R, Lebrec D. The use of vasoconstrictors in patients with cirrhosis: type 1 HRS and beyond. Hepatology 2006;43(3):385–94.

41. Israelsen M, Krag A, Allegretti AS, et al. Terlipressin versus other vasoactive drugs for hepatorenal syndrome. Cochrane Database Syst Rev 2017;(9):CD011532.

42. Nassar Junior AP, Farias AQ, LA DA, et al. Terlipressin versus norepinephrine in the treatment of hepatorenal syndrome: a systematic review and meta-analysis. PLoS One 2014;9(9):e107466.

43. Cavallin M, Kamath PS, Merli M, et al. Terlipressin plus albumin versus midodrine and octreotide plus albumin in the treatment of hepatorenal syndrome: a randomized trial. Hepatology 2015;62(2):567–74.

44. Reiberger T, Ferlitsch A, Payer BA, et al. Non-selective betablocker therapy decreases intestinal permeability and serum levels of LBP and IL-6 in patients with cirrhosis. J Hepatol 2013;58(5):911–21.

45. Thiele M, Albillos A, Abazi R, et al. Non-selective beta-blockers may reduce risk of hepatocellular carcinoma: a meta-analysis of randomized trials. Liver Int 2015;35(8):2009–16.
46. Madsen BS, Havelund T, Krag A. Targeting the gut-liver axis in cirrhosis: antibiotics and non-selective beta-blockers. Adv Ther 2013;30(7):659–70.
47. Lebrec D, Nouel O, Corbic M, et al. Propranolol–a medical treatment for portal hypertension? Lancet 1980;2(8187):180–2.
48. Lebrec D, Poynard T, Hillon P, et al. Propranolol for prevention of recurrent gastrointestinal bleeding in patients with cirrhosis: a controlled study. N Engl J Med 1981;305(23):1371–4.
49. Wong F, Salerno F. Beta-blockers in cirrhosis: friend and foe? Hepatology 2010; 52(3):811–3.
50. Gluud LL, Krag A. Banding ligation versus beta-blockers for primary prevention in oesophageal varices in adults. Cochrane Database Syst Rev 2012;(8):CD004544.
51. Hernandez-Gea V, Aracil C, Colomo A, et al. Development of ascites in compensated cirrhosis with severe portal hypertension treated with beta-blockers. Am J Gastroenterol 2012;107(3):418–27.
52. Villanueva C, Albillos A, Genescà J, et al. β blockers to prevent decompensation of cirrhosis in patients with clinically significant portal hypertension (PREDESCI): a randomised, double-blind, placebo-controlled, multicentre trial. Lancet 2019; 393(10181):1597–608.
53. Villanueva C, Albillos A, Genesca J, et al. Development of hyperdynamic circulation and response to beta-blockers in compensated cirrhosis with portal hypertension. Hepatology 2016;63(1):197–206.
54. Serste T, Melot C, Francoz C, et al. Deleterious effects of beta-blockers on survival in patients with cirrhosis and refractory ascites. Hepatology 2010;52(3): 1017–22.
55. Chirapongsathorn S, Valentin N, Alahdab F, et al. Nonselective beta-blockers and survival in patients with cirrhosis and ascites: a systematic review and meta-analysis. Clin Gastroenterol Hepatol 2016;14(8):1096–104.e9.
56. Banares R, Moitinho E, Piqueras B, et al. Carvedilol, a new nonselective beta-blocker with intrinsic anti- Alpha1-adrenergic activity, has a greater portal hypotensive effect than propranolol in patients with cirrhosis. Hepatology 1999;30(1): 79–83.
57. Sinagra E, Perricone G, D'Amico M, et al. Systematic review with meta-analysis: the haemodynamic effects of carvedilol compared with propranolol for portal hypertension in cirrhosis. Aliment Pharmacol Ther 2014;39(6):557–68.
58. Li T, Ke W, Sun P, et al. Carvedilol for portal hypertension in cirrhosis: systematic review with meta-analysis. BMJ Open 2016;6(5):e010902.
59. Shah HA, Azam Z, Rauf J, et al. Carvedilol vs. esophageal variceal band ligation in the primary prophylaxis of variceal hemorrhage: a multicentre randomized controlled trial. J Hepatol 2014;60(4):757–64.
60. Tripathi D, Ferguson JW, Kochar N, et al. Randomized controlled trial of carvedilol versus variceal band ligation for the prevention of the first variceal bleed. Hepatology 2009;50(3):825–33.
61. Lo GH, Chen WC, Wang HM, et al. Randomized, controlled trial of carvedilol versus nadolol plus isosorbide mononitrate for the prevention of variceal rebleeding. J Gastroenterol Hepatol 2012;27(11):1681–7.
62. Stanley AJ, Dickson S, Hayes PC, et al. Multicentre randomised controlled study comparing carvedilol with variceal band ligation in the prevention of variceal rebleeding. J Hepatol 2014;61(5):1014–9.

63. Garcia-Pagan JC, Feu F, Navasa M, et al. Long-term haemodynamic effects of isosorbide 5-mononitrate in patients with cirrhosis and portal hypertension. J Hepatol 1990;11(2):189–95.
64. Navasa M, Chesta J, Bosch J, et al. Reduction of portal pressure by isosorbide-5-mononitrate in patients with cirrhosis. Effects on splanchnic and systemic hemodynamics and liver function. Gastroenterology 1989;96(4):1110–8.
65. Gluud LL, Langholz E, Krag A. Meta-analysis: isosorbide-mononitrate alone or with either beta-blockers or endoscopic therapy for the management of oesophageal varices. Aliment Pharmacol Ther 2010;32(7):859–71.
66. Bureau C, Peron JM, Alric L, et al. "A La Carte" treatment of portal hypertension: adapting medical therapy to hemodynamic response for the prevention of bleeding. Hepatology 2002;36(6):1361–6.
67. Albillos A, Lledo JL, Rossi I, et al. Continuous prazosin administration in cirrhotic patients: effects on portal hemodynamics and on liver and renal function. Gastroenterology 1995;109(4):1257–65.
68. Albillos A, Lledo JL, Banares R, et al. Hemodynamic effects of alpha-adrenergic blockade with prazosin in cirrhotic patients with portal hypertension. Hepatology 1994;20(3):611–7.
69. Bataller R, Gines P, Nicolas JM, et al. Angiotensin II induces contraction and proliferation of human hepatic stellate cells. Gastroenterology 2000;118(6): 1149–56.
70. Casey S, Herath C, Rajapaksha I, et al. Effects of angiotensin-(1-7) and angiotensin II on vascular tone in human cirrhotic splanchnic vessels. Peptides 2018; 108:25–33.
71. Tandon P, Abraldes JG, Berzigotti A, et al. Renin-angiotensin-aldosterone inhibitors in the reduction of portal pressure: a systematic review and meta-analysis. J Hepatol 2010;53(2):273–82.
72. Kim JH, Kim JM, Cho YZ, et al. Effects of candesartan and propranolol combination therapy versus propranolol monotherapy in reducing portal hypertension. Clin Mol Hepatol 2014;20(4):376–83.
73. Yao H, Zhang C. Angiotensin II receptor blockers for the treatment of portal hypertension in patients with liver cirrhosis: a systematic review and meta-analysis of randomized controlled trials. Ir J Med Sci 2018;187(4):925–34.
74. Pose E, Trebicka J, Mookerjee RP, et al. Statins: old drugs as new therapy for liver diseases? J Hepatol 2019;70(1):194–202.
75. Janicko M, Drazilova S, Pella D, et al. Pleiotropic effects of statins in the diseases of the liver. World J Gastroenterol 2016;22(27):6201–13.
76. Liao JK, Laufs U. Pleiotropic effects of statins. Annu Rev Pharmacol Toxicol 2005;45:89–118.
77. Marrone G, Maeso-Diaz R, Garcia-Cardena G, et al. KLF2 exerts antifibrotic and vasoprotective effects in cirrhotic rat livers: behind the molecular mechanisms of statins. Gut 2015;64(9):1434–43.
78. Trebicka J, Hennenberg M, Laleman W, et al. Atorvastatin lowers portal pressure in cirrhotic rats by inhibition of RhoA/Rho-kinase and activation of endothelial nitric oxide synthase. Hepatology 2007;46(1):242–53.
79. Abraldes JG, Rodriguez-Vilarrupla A, Graupera M, et al. Simvastatin treatment improves liver sinusoidal endothelial dysfunction in CCl4 cirrhotic rats. J Hepatol 2007;46(6):1040–6.
80. Tripathi DM, Vilaseca M, Lafoz E, et al. Simvastatin prevents progression of acute on chronic liver failure in rats with cirrhosis and portal hypertension. Gastroenterology 2018;155(5):1564–77.

81. Pollo-Flores P, Soldan M, Santos UC, et al. Three months of simvastatin therapy vs. placebo for severe portal hypertension in cirrhosis: a randomized controlled trial. Dig Liver Dis 2015;47(11):957–63.

82. Zafra C, Abraldes JG, Turnes J, et al. Simvastatin enhances hepatic nitric oxide production and decreases the hepatic vascular tone in patients with cirrhosis. Gastroenterology 2004;126(3):749–55.

83. Bishnu S, Ahammed SM, Sarkar A, et al. Effects of atorvastatin on portal hemodynamics and clinical outcomes in patients with cirrhosis with portal hypertension: a proof-of-concept study. Eur J Gastroenterol Hepatol 2018;30(1):54–9.

84. Bang UC, Benfield T, Bendtsen F. Reduced risk of decompensation and death associated with use of statins in patients with alcoholic cirrhosis. A nationwide case-cohort study. Aliment Pharmacol Ther 2017;46(7):673–80.

85. Chang FM, Wang YP, Lang HC, et al. Statins decrease the risk of decompensation in hepatitis B virus- and hepatitis C virus-related cirrhosis: a population-based study. Hepatology 2017;66(3):896–907.

86. Kumar S, Grace ND, Qamar AA. Statin use in patients with cirrhosis: a retrospective cohort study. Dig Dis Sci 2014;59(8):1958–65.

87. Mohanty A, Tate JP, Garcia-Tsao G. Statins are associated with a decreased risk of decompensation and death in veterans with hepatitis C-related compensated cirrhosis. Gastroenterology 2016;150(2):430–40.e1.

88. Abraldes JG, Villanueva C, Aracil C, et al. Addition of simvastatin to standard therapy for the prevention of variceal rebleeding does not reduce rebleeding but increases survival in patients with cirrhosis. Gastroenterology 2016;150(5): 1160–70.e3.

89. Selva-O'Callaghan A, Alvarado-Cardenas M, Pinal-Fernandez I, et al. Statin-induced myalgia and myositis: an update on pathogenesis and clinical recommendations. Expert Rev Clin Immunol 2018;14(3):215–24.

90. Bjornsson E, Jacobsen EI, Kalaitzakis E. Hepatotoxicity associated with statins: reports of idiosyncratic liver injury post-marketing. J Hepatol 2012;56(2):374–80.

91. Jose J. Statins and its hepatic effects: newer data, implications, and changing recommendations. J Pharm Bioallied Sci 2016;8(1):23–8.

92. Souk K, Al-Badri M, Azar ST. The safety and benefit of statins in liver cirrhosis: a review. Exp Clin Endocrinol Diabetes 2015;123(10):577–80.

93. Rzouq FS, Volk ML, Hatoum HH, et al. Hepatotoxicity fears contribute to under-utilization of statin medications by primary care physicians. Am J Med Sci 2010; 340(2):89–93.

94. Leonardi F, Maria N, Villa E. Anticoagulation in cirrhosis: a new paradigm? Clin Mol Hepatol 2017;23(1):13–21.

95. Loffredo L, Pastori D, Farcomeni A, et al. Effects of anticoagulants in patients with cirrhosis and portal vein thrombosis: a systematic review and meta-analysis. Gastroenterology 2017;153(2):480–7.e1.

96. Bunchorntavakul C, Reddy KR. Drug hepatotoxicity: newer agents. Clin Liver Dis 2017;21(1):115–34.

97. Weinberg EM, Palecki J, Reddy KR. Direct-acting oral anticoagulants in cirrhosis and cirrhosis-associated portal vein thrombosis. Semin Liver Dis 2019;39(2):195–208.

98. Steffel J, Verhamme P, Potpara TS, et al. The 2018 European Heart Rhythm Association Practical Guide on the use of non-vitamin K antagonist oral anticoagulants in patients with atrial fibrillation. Eur Heart J 2018;39(16):1330–93.

99. Nair H, Berzigotti A, Bosch J. Emerging therapies for portal hypertension in cirrhosis. Expert Opin Emerg Drugs 2016;21(2):167–81.

100. Vilaseca M, Guixe-Muntet S, Fernandez-Iglesias A, et al. Advances in therapeutic options for portal hypertension. Therap Adv Gastroenterol 2018;11. 1756284818811294.

101. Gracia-Sancho J, Lavina B, Rodriguez-Vilarrupla A, et al. Increased oxidative stress in cirrhotic rat livers: a potential mechanism contributing to reduced nitric oxide bioavailability. Hepatology 2008;47(4):1248–56.

102. Verbeke L, Mannaerts I, Schierwagen R, et al. FXR agonist obeticholic acid reduces hepatic inflammation and fibrosis in a rat model of toxic cirrhosis. Sci Rep 2016;6:33453.

103. Mookerjee R, Rosselli M, Pieri G, et al. Effect of the FXR Agonist Obeticholic acid on portal pressure in alcoholic cirrhosis: a proof of concept Phase 2a study. J Hepatol 2014;60(S1):S7–8.

104. Reverter E, Mesonero F, Seijo S, et al. Effects of sapropterin on portal and systemic hemodynamics in patients with cirrhosis and portal hypertension: a bicentric double-blind placebo-controlled study. Am J Gastroenterol 2015;110(7):985–92.

105. Tandon P, Inayat I, Tal M, et al. Sildenafil has no effect on portal pressure but lowers arterial pressure in patients with compensated cirrhosis. Clin Gastroenterol Hepatol 2010;8(6):546–9.

106. Kreisel W, Deibert P, Kupcinskas L, et al. The phosphodiesterase-5-inhibitor udenafil lowers portal pressure in compensated preascitic liver cirrhosis. A dose-finding phase-II-study. Dig Liver Dis 2015;47(2):144–50.

107. Snowdon VK, Lachlan NJ, Hoy AM, et al. Serelaxin as a potential treatment for renal dysfunction in cirrhosis: preclinical evaluation and results of a randomized phase 2 trial 2017;14(2):e1002248.

108. De Gottardi A, Berzigotti A, Seijo S, et al. Postprandial effects of dark chocolate on portal hypertension in patients with cirrhosis: results of a phase 2, double-blind, randomized controlled trial. Am J Clin Nutr 2012;96(3):584–90.

109. Hernandez-Guerra M, Garcia-Pagan JC, Turnes J, et al. Ascorbic acid improves the intrahepatic endothelial dysfunction of patients with cirrhosis and portal hypertension. Hepatology 2006;43(3):485–91.

110. Garcia-Caldero H, Rodriguez-Vilarrupla A, Gracia-Sancho J, et al. Tempol administration, a superoxide dismutase mimetic, reduces hepatic vascular resistance and portal pressure in cirrhotic rats. J Hepatol 2011;54(4):660–5.

111. Guillaume M, Rodriguez-Vilarrupla A, Gracia-Sancho J, et al. Recombinant human manganese superoxide dismutase reduces liver fibrosis and portal pressure in CCl4-cirrhotic rats. J Hepatol 2013;58(2):240–6.

112. Lavina B, Gracia-Sancho J, Rodriguez-Vilarrupla A, et al. Superoxide dismutase gene transfer reduces portal pressure in CCl4 cirrhotic rats with portal hypertension. Gut 2009;58(1):118–25.

113. Di Pascoli M, Divi M, Rodriguez-Vilarrupla A, et al. Resveratrol improves intrahepatic endothelial dysfunction and reduces hepatic fibrosis and portal pressure in cirrhotic rats. J Hepatol 2013;58(5):904–10.

114. Rosado E, Rodriguez-Vilarrupla A, Gracia-Sancho J, et al. Terutroban, a TP-receptor antagonist, reduces portal pressure in cirrhotic rats. Hepatology 2013;58(4):1424–35.

115. Di Pascoli M, Zampieri F, Verardo A, et al. Inhibition of epoxyeicosatrienoic acid production in rats with cirrhosis has beneficial effects on portal hypertension by reducing splanchnic vasodilation. Hepatology 2016;64(3):923–30.

116. Steib CJ, Bilzer M, op den Winkel M, et al. Treatment with the leukotriene inhibitor montelukast for 10 days attenuates portal hypertension in rat liver cirrhosis. Hepatology 2010;51(6):2086–96.
117. Hsu SJ, Lin TY, Wang SS, et al. Endothelin receptor blockers reduce shunting and angiogenesis in cirrhotic rats. Eur J Clin Invest 2016;46(6):572–80.
118. Lebrec D, Bosch J, Jalan R, et al. Hemodynamics and pharmacokinetics of tezosentan, a dual endothelin receptor antagonist, in patients with cirrhosis. Eur J Clin Pharmacol 2012;68(5):533–41.
119. Tripathi D, Therapondos G, Ferguson JW, et al. Endothelin-1 contributes to maintenance of systemic but not portal haemodynamics in patients with early cirrhosis: a randomised controlled trial. Gut 2006;55(9):1290–5.
120. Heller J, Schepke M, Neef M, et al. Increased urotensin II plasma levels in patients with cirrhosis and portal hypertension. J Hepatol 2002;37(6):767–72.
121. Trebicka J, Leifeld L, Hennenberg M, et al. Hemodynamic effects of urotensin II and its specific receptor antagonist palosuran in cirrhotic rats. Hepatology 2008; 47(4):1264–76.
122. Coll M, Rodriguez S, Raurell I, et al. Droxidopa, an oral norepinephrine precursor, improves hemodynamic and renal alterations of portal hypertensive rats. Hepatology 2012;56(5):1849–60.
123. Coriat R, Gouya H, Mir O, et al. Reversible decrease of portal venous flow in cirrhotic patients: a positive side effect of sorafenib. PLoS One 2011;6(2): e16978.
124. Pinter M, Sieghart W, Reiberger T, et al. The effects of sorafenib on the portal hypertensive syndrome in patients with liver cirrhosis and hepatocellular carcinoma–a pilot study. Aliment Pharmacol Ther 2012;35(1):83–91.
125. D'Amico M, Mejias M, Garcia-Pras E, et al. Effects of the combined administration of propranolol plus sorafenib on portal hypertension in cirrhotic rats. Am J Physiol Gastrointest Liver Physiol 2012;302(10):G1191–8.
126. Tugues S, Fernandez-Varo G, Munoz-Luque J, et al. Antiangiogenic treatment with sunitinib ameliorates inflammatory infiltrate, fibrosis, and portal pressure in cirrhotic rats. Hepatology 2007;46(6):1919–26.
127. Lin HC, Huang YT, Yang YY, et al. Beneficial effects of dual vascular endothelial growth factor receptor/fibroblast growth factor receptor inhibitor brivanib alaninate in cirrhotic portal hypertensive rats. J Gastroenterol Hepatol 2014;29(5): 1073–82.
128. Kang SH, Lee YB, Lee JH. Rifaximin treatment is associated with reduced risk of cirrhotic complications and prolonged overall survival in patients experiencing hepatic encephalopathy. Aliment Pharmacol Ther 2017;46(9):845–55.
129. Vlachogiannakos J, Saveriadis AS, Viazis N, et al. Intestinal decontamination improves liver haemodynamics in patients with alcohol-related decompensated cirrhosis. Aliment Pharmacol Ther 2009;29(9):992–9.
130. Vlachogiannakos J, Viazis N, Vasianopoulou P, et al. Long-term administration of rifaximin improves the prognosis of patients with decompensated alcoholic cirrhosis. J Gastroenterol Hepatol 2013;28(3):450–5.
131. Dhiman RK, Rana B, Agrawal S, et al. Probiotic VSL#3 reduces liver disease severity and hospitalization in patients with cirrhosis: a randomized, controlled trial. Gastroenterology 2014;147(6):1327–37.e3.
132. Rincon D, Vaquero J, Hernando A, et al. Oral probiotic VSL#3 attenuates the circulatory disturbances of patients with cirrhosis and ascites. Liver Int 2014; 34(10):1504–12.

133. Tripathi DM, Erice E, Lafoz E, et al. Metformin reduces hepatic resistance and portal pressure in cirrhotic rats. Am J Physiol Gastrointest Liver Physiol 2015; 309(5):G301–9.

134. de Mesquita FC, Guixe-Muntet S, Fernandez-Iglesias A, et al. Liraglutide improves liver microvascular dysfunction in cirrhosis: evidence from translational studies. Sci Rep 2017;7(1):3255.

135. Rodriguez-Vilarrupla A, Lavina B, Garcia-Caldero H, et al. PPARalpha activation improves endothelial dysfunction and reduces fibrosis and portal pressure in cirrhotic rats. J Hepatol 2012;56(5):1033–9.

136. Delgado MG, Gracia-Sancho J, Marrone G, et al. Leptin receptor blockade reduces intrahepatic vascular resistance and portal pressure in an experimental model of rat liver cirrhosis. Am J Physiol Gastrointest Liver Physiol 2013; 305(7):G496–502.

137. Garcia-Tsao G, Fuchs M, Shiffman M, et al. Emricasan (IDN-6556) lowers portal pressure in patients with compensated cirrhosis and severe portal hypertension. Hepatology 2019;69(2):717–28.

138. Barreyro FJ, Holod S, Finocchietto PV, et al. The pan-caspase inhibitor Emricasan (IDN-6556) decreases liver injury and fibrosis in a murine model of non-alcoholic steatohepatitis. Liver Int 2015;35(3):953–66.

139. Schwarzer R, Kivaranovic D, Mandorfer M. Randomised clinical study: the effects of oral taurine 6g/day vs placebo on portal hypertension. Aliment Pharmacol Ther 2018;47(1):86–94.

140. Hsu SJ, Lee FY, Wang SS, et al. Caffeine ameliorates hemodynamic derangements and portosystemic collaterals in cirrhotic rats. Hepatology 2015;61(5): 1672–84.

141. Hsu SJ, Lee JY, Lin TY, et al. The beneficial effects of curcumin in cirrhotic rats with portal hypertension. Biosci Rep 2017;37(6) [pii:BSR20171015].

Role of Transjugular Intrahepatic Portosystemic Shunt in the Management of Portal Hypertension

Review and Update of the Literature

Matthew L. Hung, MD[a], Edward Wolfgang Lee, MD, PhD[a,b],*

KEYWORDS

- Transjugular intrahepatic portosystemic shunt • TIPS • Esophageal varices • Ascites
- Portal hypertension

KEY POINTS

- Transjugular intrahepatic portosystemic shunt (TIPS) is effective as a salvage therapy in acute variceal hemorrhage and prevents rebleeding more effectively compared with endoscopic and medical therapy.
- Early placement of TIPS within 3 days of esophageal variceal bleeding in high-risk patients with cirrhosis leads to improved survival depending on patient selection.
- The contemporary use of covered stents in TIPS may improve survival compared with repeated large-volume paracentesis in the setting of refractory ascites, although prospective data are limited.
- TIPS may also be beneficial in cases of hepatic hydrothorax, hepatorenal syndrome, and Budd-Chiari syndrome, although comparative studies are limited.

INTRODUCTION

Portal hypertension is one of the main complications of cirrhosis and is characterized by an increase in splanchnic blood flow and the formation of portosystemic collaterals.

Disclosure Statement: The authors have nothing to disclose.
[a] Division of Interventional Radiology, Department of Radiology, UCLA Medical Center, David Geffen School of Medicine at UCLA, Ronald Reagan Medical Center at UCLA, 757 Westwood Plaza, Suite 2125, Los Angeles, CA 90095, USA; [b] Department of Surgery, Division of Liver and Pancreas Transplant Surgery, Ronald Reagan Medical Center at UCLA, 757 Westwood Plaza, Los Angeles, CA 90095, USA
* Corresponding author. Division of Interventional Radiology, Department of Radiology, UCLA Medical Center, David Geffen School of Medicine at UCLA, Ronald Reagan Medical Center at UCLA, 757 Westwood Plaza, Suite 2125, Los Angeles, CA 90095.
E-mail address: edwardlee@mednet.ucla.edu

Clinically significant portal hypertension is diagnosed when the hepatic venous pressure gradient (HVPG) exceeds 10 mm Hg.[1,2] Sequelae of portal hypertension include variceal hemorrhage, ascites, hepatic encephalopathy, hepatic hydrothorax, and hepatorenal syndrome. The development of any of these complications marks the transition from compensated to decompensated cirrhosis and portends a worse prognosis.[3]

Although medical therapy may be sufficient when portal hypertension is clinically indolent, interventional procedures play an important role when complications of portal hypertension become refractory or severe. A transjugular intrahepatic portosystemic shunt (TIPS) is a stent placed percutaneously using image guidance that diverts blood from the portal vein to the hepatic vein, effectively reducing the pressure within the portal circulation. Although TIPS was initially used as salvage therapy in acute variceal hemorrhage,[4] multiple clinical studies have since demonstrated the efficacy and safety of TIPS in other settings, particularly for secondary prevention of variceal bleeding and refractory ascites. The purpose of this article is to review the indications for TIPS as well as the supporting evidence. The authors also discuss contraindications to the procedure, adequate patient selection, classic technique for TIPS placement, and TIPS-related complications.

INDICATIONS
Primary Prophylaxis of Variceal Bleeding

Half of the patients with cirrhosis are found to have varices at the time of diagnosis,[5] and 25% to 40% of these patients experience a hemorrhagic episode.[6] Higher portal pressures (particularly greater than 12 mm Hg) are strongly associated with the development and bleeding of varices.[7] Early trials of prophylactic surgical shunt placement for esophageal varices demonstrated high rates of encephalopathy and mortality in patients randomized to surgery.[8] Therefore, TIPS has not been tested for primary prophylaxis of esophageal or gastric variceal bleeding, and it is not recommended in this setting.

Salvage Therapy for Acute Esophageal Variceal Hemorrhage

Current guidelines recommend medical resuscitation, correction of thrombocytopenia and coagulopathy, early vasoactive drug administration, endoscopic therapy, and prophylactic antibiotics for patients presenting with acute variceal bleeding.[9] However, 10% to 20% of patients fail to achieve hemostasis with this first-line therapy.[10] For these patients, TIPS can be used as an effective rescue therapy.[11–13] In this setting, TIPS controls variceal hemorrhage in 90% of patients,[11] but 15% of patients experience recurrent bleeding at 1 month.[14] Mortality remains high even after successful TIPS placement, as a recent case series by Mainmone and colleagues[15] reports 6-week and 12-month mortality rates of 36% and 42%, respectively.

Early Transjugular Intrahepatic Portosystemic Shunt After Esophageal Variceal Hemorrhage

Patients who recover from the first episode of variceal hemorrhage can have up to a 60% risk of rebleeding in the first year.[9] The concept of early TIPS, usually defined as TIPS performed within 72 hours of presentation with variceal bleeding, was first introduced by Monescillo and colleagues.[16] In this randomized controlled trial (RCT), patients with high-risk bleeding esophageal varices (HVPG >20 mm Hg measured within 24 hours after admission) who received standard medical therapy experienced more treatment failures (50% vs 12%) and higher 1-year mortality (65% vs 31%) compared with patients who underwent early TIPS. A more contemporaneous trial[17] randomized 63 high-risk patients (Child-Pugh Class C10–13 or Child-Pugh Class B with active bleeding on endoscopy) to receive early TIPS with polytetrafluoroethylene (PTFE)-covered stents or ongoing vasoactive drug therapy followed by beta-blockers and long-term endoscopic band ligation (EBL). Rebleeding or failure to control bleeding occurred in 45% of patients in the pharmacotherapy-EBL group compared with 3% of patients in the early-TIPS group. The 1-year actuarial survival was 61% in the pharmacotherapy-EBL group versus 86% in the early-TIPS group. Interestingly, rates of hepatic encephalopathy were similar between the 2 groups. The same investigators corroborated their findings in a posttrial surveillance study.[18]

Similar findings were reported in different patient populations. A prospective study by Rudler and colleagues[19] of 31 patients who underwent early TIPS reported a 97% 1-year probability of being free of rebleeding compared with 51% in historical control patients. However, TIPS did not significantly influence 1-year survival in this study. Njei and colleagues[20] conducted a retrospective analysis using the United States Nationwide Inpatient Sample database and found that compared with no TIPS, early TIPS was associated with decreased inpatient mortality (risk ratio [RR] = 0.87; 95% confidence interval [CI], 0.84 to 0.90) and rebleeding (RR = 0.56; 95% CI, 0.45–0.71). In their multivariate regression, early TIPS did not increase rates of hepatic encephalopathy, similar to the findings reported by Garcia-Pagan and colleagues.[17]

Results from the largest prospective study of early TIPS were recently reported by Hernández-Gea and colleagues.[21] In this cohort of 671 patients (high-risk as defined by García-Pagán and colleagues[17]) from 34 centers, early TIPS reduced the 1-year probability of treatment failure and rebleeding compared with standard drug and endoscopy therapy (92% vs 74%; $P = .017$) as well as the development of de novo or worsening of previous ascites without affecting rates of hepatic encephalopathy. One-year mortality was also lower in Child-Pugh C patients who received early TIPS compared with patients who received drug and endoscopy therapy (22% vs 47%). Mortality rates did not differ in Child-Pugh B patients who exhibited active bleeding at endoscopy.

Despite these promising findings, adherence to early TIPS is low. In a recent study by Thabut and colleagues,[22] only 6.8% of patients with variceal bleeding eligible for early TIPS actually underwent the procedure. In 45% of cases, there was no local availability of TIPS. An additional 34% of potential early TIPS candidates did not get shunt placement because the physician did not believe in the beneficial effects of early TIPS.

Secondary Prophylaxis of Esophageal Variceal Bleeding

Multiple clinical trials have also examined the utility of TIPS in preventing recurrent variceal hemorrhage outside the time window of early TIPS.[23–36] The results of early meta-analyses[37] comparing TIPS with endoscopic therapy reported a 3-fold decreased incidence in both variceal rebleeding and deaths due to rebleeding and an increased rate of posttreatment encephalopathy in patients who received TIPS. Overall survival was not influenced by therapeutic modality. However, many of the early trials used sclerotherapy in the endoscopy arm, which is inferior in terms of both safety and efficacy compared with endoscopic variceal ligation.[38] Furthermore, these early trials also used bare metal stents, which demonstrate higher rates of dysfunction,[39,40] variceal rebleeding, and mortality[41] compared with covered stents. Several RCTs in recent years have examined the efficacy of TIPS in the secondary prophylaxis of esophageal variceal bleeding with the use of covered stents (**Table 1**).

Holster and colleagues[36] performed a multicenter RCT comparing TIPS (using covered stents) with endoscopic variceal ligation (EVL) or glue injection plus

Table 1
Randomized controlled trials examining transjugular intrahepatic portosystemic shunt for variceal hemorrhage with the use of covered stents

Author, Year	Patients	Rebleeding Incidence (TIPS vs Endoscopy)	Mortality (TIPS vs Endoscopy)	HE Incidence (TIPS vs Endoscopy)
García-Pagán et al,[17] 2010	63	3% vs 50%[a,b]	14% vs 39%[a,b]	25% vs 39%[d]
Luo et al,[34] 2015	73	22.2% vs 57.1%[a,c]	27.1% vs 42.8%[c]	48% vs 44%[d]
Sauerbruch et al,[35] 2015	185	7% vs 26%[a,c]	30% vs 26%[d]	18% vs 8%[a,d]
Holster et al,[36] 2016	72	0% vs 29%[a,d]	32% vs 26%[d]	38% vs 23%[d]

Abbreviation: HE, hepatic encephalopathy.
[a] Significant difference was observed between groups.
[b] Assessed at 1 y.
[c] Assessed at 2 y.
[d] Cumulative for the study period.

beta-blockers. Patients who received TIPS experienced a lower rate of variceal rebleeding (0% vs 29%) and a higher rate of early hepatic encephalopathy (35% vs 14%) in a median follow-up of 23 months. There was no difference in mortality and the prevalence of hepatic encephalopathy was similar between the 2 groups beyond 1 year from the index bleed.

Another recent RCT by Sauerbruch and colleagues[35] compared covered TIPS with HVPG-guided therapy. Patients randomized to HVPG-guided therapy were started on propranolol and isosorbide-5-mononitrate and underwent variceal band ligation if 2 weeks of medical therapy did not decrease the HVPG by more than 20% from baseline measurement. TIPS demonstrated lower rebleeding rates (7% vs 26%) and a higher incidence of encephalopathy without differences in survival.

Luo and colleagues[34] compared covered TIPS with EVL plus propranolol in patients who presented with variceal hemorrhage as well as portal vein thrombosis. Although the patient cohort experienced higher rates of rebleeding compared with other trials, patients who received TIPS experienced a 22.2% 2-year probability of recurrent variceal bleeding compared with 57.1% of patients in the EVL group. Hepatic encephalopathy rates and mortality did not differ between the 2 groups.

Qi and colleagues[42] performed a meta-analysis of these 3 recent trials, again demonstrating a significantly lower risk of variceal rebleeding in patients who received covered TIPS compared with endoscopic and medical therapy. Overall survival and the risk of hepatic encephalopathy were similar between the 2 groups. Although this may suggest that the balance of risks and benefits is in favor of TIPS, more studies comparing covered TIPS with current optimal endoscopic and medical therapy are needed to clearly quantify the risk of hepatic encephalopathy. For now, current guidelines[9] suggest beta-blockers and EVL as first-line therapy in the prevention of rebleeding outside the window for early TIPS. TIPS is the recommended rescue therapy in patients who experience recurrent hemorrhage despite beta-blockers and EVL.

Gastric Varices

Gastric varices are found in 20% of patients with portal hypertension. Compared with esophageal varices, gastric varices are at lower risk of hemorrhage, but require significantly more blood transfusions once they do bleed.[43] The risk of bleeding is higher with fundal varices (type 1 isolated gastric varices [IGV1] and type 2 gastroesophageal

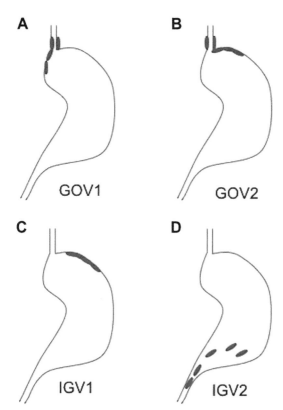

Fig. 1. Sarin classification of gastric varices. (*A*) GOV1 involve the esophagus and extend along the lesser curvature. (*B*) GOV2 involve the esophagus and extend toward the gastric fundus. (*C*) IGV1 are found in isolation in the fundus alone. (*D*) IGV2 are found in isolation in the gastric body, antrum, or prepyloric region.

varices [GOV2] according to Sarin classification;[43] **Fig. 1**), larger size, presence of red spots, and severe liver dysfunction.[44]

In the setting of acute hemorrhage, TIPS is effective in achieving hemostasis in 90% to 96% of cases refractory to vasoconstrictor and endoscopic therapy.[45,46] There are limited studies comparing TIPS with endoscopic interventions for gastric varices. In a retrospective cohort analysis by Procaccini and colleagues,[47] patients who underwent TIPS for acute gastric variceal hemorrhage had comparable rebleeding rates and mortality up to 1 year compared with patients who underwent endoscopic therapy with cyanoacrylate glue. However, the TIPS group had much higher long-term morbidity (41% vs 1.6%), defined as adverse events related to the procedural intervention that prolonged or caused a patient to be hospitalized. In another study comparing TIPS with cyanoacrylate for acute gastric variceal bleeding,[48] there was no difference in 30-day rebleeding rates, duration of hospitalization, or in-hospital mortality. However, follow-up was extremely limited. Current guidelines recommend TIPS as the treatment of choice for bleeding from cardiofundal varices (IGV1 or GOV2), as these are the gastric varices at highest risk for rebleeding.[9]

Only one randomized trial studied the efficacy of TIPS in the prevention of rebleeding following stabilization of the acute hemorrhage.[49] Patients who underwent TIPS insertion experienced lower rates of gastric variceal rebleeding (11% vs 38%) but higher rates of hepatic encephalopathy (25.7% vs 2.7%) compared with patients who received cyanoacrylate treatment. Other complications and survival were similar between the 2 groups.

Balloon retrograde transvenous obliteration of gastric varices (BRTO) is also a treatment option that has been compared with TIPS in several studies. In BRTO, portosystemic collaterals (usually gastrorenal shunts) are occluded by a balloon and a sclerosant agent is injected to obliterate the varices. In contrast to TIPS, BRTO increases the portal pressure and consequently aggravates complications related to portal hypertension. However, because the diversion of portal venous blood is avoided, the risk of encephalopathy is lower with BRTO.[50] Studies comparing BRTO with TIPS have had conflicting results. A retrospective review by Kim and colleagues[51] found that patients with isolated gastric varices who underwent BRTO had lower rates of hepatic encephalopathy (0% vs 22%) but similar rebleeding rates (8% vs 7%), de novo ascites (4% vs 4%), and mean survival (24 months vs 30 months) compared with patients who received TIPS. Sabri and colleagues[52] observed lower rates of rebleeding (0% vs 11%) and hepatic encephalopathy (0% vs 15%) in the BRTO group, but these differences were nonsignificant. In contrast, Gimm and colleagues[53] found in a retrospective analysis that BRTO provided better bleeding control, rebleeding-free survival, and overall survival after adjusting for confounding factors in multivariate regression. Further prospective, controlled studies are warranted.

Refractory Ascites

Up to 60% of the patients with cirrhosisdevelop ascites within 10 years of diagnosis.[54] Initial therapy consists of dietary sodium restriction and diuretics. However, 5% to 10% of cases become refractory to medical therapy. In such instances, large-volume paracentesis (LVP) and TIPS are therapeutic options.

To date, 7 RCTs have been published comparing the outcomes of TIPS versus LVP in the treatment of refractory ascites[55-61] (Table 2). TIPS clearly offers superior control of ascites; rates of complete resolution of ascites in 6 months to 1 year are 30% to 60% with TIPS and 0% to 16% with LVP. On the other hand, 4 out of the 7 trials

Table 2
Randomized controlled trials examining transjugular intrahepatic portosystemic shunt versus LVP for refractory ascites

Author, Year	Stent Used	Patients	Survival Rate (TIPS vs LVP)	Newly Developed or Severe HE at Follow-up (TIPS vs LVP)
Lebrec et al,[55] 1996	Bare	25	29% vs 56%[a,b]	45% vs 0%[a]
Rössle et al,[56] 2000	Bare	60	58% vs 32%[b]	23% vs 13%
Ginès et al,[57] 2002	Bare	70	26% vs 30%[b]	60% vs 34%[a]
Sanyal et al,[58] 2003	Bare	109	35% vs 33%[b]	38% vs 21%[a]
Salerno et al,[59] 2004	Bare	66	59% vs 29%[a,b]	61% vs 39%
Narahara et al,[60] 2011	Bare	60	64% vs 35%[a,b]	67% vs 17%[a]
Bureau et al,[61] 2017	Covered	62	93% vs 52%[a,c]	34% vs 33%

Abbreviation: HE, hepatic encephalopathy.
[a] Significant difference was observed between groups.
[b] Assessed at 2 y.
[c] Assessed at 1 y.

demonstrate a statistically significant increase in the incidence of hepatic encephalopathy with TIPS. The effect of TIPS on survival is less clear. The earliest trial by Lebrec and colleagues[55] observed a 2-year survival of 29% in the TIPS group and 60% in the LVP group. The remaining trials either found TIPS to significantly prolong survival or found a nonsignificant difference.

Multiple meta-analyses have been performed over the past several years,[62–65] but again, produce conflicting results. In order to address heterogeneity across studies and account for time to death (a flaw of earlier meta-analyses), Salerno and colleagues[64] conducted a meta-analysis by pooling individual patient data from 4 of the RCTs. Patients who were allocated to receive TIPS had improved 1- and 2-year liver transplant-free survival compared with patients who received LVP (63.1% and 49.0% vs 52.5% and 35.2%, respectively). In multivariate analysis, allocation to TIPS also was associated with improved mortality (HR = 0.61; 95% CI, 0.41–0.91). There were more cases of hepatic encephalopathy per patient for those assigned to TIPS compared with LVP (1.13 ± 1.93 vs 0.63 ± 1.18). Bai and colleagues[65] performed a meta-analysis examining all but the most recent RCT and also accounted for time to death by pooling hazard ratios. In this study, TIPS significantly improved liver transplant–free survival (HR = 0.61; 95% CI, 0.46–0.82) and decreased liver disease–related death (odds ratio [OR] = 0.62; 95% CI, 0.39–0.98), recurrent ascites (OR = 0.15; 95% CI, 0.09–0.24), and hepatorenal syndrome (OR = 0.32; 95% CI, 0.12–0.86).

It is worth noting that aside from the most recent RCT, trials studying the use of TIPS for refractory ascites have used bare metal stents. Recent evidence suggests that as is the case with variceal bleeding, the use of covered stents offers better patency and survival benefits compared with the use of bare metal stents for refractory ascites. Bercu and colleagues[66] studied 61 patients who underwent TIPS placement with a covered stent for refractory ascites and found overall survival of 78.7% at 1 year. Improved or complete resolution of ascites was observed in 90.2% of patients. Only 13% of patients required a TIPS revision. Parvinian and colleagues[67] conducted a retrospective study assessing outcomes in 80 patients with refractory ascites who underwent TIPS placement, 70 of whom received covered stents and 10 received bare metal stents. Although statistical comparisons were not made based on stent type, the investigators noted that 40% of patients with a bare metal stent required TIPS revision compared with 24% of patients who received a covered stent. Tan and colleagues[68] retrospectively analyzed long-term outcomes for patients who underwent TIPS for refractory ascites with a covered stent versus a bare metal stent. Covered stent recipients experienced shunt dysfunction less frequently (25% vs 74%), had a higher 1-year patency rate (79.9% vs 23.1%), and had higher 2-year survival (85.9% vs 69.5%) compared with patients who received bare metal stents.

Bureau and colleagues[61] conducted the only RCT to date that compared LVP (n = 33) with TIPS (n = 29) with covered stents in the treatment of refractory ascites. The 1-year liver transplant–free survival was significantly higher in the TIPS group compared with the LVP group (93% vs 52%, P = .003). Furthermore, patients in the LVP group had twice as many days of hospitalization as the TIPS group in follow-up (35 days vs 17 days). Interestingly, the 1-year incidence of encephalopathy was 35% in each group. Gaba and colleagues[69] retrospectively evaluated survival in 150 patients with refractory ascites who underwent TIPS with covered stents (n = 70) versus LVP (n = 80). After propensity score weighting, patients in the TIPS group demonstrated a trend toward enhanced survival compared with patients in the LVP group (median survival 1037 vs 262 days, P = .074). TIPS also conferred significantly improved survival at 1 year (66% vs 44%, P = .018).

Collectively, the current body of evidence suggests that even the use of bare metal stents in TIPS may improve survival compared with LVP. Covered stents are the contemporary standard of care, demonstrate improved mortality and patency rates compared with bare metal stents, and have thus far demonstrated promising results. More prospective studies and meta-analyses restricted to the use of covered stents are needed to show a definitive survival advantage of TIPS compared with LVP for the treatment of refractory ascites.

Refractory Hepatic Hydrothorax

Hepatic hydrothorax (HH) is defined as the accumulation of greater than 500 mL of transudative fluid in the pleural cavity of patients with cirrhosis.[70] It is postulated that this pleural fluid collects as a result of transdiaphragmatic migration of ascitic fluid, usually on the right side. HH is initially managed with the same strategy as ascites—salt restriction and diuretics. HH becomes refractory to medical therapy in approximately 25% of cases. Although no RCTs have been performed to study TIPS for this indication, several retrospective studies suggest that TIPS is beneficial for refractory HH.

Dhanasekaran and colleagues[71] reported the largest cohort, which included 73 patients who underwent TIPS for refractory HH. The 1-month and 6-month complete response rates, defined as absence of symptoms related to HH and no further requirement for thoracentesis, were 58.9% and 60%, respectively. Survival rates at 90 days, 1 year, 3 years, and 5 years were 72%, 48%, 26%, and 15%, respectively. The rate of hepatic encephalopathy in this cohort was 15.1%. Ditah and colleagues[72] recently reported the first meta-analysis for TIPS in the setting of refractory HH. A complete response was observed in 55.8% (95% CI: 44.7–66.9) of patients and a partial response, defined as improvement in symptoms with less frequent thoracentesis, was observed in an additional 17.6% (95% CI: 10.9–24.2). The incidence of hepatic encephalopathy and 45-day mortality were 11.7% and 17.7%, respectively. Both of these figures are comparable to those observed with TIPS for other indications, such as variceal bleeding and refractory ascites.

Hepatorenal Syndrome

Hepatorenal syndrome (HRS) is the development of renal dysfunction in a patient with cirrhosis in the absence of another cause. It is the result of splanchnic vasodilation and circulatory dysfunction, leading to renal vasoconstriction and upregulation of the renin-angiotensin-aldosterone system.[73] Type 1 HRS is a severe variant characterized by rapid decompensation, whereas type 2 HRS is insidious and causes a more gradual decline in renal function.

TIPS has been shown to improve the glomerular filtration rate and urinary sodium excretion while decreasing plasma renin and aldosterone levels.[74,75] In the largest prospective study reported by Brensing and colleagues,[76] 31 nontransplantable patients underwent TIPS for HRS (14 type 1, 17 type 2) and were compared with 10 nontransplantable patients with HRS who had advanced liver failure that precluded TIPS placement. The survival rates at 3 months were 81% in the TIPS group and 10% for patients who were ineligible for TIPS. Although this comparison is fraught with selection bias, the survival rates for patients with type 1 HRS who underwent TIPS were nonetheless encouraging. Whereas the median survival of untreated type 1 HRS is less than 2 weeks,[77] patients with type 1 HRS who underwent TIPS in this study had 3-, 6-, and 12-month survival rates of 64%, 50%, and 20%, respectively. Song and colleagues[78] recently performed a meta-analysis of 128 patients with HRS who were treated with TIPS. Pooled short-term and 1-year survival rates were 72% and 47%

in type 1 HRS and 86% and 64% in type 2 HRS. Renal function improved in 83% of the entire cohort. The rate of hepatic encephalopathy was high at 49%. Based on this limited evidence, there may be a potential survival benefit of TIPS in properly selected patients with HRS, but no studies to date have compared it to a suitable control. Therefore, TIPS is not routinely recommended for HRS.

Budd-Chiari Syndrome

Budd-Chiari syndrome (BCS) is characterized by hepatic venous outflow obstruction from thrombosis of the hepatic veins and/or hepatic portion of the inferior vena cava, which can lead to portal hypertension and its complications. Medical therapy, usually anticoagulation, is offered in all cases. However, Seijo and colleagues[79] demonstrated in a prospective study of 157 patients with BCS that 30% of patients who managed with medical therapy alone died in a median follow-up of 50 months. Therefore, if there are any signs of portal hypertension, decompressive therapies are offered. A step-wise management protocol is currently favored,[80] where hepatic vein interventions (eg, angioplasty ± stenting) are attempted before TIPS, unless there is diffuse hepatic vein obstruction or the patient has a high Rotterdam score, which is used to predict intervention-free survival.[79]

In a retrospective study of 124 patients with BCS who underwent TIPS, by Garcia-Pagán and colleagues,[81] 1- and 5-year liver transplant–free survival rates were 88% and 78%, respectively. Furthermore, in patients identified as high-risk by the Rotterdam score, 5-year liver transplant–free survival was much better than predicted (71% vs 42%). Qi and colleagues[82] retrospectively analyzed the outcomes of 51 patients with BCS in whom percutaneous recanalization was either ineffective or inappropriate. Patients were further classified as early TIPS (no prior recanalization or recanalization within 3 days before TIPS, n = 19) or converted TIPS (TIPS performed more than 3 days after recanalization, n = 32). Cumulative 1-, 2-, and 3-year survival rates were 83.8%, 81.2%, and 76.9%, respectively. Survival was similar between the early and converted TIPS groups.

There are no prospective trials comparing TIPS with other hepatic vein interventions due to the rarity of BCS. However, Tripathi and colleagues[83] performed a retrospective analysis that demonstrated that hepatic vein interventions resulted in similar patency and survival rates compared with TIPS but resulted in lower rates of procedural complications (9.5% vs 27.1%) and hepatic encephalopathy (0% vs 18%). These results support the current stepwise approach to treatment.

CONTRAINDICATIONS AND PATIENT SELECTION

Absolute and relative contraindications to TIPS are listed in **Table 3**.[84] The increased volume load shunted to the heart after TIPS results in increased central venous pressure, pulmonary capillary wedge pressure, and ultimately could exceed the preload reserve of the ventricles in the setting of preexisting cardiopulmonary dysfunction. Thus, congestive heart failure, severe pulmonary hypertension, and severe tricuspid regurgitation are absolute contraindications to TIPS. Relative contraindications include anatomic issues (eg, central masses or cysts, venous thrombosis) that may complicate the creation of the shunt and history of hepatic encephalopathy, which puts patients at risk for exacerbation of hepatic encephalopathy after TIPS.[85]

Several prognostic factors have been identified in retrospective analyses that may help the clinician weigh risks and benefits of TIPS for a given patient. Child-Pugh Class C status,[86] bilirubin level greater than 3.0 mg/dL, alanine aminotransferase level greater than 100 IU/L, and pre-TIPS encephalopathy[87] have all been shown to

Table 3
Contraindications to transjugular intrahepatic portosystemic shunt placement

Absolute	Relative
Congestive heart failure	Portal vein thrombosis
Severe tricuspid regurgitation	Severe coagulopathy
Severe pulmonary hypertension	Severe thrombocytopenia
Uncontrolled sepsis	Hepatic encephalopathy
Unrelieved biliary obstruction	Hepatic vein obstruction
Multiple hepatic cysts	Moderate pulmonary hypertension
Primary prophylaxis of variceal bleeding	Centrally located liver mass

independently predict mortality after TIPS. The model of end-stage liver disease (MELD) score is the most widely used score to predict post-TIPS mortality and has been shown to be superior to the Child-Pugh score.[88,89] Patients with a MELD score greater than 18 carry a significantly higher mortality 3 months after TIPS compared with patients with MELD scores of 18 or less.[90,91] Because prospective studies are limited, it is difficult to determine how much of the discrepancy in mortality is due to the TIPS procedure itself versus the generally poor prognosis of patients with high MELD scores.[92] Recent studies suggest that there could be a survival benefit of TIPS, even in patients with high MELD scores. Ascha and colleagues[93] retrospectively analyzed 144 patients with an MELD score greater than or equal to 15 who had TIPS placement and matched them by age and MELD score to 144 patients who did not undergo TIPS. Beyond 2 months post-TIPS, patients who received TIPS had a 56% lower risk of dying or needing liver transplantation ($P<.01$) than cirrhotic patients who did not undergo TIPS.

TECHNIQUE
Patient Assessment

Preprocedural assessment includes a complete history and physical and routine laboratory studies, including a complete blood count, coagulation panel, and metabolic panel to assess kidney and liver function. Severe anemia, thrombocytopenia, and coagulopathy should be corrected before TIPS. Cross-sectional imaging within 1 month before TIPS is ideal to evaluate for vascular patency, hepatic masses, or other anatomic findings that may complicate the procedure. If recent imaging is not available, an ultrasound with doppler evaluation should be performed to assess for portal vein patency. Patients with suspected or known cardiopulmonary disease should be evaluated with an echocardiogram to exclude underlying heart failure, tricuspid valve disease, or severe pulmonary hypertension. If TIPS is performed for refractory ascites, an LVP should be performed before the procedure.

Conventional Technique

TIPS can be performed under conscious sedation or under general anesthesia with endotracheal intubation. After the patient is positioned and draped in a sterile fashion, venous access is usually obtained via the right internal jugular vein. A catheter is then advanced from the site of venous access to a hepatic vein. Usually the right hepatic vein is chosen to allow for an anterior inferior transhepatic puncture of the right portal vein. After a hepatic vein has been selected, a wedged or balloon-occluded hepatic venogram is obtained using carbon dioxide in order to delineate the portal venous anatomy. A needle is then fluoroscopically guided from the hepatic vein to the portal vein. If the site of portal venous access is large enough and without severe angulation, a guidewire is introduced through the needle and passed into the portal venous system. Once transportal access is secured with the stiff guidewire, a catheter is passed over the wire and portal venography and pressure measurements are performed. The hepatic parenchymal track is subsequently dilated with an angioplasty balloon. The 10-French TIPS sheath can then be placed across this track in order to deploy and dilate the polytetrafluoroethylene-covered stent (Viatorr, W.L. Gore), which is the standard TIPS stent. The stent is initially dilated to 8 mm, and post-TIPS portal venography and pressure measurements are repeated. Further stent dilation can be performed to achieve the desired portosystemic pressure gradient, which should be less than 12 mm Hg in patients with a history of variceal bleeding.[94] The goal of portosystemic pressure gradient in patients with refractory ascites is less clear, with some investigators advocating for a threshold of 8 mm Hg.[58]

Patients with a history of variceal bleeding may benefit from concomitant variceal embolization at the time of TIPS placement. Qi and colleagues[95] recently performed a meta-analysis of 6 studies comparing outcomes of a total of 662 patients with variceal bleeding who underwent TIPS with or without variceal embolization. Adjunctive embolotherapy was associated with a lower rate of rebleeding (OR 2.02, $P = .002$) with similar incidence of shunt dysfunction, encephalopathy, and mortality when compared with TIPS alone.

Postprocedural Care

Patients are monitored for a minimum of 24 hours following TIPS placement. Laboratory studies, including hemoglobin, kidney, and liver function tests, are monitored regularly. A liver ultrasound with doppler should be obtained 2 to 3 weeks after TIPS placement to assess for shunt patency. Then, Doppler ultrasonography should be performed every 6 or 12 months. Elevated shunt velocities are associated with shunt dysfunction. Patients with suspected shunt dysfunction or those who develop significant encephalopathy are eligible for TIPS venography, at which time TIPS revision may be performed.

COMPLICATIONS

Potential adverse events that may happen during or after TIPS are listed in **Table 4**. Hepatic encephalopathy and shunt dysfunction are common complications that have been discussed at length in previous sections. Independent factors that predict post-TIPS encephalopathy include increased age, prior hepatic encephalopathy, higher Child-Pugh score, high creatinine levels, and low serum sodium or albumin values.[96,97] Puncture of the liver capsule occurs in up to 33% of patients, with intraperitoneal hemorrhage occurring in 1% to 2% of cases.[98] Biliary puncture with resultant fistula formation can lead to hemobilia, cholangitis, or early stent occlusion.

Table 4
Complications of transjugular intrahepatic portosystemic shunt

Related to Needle Puncture or Access	Stent-Related	Related to Portosystemic Shunting
Liver capsule puncture	Thrombosis	Hepatic encephalopathy
Intraperitoneal bleeding	Migration	Hepatic ischemia
Hemobilia	Occlusion	
Biliary Fistula	Hemolysis	
	Tipsitis	

Minimizing the number of needle passes will reduce the probability of liver capsule or biliary puncture. Diversion of portal venous flow not only increases the chance of hepatic encephalopathy but also can lead to hepatic ischemia or deterioration of hepatic function in approximately 10% of patients.[37] TIPS can cause intravascular hemolysis in 10% of patients (particularly in those who received bare metal stents), but this is usually self-limited and rarely requires treatment.[99] Lastly, the stent is subject to microbial seeding and infection, known as tipsitis. It occurs in about 1% of patients and should be treated aggressively with prolonged antibiotics.[100]

SUMMARY

TIPS is a well-established intervention that is valuable in the management for complications of portal hypertension. The strongest evidence for TIPS is for secondary prophylaxis of esophageal variceal bleeding and treatment of refractory ascites. Recent data provide a compelling argument for the early use of TIPS after variceal bleeding and that TIPS may confer a survival benefit in the setting of refractory ascites. As more prospective data are collected with the contemporary use of covered stents and optimal medical therapy, the role of TIPS will be more clearly defined and may be supported for other indications, such as hepatic hydrothorax, hepatorenal syndrome, and BCS.

REFERENCES

1. Bosch J, Garcia-Pagán JC, Berzigotti A, et al. Measurement of portal pressure and its role in the management of chronic liver disease. Semin Liver Dis 2006; 26(4):348–62.
2. Bosch J, Berzigotti A, Garcia-Pagan JC, et al. The management of portal hypertension: rational basis, available treatments and future options. J Hepatol 2008; 48(Suppl 1):S68–92.
3. D'Amico G, Garcia-Tsao G, Pagliaro L. Natural history and prognostic indicators of survival in cirrhosis: a systematic review of 118 studies. J Hepatol 2006;44(1): 217–31.
4. Gordon JD, Colapinto RF, Abecassis M, et al. Transjugular intrahepatic portosystemic shunt: a nonoperative approach to life-threatening variceal bleeding. Can J Surg 1987;30(1):45–9.
5. Kovalak M, Lake J, Mattek N, et al. Endoscopic screening for varices in cirrhotic patients: data from a national endoscopic database. Gastrointest Endosc 2007; 65(1):82–8.
6. Grace ND. Prevention of initial variceal hemorrhage. Gastroenterol Clin North Am 1992;21(1):149–61.
7. Garcia-Tsao G, Groszmann RJ, Fisher RL, et al. Portal pressure, presence of gastroesophageal varices and variceal bleeding. Hepatology 1985;5(3): 419–24.
8. Conn HO, Lindenmuth WW, May CJ, et al. Prophylactic portacaval anastomosis. Medicine 1972;51(1):27–40.
9. Garcia-Tsao G, Abraldes JG, Berzigotti A, et al. Portal hypertensive bleeding in cirrhosis: risk stratification, diagnosis, and management: 2016 practice guidance by the American Association for the study of liver diseases. Hepatology 2017;65(1):310–35.
10. Garcia-Tsao G, Bosch J. Management of varices and variceal hemorrhage in cirrhosis. N Engl J Med 2010;362(9):823–32.

11. Azoulay D, Castaing D, Majno P, et al. Salvage transjugular intrahepatic porto-systemic shunt for uncontrolled variceal bleeding in patients with decompensated cirrhosis. J Hepatol 2001;35(5):590–7.

12. Vangeli M, Patch D, Burroughs AK. Salvage tips for uncontrolled variceal bleeding. J Hepatol 2002;37:703–4.

13. Sanyal AJ, Freedman AM, Luketic VA, et al. Transjugular intrahepatic portosystemic shunts for patients with active variceal hemorrhage unresponsive to sclerotherapy. Gastroenterology 1996;111(1):138–46.

14. Banares R, Casado M, Rodriguez-Laiz JM, et al. Urgent transjugular intrahepatic portosystemic shunt for control of acute variceal bleeding. Am J Gastroenterol 1998;93(1):75–9.

15. Maimone S, Saffioti F, Filomia R, et al. Predictors of Re-bleeding and mortality among patients with refractory variceal bleeding undergoing salvage transjugular intrahepatic portosystemic shunt (TIPS). Dig Dis Sci 2019;64(5):1335–45.

16. Monescillo A, Martínez-Lagares F, Ruiz-del-Arbol L, et al. Influence of portal hypertension and its early decompression by TIPS placement on the outcome of variceal bleeding. Hepatology 2004;40(4):793–801.

17. García-Pagán JC, Caca K, Bureau C, et al. Early use of TIPS in patients with cirrhosis and variceal bleeding. N Engl J Med 2010;362(25):2370–9.

18. Garcia-Pagán JC, Di Pascoli M, Caca K, et al. Use of early-TIPS for high-risk variceal bleeding: results of a post-RCT surveillance study. J Hepatol 2013;58(1):45–50.

19. Rudler M, Cluzel P, Corvec TL, et al. Early-TIPSS placement prevents rebleeding in high-risk patients with variceal bleeding, without improving survival. Aliment Pharmacol Ther 2014;40(9):1074–80.

20. Njei B, McCarty TR, Laine L. Early transjugular intrahepatic portosystemic shunt in US patients hospitalized with acute esophageal variceal bleeding. J Gastroenterol Hepatol 2017;32(4):852–8.

21. Hernández-Gea V, Procopet B, Giráldez Á, et al. Preemptive-TIPS improves outcome in high-risk variceal bleeding: an observational study. Hepatology 2019;69(1):282–93.

22. Thabut D, Pauwels A, Carbonell N, et al. Cirrhotic patients with portal hypertension-related bleeding and an indication for early-TIPS: a large multicentre audit with real-life results. J Hepatol 2017;68(1):73–81.

23. Rössle M, Haag K, Ochs A, et al. The transjugular intrahepatic portosystemic stent-shunt procedure for variceal bleeding. N Engl J Med 1994;330(3):165–71.

24. Cello JP, Ring EJ, Olcott EW, et al. Endoscopic sclerotherapy compared with percutaneous transjugular intrahepatic portosystemic shunt after initial sclerotherapy in patients with acute variceal hemorrhage. A randomized, controlled trial. Ann Intern Med 1997;126(11):858–65.

25. Sanyal AJ, Freedman AM, Luketic VA, et al. Transjugular intrahepatic portosystemic shunts compared with endoscopic sclerotherapy for the prevention of recurrent variceal hemorrhage. A randomized, controlled trial. Ann Intern Med 1997;126(11):849–57.

26. Cabrera J, Maynar M, Granados R, et al. Transjugular intrahepatic portosystemic shunt versus sclerotherapy in the elective treatment of variceal hemorrhage. Gastroenterology 1996;110(3):832–9.

27. Sauer P, Theilmann L, Stremmel W, et al. Transjugular intrahepatic portosystemic stent shunt versus sclerotherapy plus propranolol for variceal rebleeding. Gastroenterology 1997;113(5):1623–31.

28. Jalan R, Forrest EH, Stanley AJ, et al. A randomized trial comparing transjugular intrahepatic portosystemic stent-shunt with variceal band ligation in the prevention of rebleeding from esophageal varices. Hepatology 1997;26(5):1115–22.

29. Merli M, Salerno F, Riggio O, et al. Transjugular intrahepatic portosystemic shunt versus endoscopic sclerotherapy for the prevention of variceal bleeding in cirrhosis: a randomized multicenter trial. Gruppo Italiano Studio TIPS (G.I.S.T.). Hepatology 1998;27(1):48–53.

30. García-Villarreal L, Martínez-Lagares F, Sierra A, et al. Transjugular intrahepatic portosystemic shunt versus endoscopic sclerotherapy for the prevention of variceal rebleeding after recent variceal hemorrhage. Hepatology 1999;29(1): 27–32.

31. Pomier-Layrargues G, Villeneuve JP, Deschênes M, et al. Transjugular intrahepatic portosystemic shunt (TIPS) versus endoscopic variceal ligation in the prevention of variceal rebleeding in patients with cirrhosis: a randomised trial. Gut 2001;48(3):390–6.

32. Narahara Y, Kanazawa H, Kawamata H, et al. A randomized clinical trial comparing transjugular intrahepatic portosystemic shunt with endoscopic sclerotherapy in the long-term management of patients with cirrhosis after recent variceal hemorrhage. Hepatol Res 2001;21(3):189–98.

33. Gülberg V, Schepke M, Geigenberger G, et al. Transjugular intrahepatic portosystemic shunting is not superior to endoscopic variceal band ligation for prevention of variceal rebleeding in cirrhotic patients: a randomized, controlled trial. Scand J Gastroenterol 2002;37(3):338–43.

34. Luo X, Wang Z, Tsauo J, et al. Advanced cirrhosis combined with portal vein thrombosis: a randomized trial of TIPS versus endoscopic band ligation plus propranolol for the prevention of recurrent esophageal variceal bleeding. Radiology 2015;276(1):286–93.

35. Sauerbruch T, Mengel M, Dollinger M, et al. Prevention of rebleeding from esophageal varices in patients with cirrhosis receiving small-diameter stents versus hemodynamically controlled medical therapy. Gastroenterology 2015; 149(3):660–8.e1.

36. Holster IL, Tjwa ET, Moelker A, et al. Covered transjugular intrahepatic portosystemic shunt versus endoscopic therapy + β-blocker for prevention of variceal rebleeding. Hepatology 2016;63(2):581–9.

37. Zheng M, Chen Y, Bai J, et al. Transjugular intrahepatic portosystemic shunt versus endoscopic therapy in the secondary prophylaxis of variceal rebleeding in cirrhotic patients: meta-analysis update. J Clin Gastroenterol 2008;42(5): 507–16.

38. Dai C, Liu WX, Jiang M, et al. Endoscopic variceal ligation compared with endoscopic injection sclerotherapy for treatment of esophageal variceal hemorrhage: a meta-analysis. World J Gastroenterol 2015;21(8):2534–41.

39. Perarnau JM, Le Gouge A, Nicolas C, et al. Covered vs. uncovered stents for transjugular intrahepatic portosystemic shunt: a randomized controlled trial. J Hepatol 2014;60(5):962–8.

40. Qi X, Tian Y, Zhang W, et al. Covered. Therap Adv Gastroenterol 2017;10(1): 32–41.

41. Bucsics T, Schoder M, Diermayr M, et al. Transjugular intrahepatic portosystemic shunts (TIPS) for the prevention of variceal re-bleeding - a two decades experience. PLoS One 2018;13(1):e0189414.

42. Qi X, Tian Y, Zhang W, et al. Covered TIPS for secondary prophylaxis of variceal bleeding in liver cirrhosis: a systematic review and meta-analysis of randomized controlled trials. Medicine 2016;95(50):e5680.

43. Sarin SK, Lahoti D, Saxena SP, et al. Prevalence, classification and natural history of gastric varices: a long-term follow-up study in 568 portal hypertension patients. Hepatology 1992;16(6):1343–9.

44. Kim T, Shijo H, Kokawa H, et al. Risk factors for hemorrhage from gastric fundal varices. Hepatology 1997;25(2):307–12.

45. Barange K, Péron JM, Imani K, et al. Transjugular intrahepatic portosystemic shunt in the treatment of refractory bleeding from ruptured gastric varices. Hepatology 1999;30(5):1139–43.

46. Chau TN, Patch D, Chan YW, et al. "Salvage" transjugular intrahepatic portosystemic shunts: gastric fundal compared with esophageal variceal bleeding. Gastroenterology 1998;114(5):981–7.

47. Procaccini NJ, Al-Osaimi AM, Northup P, et al. Endoscopic cyanoacrylate versus transjugular intrahepatic portosystemic shunt for gastric variceal bleeding: a single-center U.S. analysis. Gastrointest Endosc 2009;70(5):881–7.

48. Kochhar GS, Navaneethan U, Hartman J, et al. Comparative study of endoscopy vs. transjugular intrahepatic portosystemic shunt in the management of gastric variceal bleeding. Gastroenterol Rep (Oxf) 2015;3(1):75–82.

49. Lo GH, Liang HL, Chen WC, et al. A prospective, randomized controlled trial of transjugular intrahepatic portosystemic shunt versus cyanoacrylate injection in the prevention of gastric variceal rebleeding. Endoscopy 2007;39(8):679–85.

50. Wang YB, Zhang JY, Gong JP, et al. Balloon-occluded retrograde transvenous obliteration versus transjugular intrahepatic portosystemic shunt for treatment of gastric varices due to portal hypertension: a meta-analysis. J Gastroenterol Hepatol 2016;31(4):727–33.

51. Kim SK, Lee KA, Sauk S, et al. Comparison of transjugular intrahepatic portosystemic shunt with covered stent and balloon-occluded retrograde transvenous obliteration in managing isolated gastric varices. Korean J Radiol 2017;18(2):345–54.

52. Sabri SS, Abi-Jaoudeh N, Swee W, et al. Short-term rebleeding rates for isolated gastric varices managed by transjugular intrahepatic portosystemic shunt versus balloon-occluded retrograde transvenous obliteration. J Vasc Interv Radiol 2014;25(3):355–61.

53. Gimm G, Chang Y, Kim HC, et al. Balloon-occluded retrograde transvenous obliteration versus transjugular intrahepatic portosystemic shunt for the management of gastric variceal bleeding. Gut Liver 2018;12(6):704–13.

54. Wong F. Management of ascites in cirrhosis. J Gastroenterol Hepatol 2012;27(1):11–20.

55. Lebrec D, Giuily N, Hadengue A, et al. Transjugular intrahepatic portosystemic shunts: comparison with paracentesis in patients with cirrhosis and refractory ascites: a randomized trial. French Group of Clinicians and a Group of Biologists. J Hepatol 1996;25(2):135–44.

56. Rössle M, Ochs A, Gülberg V, et al. A comparison of paracentesis and transjugular intrahepatic portosystemic shunting in patients with ascites. N Engl J Med 2000;342(23):1701–7.

57. Ginès P, Uriz J, Calahorra B, et al. Transjugular intrahepatic portosystemic shunting versus paracentesis plus albumin for refractory ascites in cirrhosis. Gastroenterology 2002;123(6):1839–47.

58. Sanyal AJ, Genning C, Reddy KR, et al. The North American study for the treatment of refractory ascites. Gastroenterology 2003;124(3):634–41.

59. Salerno F, Merli M, Riggio O, et al. Randomized controlled study of TIPS versus paracentesis plus albumin in cirrhosis with severe ascites. Hepatology 2004; 40(3):629–35.

60. Narahara Y, Kanazawa H, Fukuda T, et al. Transjugular intrahepatic portosystemic shunt versus paracentesis plus albumin in patients with refractory ascites who have good hepatic and renal function: a prospective randomized trial. J Gastroenterol 2011;46(1):78–85.

61. Bureau C, Thabut D, Oberti F, et al. Transjugular intrahepatic portosystemic shunts with covered stents increase transplant-free survival of patients with cirrhosis and recurrent ascites. Gastroenterology 2017;152(1):157–63.

62. D'Amico G, Luca A, Morabito A, et al. Uncovered transjugular intrahepatic portosystemic shunt for refractory ascites: a meta-analysis. Gastroenterology 2005; 129(4):1282–93.

63. Saab S, Nieto JM, Lewis SK, et al. TIPS versus paracentesis for cirrhotic patients with refractory ascites. Cochrane Database Syst Rev 2006;(4):CD004889.

64. Salerno F, Cammà C, Enea M, et al. Transjugular intrahepatic portosystemic shunt for refractory ascites: a meta-analysis of individual patient data. Gastroenterology 2007;133(3):825–34.

65. Bai M, Qi XS, Yang ZP, et al. TIPS improves liver transplantation-free survival in cirrhotic patients with refractory ascites: an updated meta-analysis. World J Gastroenterol 2014;20(10):2704–14.

66. Bercu ZL, Fischman AM, Kim E, et al. TIPS for refractory ascites: a 6-year single-center experience with expanded polytetrafluoroethylene-covered stent-grafts. AJR Am J Roentgenol 2015;204(3):654–61.

67. Parvinian A, Bui JT, Knuttinen MG, et al. Transjugular intrahepatic portosystemic shunt for the treatment of medically refractory ascites. Diagn Interv Radiol 2014; 20(1):58–64.

68. Tan HK, James PD, Sniderman KW, et al. Long-term clinical outcome of patients with cirrhosis and refractory ascites treated with transjugular intrahepatic portosystemic shunt insertion. J Gastroenterol Hepatol 2015;30(2):389–95.

69. Gaba RC, Parvinian A, Casadaban LC, et al. Survival benefit of TIPS versus serial paracentesis in patients with refractory ascites: a single institution case-control propensity score analysis. Clin Radiol 2015;70(5):e51–7.

70. Garbuzenko DV, Arefyev NO. Hepatic hydrothorax: an update and review of the literature. World J Hepatol 2017;9(31):1197–204.

71. Dhanasekaran R, West JK, Gonzales PC, et al. Transjugular intrahepatic portosystemic shunt for symptomatic refractory hepatic hydrothorax in patients with cirrhosis. Am J Gastroenterol 2010;105(3):635–41.

72. Ditah IC, Al Bawardy BF, Saberi B, et al. Transjugular intrahepatic portosystemic stent shunt for medically refractory hepatic hydrothorax: a systematic review and cumulative meta-analysis. World J Hepatol 2015;7(13):1797–806.

73. Runyon BA, AASLD. Introduction to the revised American Association for the Study of Liver Diseases Practice Guideline management of adult patients with ascites due to cirrhosis 2012. Hepatology 2013;57(4):1651–3.

74. Wong F, Pantea L, Sniderman K. Midodrine, octreotide, albumin, and TIPS in selected patients with cirrhosis and type 1 hepatorenal syndrome. Hepatology 2004;40(1):55–64.

75. Guevara M, Ginès P, Bandi JC, et al. Transjugular intrahepatic portosystemic shunt in hepatorenal syndrome: effects on renal function and vasoactive systems. Hepatology 1998;28(2):416–22.

76. Brensing KA, Textor J, Perz J, et al. Long term outcome after transjugular intrahepatic portosystemic stent-shunt in non-transplant cirrhotics with hepatorenal syndrome: a phase II study. Gut 2000;47(2):288–95.

77. Ng CK, Chan MH, Tai MH, et al. Hepatorenal syndrome. Clin Biochem Rev 2007; 28(1):11–7.

78. Song T, Rössle M, He F, et al. Transjugular intrahepatic portosystemic shunt for hepatorenal syndrome: a systematic review and meta-analysis. Dig Liver Dis 2018;50(4):323–30.

79. Seijo S, Plessier A, Hoekstra J, et al. Good long-term outcome of Budd-Chiari syndrome with a step-wise management. Hepatology 2013;57(5):1962–8.

80. Khan F, Mehrzad H, Tripathi D. Timing of transjugular intrahepatic portosystemic stent-shunt in Budd-Chiari syndrome: a Uk hepatologist's perspective. J Transl Int Med 2018;6(3):97–104.

81. Garcia-Pagán JC, Heydtmann M, Raffa S, et al. TIPS for Budd-Chiari syndrome: long-term results and prognostics factors in 124 patients. Gastroenterology 2008;135(3):808–15.

82. Qi X, Guo W, He C, et al. Transjugular intrahepatic portosystemic shunt for Budd-Chiari syndrome: techniques, indications and results on 51 Chinese patients from a single centre. Liver Int 2014;34(8):1164–75.

83. Tripathi D, Sunderraj L, Vemala V, et al. Long-term outcomes following percutaneous hepatic vein recanalization for Budd-Chiari syndrome. Liver Int 2017; 37(1):111–20.

84. Boyer TD, Haskal ZJ, Diseases AAftSoL. The role of transjugular intrahepatic portosystemic shunt (TIPS) in the management of portal hypertension: update 2009. Hepatology 2010;51(1):306.

85. Riggio O, Nardelli S, Moscucci F, et al. Hepatic encephalopathy after transjugular intrahepatic portosystemic shunt. Clin Liver Dis 2012;16(1):133–46.

86. Jalan R, Elton RA, Redhead DN, et al. Analysis of prognostic variables in the prediction of mortality, shunt failure, variceal rebleeding and encephalopathy following the transjugular intrahepatic portosystemic stent-shunt for variceal haemorrhage. J Hepatol 1995;23(2):123–8.

87. Chalasani N, Clark WS, Martin LG, et al. Determinants of mortality in patients with advanced cirrhosis after transjugular intrahepatic portosystemic shunting. Gastroenterology 2000;118(1):138–44.

88. Kamath PS, Wiesner RH, Malinchoc M, et al. A model to predict survival in patients with end-stage liver disease. Hepatology 2001;33(2):464–70.

89. Salerno F, Merli M, Cazzaniga M, et al. MELD score is better than Child-Pugh score in predicting 3-month survival of patients undergoing transjugular intrahepatic portosystemic shunt. J Hepatol 2002;36(4):494–500.

90. Ferral H, Gamboa P, Postoak DW, et al. Survival after elective transjugular intrahepatic portosystemic shunt creation: prediction with model for end-stage liver disease score. Radiology 2004;231(1):231–6.

91. Angermayr B, Cejna M, Karnel F, et al. Child-Pugh versus MELD score in predicting survival in patients undergoing transjugular intrahepatic portosystemic shunt. Gut 2003;52(6):879–85.

92. Said A, Williams J, Holden J, et al. Model for end stage liver disease score predicts mortality across a broad spectrum of liver disease. J Hepatol 2004;40(6): 897–903.

93. Ascha M, Hanouneh M, S Ascha M, et al. Transjugular intrahepatic porto-systemic shunt in patients with liver cirrhosis and model for end-stage liver disease ≥15. Dig Dis Sci 2017;62(2):534–42.

94. Tripathi D, Redhead D. Transjugular intrahepatic portosystemic stent-shunt: technical factors and new developments. Eur J Gastroenterol Hepatol 2006; 18(11):1127–33.

95. Qi X, Liu L, Bai M, et al. Transjugular intrahepatic portosystemic shunt in combination with or without variceal embolization for the prevention of variceal re-bleeding: a meta-analysis. J Gastroenterol Hepatol 2014;29(4):688–96.

96. Riggio O, Angeloni S, Salvatori FM, et al. Incidence, natural history, and risk factors of hepatic encephalopathy after transjugular intrahepatic portosystemic shunt with polytetrafluoroethylene-covered stent grafts. Am J Gastroenterol 2008;103(11):2738–46.

97. Bai M, Qi X, Yang Z, et al. Predictors of hepatic encephalopathy after transjugular intrahepatic portosystemic shunt in cirrhotic patients: a systematic review. J Gastroenterol Hepatol 2011;26(6):943–51.

98. Fidelman N, Kwan SW, LaBerge JM, et al. The transjugular intrahepatic porto-systemic shunt: an update. AJR Am J Roentgenol 2012;199(4):746–55.

99. Sanyal AJ, Freedman AM, Purdum PP, et al. The hematologic consequences of transjugular intrahepatic portosystemic shunts. Hepatology 1996;23(1):32–9.

100. Kochar N, Tripathi D, Arestis NJ, et al. Tipsitis: incidence and outcome-a single centre experience. Eur J Gastroenterol Hepatol 2010;22(6):729–35.

Surgery in Patients with Portal Hypertension

Melissa Wong, MD[a], Ronald W. Busuttil, MD, PhD[b],*

KEYWORDS

- Portal hypertension • Chronic liver disease and cirrhosis • Nontransplant surgery
- Perioperative risk stratification • Child-Turcotte-Pugh
- Model for End-stage Liver Disease

KEY POINTS

- Patients with portal hypertension and chronic liver disease have a syndrome of multiorgan dysfunction and are at increased risk for perioperative morbidity and mortality.
- Preoperative assessment should seek to distinguish between compensated and decompensated cirrhosis, and identify factors that increase perioperative risk, including portal hypertension, malnutrition, coagulopathy, renal dysfunction, and emergency surgery.
- The Child-Turcotte-Pugh and Model for End-stage Liver Disease scores are still the most commonly used tools for surgical risk stratification.
- Perioperative risk in patients with portal hypertension and cirrhosis may be mitigated by referral to specialized providers, nutritional optimization, use of laparoscopy, preoperative transjugular intrahepatic portosystemic shunt placement, and avoidance of surgery when imprudent.

INTRODUCTION

Portal hypertension is most commonly encountered in the context of chronic liver disease and cirrhosis, which together were the 12th leading cause of death in the United States and accounted for some 40,545 deaths in 2016.[1] The most common causes are currently hepatitis C virus (HCV) and alcohol, but are expected to transition over the next decade to alcohol and nonalcoholic fatty liver disease or nonalcoholic steatohepatitis (NASH). This epidemiologic shift is anticipated because of the success of direct-acting antivirals for HCV, the plateauing of national obesity rates during this

Disclosures: None.
[a] Division of Transplant Surgery, Department of Surgery, Medical College of Wisconsin, Transplant Center, 9200 West Wisconsin Avenue, Milwaukee, WI 53226, USA; [b] Division of Liver and Pancreas Transplantation, Department of Surgery, David Geffen School of Medicine, University of California at Los Angeles, The Dumont-UCLA Transplant Center, 757 Westwood Blvd, Suite 8236, Los Angeles, CA 90095, USA
* Corresponding author.
E-mail address: rbusuttil@mednet.ucla.edu

Clin Liver Dis 23 (2019) 755–780
https://doi.org/10.1016/j.cld.2019.07.003
1089-3261/19/© 2019 Elsevier Inc. All rights reserved.

decade, and the increase of alcohol consumption coupled with the dearth of advancements in the treatment of alcohol use disorders.[2] One recent study based on National Health and Nutrition Examination Survey (NHANES) data from 1999 to 2010 estimated that cirrhosis affects approximately 0.27% of the US population, or 633,323 adults, although experts agree that it is underrecognized and its prevalence is likely increasing.[3] More than 10% of patients with cirrhosis require surgery during the last 2 years of their lifetimes.[4] As a result, patients with portal hypertension and chronic liver disease present with indications for surgery, and often in the later stages of their disease.

Patients with portal hypertension and chronic liver disease have been historically recognized as having higher perioperative risk compared with healthy patients, proportional to the severity of their liver disease. For example, a 1982 study by Aranha and colleagues[5] of open cholecystectomy found higher mortality among cirrhotic patients compared with noncirrhotics (25% vs 1.1%). Further subdividing the cirrhotic patients by prothrombin time (PT) showed that greater liver dysfunction correlated with significantly worse outcome: mortality was 83.3% among patients with PT greater than 2.5 seconds more than normal, compared with 9.3% if PT was less than or equal to 2.5 seconds prolonged, and only 1.1% in patients with normal liver function and normal PT. Even then, complications of liver disease, namely bleeding, sepsis, and decompensated liver failure, were recognized as the major causes of postoperative death among patients with cirrhosis.

Another widely cited early study similarly reported higher mortality, wound infection, and recurrence rates after umbilical herniorrhaphy among patients with cirrhosis compared with noncirrhotics (8.3% vs 1.8% for mortality).[6] Notably, a small subgroup of cirrhotic patients with patent peritoneovenous shunts showed perioperative outcomes similar to the noncirrhotic group, an early clue that perioperative risk in these challenging patients might be mitigated by managing the complications of cirrhosis.

Subsequent studies have continued to show persistently high morbidity (30.1%–69% in studies of nonhepatic abdominal surgery) for cirrhotic patients undergoing surgery, although perioperative mortalities have generally decreased compared with those reported 20 to 30 years ago (**Table 1**).[7–11] Although risk varies by type of surgery, with higher mortality reported after cardiac surgery (17% overall in a review of modern series reporting on a range from 6% to 33% mortality)[12] and colectomy (18%–25% from recent representative studies),[13–15] decompensated cirrhosis with evidence of portal hypertension is still associated with the highest risk-adjusted perioperative mortality.[16] Improved outcomes may be attributable to advances in hepatology, surgical technique, and critical care; greater institutional experience with multidisciplinary teams dedicated to the perioperative care of patients with liver disease (often where liver transplantation is also performed); and an evolving understanding of how to appropriately risk stratify and optimize these patients, when possible.[10,13,17]

PATHOPHYSIOLOGY

Essential to understanding how portal hypertension affects patients' perioperative risk is an appreciation of the extent of systemic dysfunction present. An illustrative example is the case of presinusoidal portal hypertension, which may develop secondary to hepatosplenic schistosomiasis caused by *Schistosoma mansoni* and *Schistosoma japonicum*. In the context of intact liver function, patients develop a hyperdynamic circulation, splenomegaly, thrombocytopenia, and possibly life-threatening hemorrhage from

Table 1
Mortality after general surgery operations in patients with and without cirrhosis

Study: Operation Type	No. of Patients Cirrhotic/Non	Mortality (%) Cirrhotic/Noncirrhotic
Del Olmo et al,[9] 2003: nonhepatic abdominal surgery	135/86	16.3/3.5
Leonetti et al,[6] 1984: umbilical hernia repair	39/53	5.1/1.9
Carbonell et al,[121] 2005: abdominal wall hernia repair	1197/30,836	2.5/0.2
Gray et al,[122] 2008: umbilical hernia repair	127/1294	0.79/0.39
Oh et al, 2011,[123] inguinal hernia repair	129/651	1.6/0
Aranha et al,[5] 1982: open cholecystectomy	55/274	25.5/1.1
Fernandes et al,[124] 2000: laparoscopic cholecystectomy	48/187	0/0
Yeh et al,[125] 2002: laparoscopic cholecystectomy	226/4030	0.88/0.05
Perkins et al,[75] 2004: cholecystectomy	33/31	6/0
Al-Azzawi et al,[113] 2018: laparoscopic appendectomy	376/378	0.5/0.3
Nguyen et al,[15] 2009: colorectal surgery	4042/499,541	18/5
Warnick et al,[126] 2011: pancreatic surgery	32/32	9/0

esophageal varices.[18] Perioperative mortality for such patients undergoing surgical devascularization or shunt procedures for secondary prophylaxis of variceal bleeding is much lower than for similar procedures performed in cirrhotic patients.[19–22] Most patients with portal hypertension who present for surgery have liver cirrhosis, a syndrome of multiorgan dysfunction with implications for all aspects of perioperative care.[23]

In cirrhotic portal hypertension, the degree of hyperdynamic circulatory alteration directly correlates with the severity of liver disease (**Fig. 1**). The portal vein supplies 75% of blood flow to the liver at baseline, with the remainder supplied by the hepatic artery. In a diseased liver with increasing resistance to portal flow, relative hepatic ischemia fuels the development of mechanisms to increase hepatic blood flow by splanchnic and systemic arteriolar vasodilatation: impaired hepatocyte degradation of circulating vasoactive molecules (eg, natriuretic peptides, renin, angiotensin II, vasopressin, substance P, aldosterone), increased production of vasodilators (eg, nitric oxide, cannabinoids) in hepatic stellate cells and sinusoidal endothelium, and increased production of proinflammatory cytokines (eg, tumor necrosis factor alpha, interleukin-6) in response to diminished immune clearance by antigen-presenting Kupffer cells. Central blood volume decreases as blood is shunted preferentially to the splanchnic circulation. As portal hypertension progresses and spontaneous portosystemic shunts form, more vasodilators bypass hepatic degradation and persist in the circulation. Arterial underfilling ensues, triggering the renin-angiotensin-aldosterone system and renal sodium and water retention in an attempt to expand circulating plasma volume. Renal vasoconstriction is also directly driven by the portal flow-dependent hepatorenal reflex. Acute kidney injury affects 20% of hospitalized cirrhotics, of which two-thirds are have prerenal causes or are caused by the hepatorenal syndrome.[23]

Increased splanchnic inflow also increases filtration pressure and lymph formation, leading to the accumulation of abdominal ascites and further decreases in effective circulating volume. In postoperative patients, abdominal ascites may increase tension

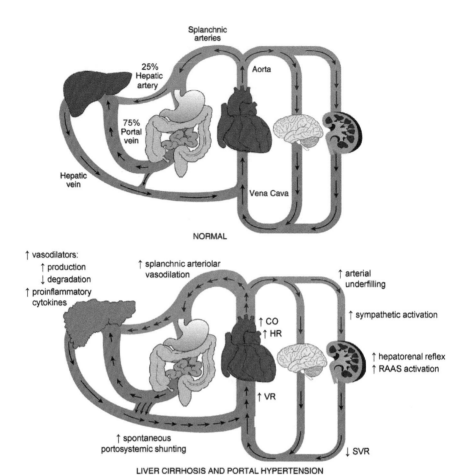

Fig. 1. Hyperdynamic circulation of portal hypertension and cirrhosis. CO, cardiac output; HR, heart rate; RAAS, renin-angiotensin-aldosterone system; SVR, systemic vascular resistance; VR, venous return. (*Adapted from* McAvoy NC, Semple S, Richards JMJ, et al. Differential visceral blood flow in the hyperdynamic circulation of patients with liver cirrhosis. *Aliment Pharmacol Ther.* 2016;43(9):952; with permission.)

on an operative incision leading to dehiscence or hernia, and leaking ascites may become secondarily infected. Counterregulatory sympathetic activation in response to intravascular hypovolemia is compounded by impaired hepatocyte clearance of epinephrine and norepinephrine, which increases venous return, heart rate, myocardial contractility, and cardiac output initially. Despite this, systemic vascular resistance remains inappropriately low, and low arterial blood pressure (particularly diastolic) develops late. With desensitized and downregulated beta-adrenergic receptors, alterations in membrane potassium and calcium ion channels, and persistent circulation of vasoactive substances and cytokines, some patients develop cirrhotic cardiomyopathy. Conditions of hemodynamic stress, such as induction of anesthesia and surgery, may unmask impaired contractility, diastolic dysfunction, and electrophysiologic changes such as QT prolongation.[23]

The complications of portal hypertension also increase the risk of hypoxemia in cirrhotic patients undergoing surgery. Abdominal ascites and hepatic hydrothorax can restrict lung expansion. The hyperdynamic circulatory changes described earlier predispose patients to developing pulmonary edema with increased pulmonary vascular resistance and impaired gas exchange. In addition, hepatopulmonary syndrome affects approximately 20% of cirrhotic patients with portal hypertension and is characterized by pulmonary alveolar capillary dilatation causing intrapulmonary shunting and progressive hypoxemia. A rarer pulmonary complication of portal hypertension, portopulmonary hypertension, affects up to 5% of cirrhotic patients and is associated with lower median survival than primary idiopathic pulmonary hypertension despite medical treatment with pulmonary vasodilators.[23]

Perioperative care in cirrhotic patients must account for the diseased liver's reduced synthetic and metabolic functions. Almost all aspects of drug metabolism may be affected: variable declines in the cytochrome P450 enzymes and other metabolic pathways in the liver impede drug elimination unpredictably, portosystemic shunting reduces first-pass effect and may greatly increase systemic absorption, and volume of distribution may be significantly altered by decreased plasma protein synthesis for protein-bound drugs and active metabolites.[24] Combined with the predisposition to multiorgan dysfunction described earlier, this altered metabolic capacity means that some drugs should be dose reduced or avoided altogether. Acetaminophen may be used judiciously (up to 2 g/d in select patients), but nonessential medications and all herbal supplements should be stopped to limit the risk of hepatotoxicity. Benzodiazepines and some opiates, particularly those with longer action or active metabolites, may exacerbate hepatic encephalopathy. Nonsteroidal antiinflammatory drugs such as ketorolac and other nephrotoxic medications should be avoided. QT prolongation, if present, may limit the use of several medications commonly applied in perioperative settings, such as ondansetron, metoclopramide, fluoroquinolones, metronidazole, and azole antifungals. Preferred drugs for anesthesia undergo minimal hepatic or renal metabolism, and include isoflurane, desflurane, or sevoflurane for volatile anesthetics; atracurium or cis-atracurium for neuromuscular blockade; and fentanyl or remifentanil for opioid analgesia.[25,26]

Liver dysfunction also affects the risks of bleeding and infection, the most common postoperative complications in patients with cirrhosis.[8] Coagulation and homeostasis rely on normal liver function because most procoagulant and anticoagulant factors are produced in the liver. Both abnormal thrombosis and bleeding may occur in chronic liver disease. For example, surgical patients with liver disease are still at increased risk for deep vein thrombosis despite conventional laboratory measures suggesting coagulopathy, and pharmacologic prophylaxis is both safe and beneficial.[27,28] Cirrhotic patients are also predisposed to developing infections because of depressed immune cell functions such as chemotaxis, phagocytosis, intracellular killing, and cytokine production; portosystemic shunting, which allows circulating bacteria and toxins to bypass clearance in the reticuloendothelial system; deficiencies in the liver-produced complement system; and intestinal bacterial overgrowth with greater gut permeability leading to translocation. Other contributors to this chronically immunocompromised state include malnutrition and, when present, alcohol use and steroids.[29]

Cirrhosis and portal hypertension is a multiorgan disease with significant neurohormonal, cardiovascular, pulmonary, renal, immune, coagulation, and metabolic consequences for surgical patients.

PREOPERATIVE ASSESSMENT

Preanesthesia assessment is guided by the patient's history and physical examination, and the anticipated risks of the planned procedure (**Box 1**). Routine screening

---

Box 1
Preoperative assessment

All patients
  History
  - Diagnosed chronic liver disease
  - Prior decompensation; for example, hepatic encephalopathy, variceal bleed, jaundice
  - Risk factors for liver disease; for example, alcohol or drug use, tattoos, blood transfusions, high-risk sexual behavior, travel history
  - Family history; for example, hemochromatosis
  - Medications and supplements
  - Surgical history
  Physical examination
  - Tachycardia, hypotension, hypoxia, hypothermia
  - Asterixis
  - Jaundice, scleral icterus
  - Spider angiomata, palmar erythema, gynecomastia
  - Ascites, hepatic hydrothorax, splenomegaly
  - Caput medusae

Select patients (as indicated by history and physical examination)
- Complete blood count, electrolytes, liver function tests, International Normalized Ratio, fibrinogen, blood gas, type and screen
- Serologic testing for cause of liver disease
- Alcohol and drug screens
- Liver duplex ultrasonography
- Transthoracic echocardiogram
- Upper endoscopy
- Hepatic vein pressure gradient

---

for liver dysfunction is not recommended.[30] Although studies based on the NHANES suggest that the prevalence of increased aminotransferase levels may be increasing, affecting up to 9.8% of US adults, asymptomatic transaminitis does not predict histopathologic severity of liver disease or postoperative outcomes.[30–33] Notably, a focused approach to preoperative assessment may increase the risk of incidentally discovering cirrhosis intraoperatively, which has been reported as from 1% to 4% of patients undergoing bariatric surgery, and up to 22% in a cohort of general surgery patients.[34,35]

A history to screen for the risk of liver disease should include alcohol use, intravenous drug use, tattoos, high-risk sexual behavior, transfusion history, travel history, and family history of liver disease. A review of current medications and over-the-counter supplements is also important. Physical examination may reveal clinical signs of chronic liver disease and portal hypertension, such as asterixis, jaundice and scleral icterus, spider angiomata, palmar erythema, gynecomastia, abdominal ascites, splenomegaly, and caput medusae. Suggestive history and physical examination findings warrant laboratory tests, including a complete blood count, liver function tests, international normalized ratio (INR), and chemistries. In the absence of a previous diagnosis of liver disease, liver ultrasonography; viral hepatitis serologies; screening for nonalcoholic fatty liver disease and alcoholic liver disease; and tests for autoimmune hepatitis, Wilson disease, and alpha-1 antitrypsin deficiency should be checked.[36]

Any history of prior hepatic decompensation should be specifically sought in patients with chronic liver disease. Commonly the first hepatic decompensation to develop is abdominal ascites, and others include hepatic encephalopathy, variceal bleeding, and jaundice.[37] Decompensation reflects the severity of portal hypertension and carries grave prognostic implications. A prospective cohort study of 213 patients with compensated cirrhosis found that hepatic venous pressure gradient (HVPG), a proxy for portal pressure gradient, independently predicted progression to decompensated cirrhosis, and HVPG less than 10 mm Hg was associated with a 90% probability of not decompensating during a 4-year median follow-up.[38] Progression from compensated to decompensated cirrhosis occurs at a rate of approximately 5% to 7% per year, and is greater in the first year after diagnosis.[37,39] Reporting on a population-based cohort of 4537 cirrhotic patients in the United Kingdom, Fleming and colleagues[40] observed significantly better overall survival for patients with compensated cirrhosis compared with decompensated (87.3% vs 75% at 1 year, and 66.5% vs 45.4% at 5 years, respectively), consistent with other studies.[41,42] Compensated cirrhotics are much more likely to experience a decompensation rather than die before or during their first decompensation, whereas patients with decompensated cirrhosis die of liver-related causes.[43]

Abnormal results of the foregoing assessment may trigger further testing or intervention with the goal of hepatic optimization before nonurgent surgery. For example, patients with acute alcoholic hepatitis should be counseled to avoid alcohol and defer surgery until liver function stabilizes and the risk of alcohol withdrawal passes.[44] Surgery during acute viral hepatitis is similarly unadvised based on early studies reporting up to 15% perioperative mortality after laparotomy and open biliary drainage for jaundice.[45,46] Certain chronic liver diseases, such as nonalcoholic steatohepatitis and hemochromatosis, are associated with increased cardiac risk and may warrant preoperative transthoracic echocardiogram. Although routine invasive testing is not recommended for preanesthesia assessment without appropriate indication, an unexpected finding of anemia on preoperative blood testing may warrant further work-up with upper endoscopy to assess for varices and portal hypertensive gastropathy. Any history of new or worsening variceal bleeding or ascites should also prompt a duplex ultrasonography scan of the liver to rule out portal vein thrombosis. Routine measurement of HVPG before surgery is also not practical or indicated, but thrombocytopenia likely indicates the presence of portal hypertension and should be noted. A study of noninvasive measures of portal hypertension found that a platelet count less than $100 \times 10^3/\mu L$ independently predicted the presence of esophageal varices.[47] Cholestatic liver tests (increased bilirubin, alkaline phosphatase, and gamma-glutamyl transferase levels) suggest screening for biliary dilatation by ultrasonography followed by magnetic resonance cholangiopancreatography. Any significant biliary obstruction should be decompressed before surgery, by endoscopic retrograde cholangiopancreatography or percutaneous transhepatic cholangiography. Electrolyte and acid-base abnormalities become more common as chronic liver disease progresses, exacerbated by comorbid renal dysfunction and by the first-line use of diuretics and lactulose in managing ascites and hepatic encephalopathy.[48] Severe abnormalities should be corrected before the administration of anesthesia. A high index of suspicion for the complications of liver disease helps direct preoperative testing.

STRATIFYING SURGICAL RISK

Early surgical experience in patients with cirrhosis and portal hypertension flourished under the search for safe and successful treatments for recurrent variceal hemorrhage. These operations, which include gastroesophageal devascularization with splenectomy, esophageal transection, and various selective and nonselective portosystemic shunts, are performed infrequently now, but the lessons of that experience remain relevant: judicious patient selection, an operative plan tailored to the patient, avoidance of emergency procedures when possible, and improved technical facility.[49–52] An ideal assessment of a patient's surgical risk would be safe and easy to perform in a variety of settings with prompt and reproducible results, and, most importantly, would accurately separate those cirrhotics who would likely benefit from an operation and should still be offered surgery, even at increased risk, from those who would likely be harmed.

Child-Turcotte-Pugh

In 1964, Child and Turcotte[53] originally described an empiric grading system for liver disease in patients undergoing portosystemic shunt surgery. Pugh and colleagues[49] modified the original components (serum albumin, total bilirubin, ascites, encephalopathy, and nutritional status) in 1973, adding PT (subsequently replaced with INR) and removing nutritional status (**Table 2**). In a cohort of patients undergoing emergency surgical ligation and esophageal transection for variceal hemorrhage, they reported 29% mortality among Child-Turcotte-Pugh (CTP) class A patients, 38% mortality for CTP B, and 88% mortality for CTP C. Since then, large studies of nontransplant surgery in cirrhotic patients spanning almost 30 years had reported comparable perioperative mortalities by CTP class, especially for CTP class B and C patients, and have only recently shown improvements for all CTP classes over the past decade.[7,35,54,55] Beyond the surgical context, the CTP score has shown value in predicting overall survival in cirrhotic patients.[56,57]

Despite being widely used even now to risk stratify and prognosticate in patients with cirrhosis, the CTP scoring system has several limitations. Its 5 included parameters, their equal weighting within the score, and the boundary values for assigning points were all chosen empirically and have not been formally validated.[13,58] A limited score range (5–15) is further simplified to only 3 classes, resulting in a considerable spectrum of disease severity being grouped together. Patients with decompensated, CTP class C disease are disproportionately affected because of a ceiling effect: although there is likely a clinically significant difference between one patient with a total bilirubin level of 3.1 mg/dL and another with a total bilirubin level of 31 mg/dL, both would be assigned the same 3 points in the CTP score. Another concern is the 2

Table 2
Child-Turcotte-Pugh score for cirrhosis[49,53]

Parameter	1 Point	2 Points	3 Points
Albumin (g/dL)	>3.5	2.8–3.5	<2.8
Bilirubin (mg/dL)	<2	2–3	>3
INR	<1.7	1.7–2.3	>2.3
Ascites	None	Mild/moderate	Severe
Hepatic Encephalopathy	None	Grade 1–2	Grade 3–4

CTP Class	Points Total
A	5–6
B	7–9
C	10–15

Abbreviation: INR, international normalized ratio.

Adapted from Pugh RN, Murray-Lyon IM, Dawson JL, Pietroni MC, Williams R. Transection of the oesophagus for bleeding oesophageal varices. *Br J Surg.* 1973;60(8):646–649; and Child CG, Turcotte JG. Surgery and portal hypertension. *Major Probl Clin Surg.* 1964;1:1-85.

clinically assessed parameters, ascites and encephalopathy, which are subject to interobserver variability in examination findings and grading. For example, hepatic encephalopathy can fluctuate quickly with treatment or with changes in the patient's clinical condition. Mild cases may be missed on examination or misinterpreted.

Model for End-Stage Liver Disease and Model for End-Stage Liver Disease–Sodium

The Model for End-stage Liver Disease (MELD), based on total bilirubin, serum creatinine, INR, and cause of liver disease, was first described in 2000 to predict 3-month mortality after elective transjugular intrahepatic portosystemic shunt (TIPS) placement in a multi-institutional US cohort.[59] Later, it was found to predict 3-month overall mortality in cirrhotic patients across a spectrum of clinical acuity, without needing to account for the cause of liver disease.[58] In 2002, the United Network for Organ Sharing (UNOS) adopted the MELD score to replace the existing system of liver allocation based on CTP, inpatient status, and complications of cirrhosis, and subsequently transitioned to the MELD-Na score in 2016, which was shown to outperform the MELD score in predicting mortality among patients awaiting liver transplant.[60,61] Compared with the shortcomings of the CTP score, the MELD score has been prospectively validated in liver transplant candidates; uses only objectively measurable laboratory values in an equation weighted to maximize the model's predictive power, and yields a continuous score capable of discriminating prognosis for a spectrum of liver disease severity, especially among patients with decompensated cirrhosis.[37,58,62] In contrast, unlike CTP, the MELD score does not include any components of portal hypertension, and in most cases their addition (eg, spontaneous bacterial peritonitis, variceal hemorrhage) does not improve the model's predictive power.[58,63]

Surgical outcomes analyses have generally shown a correlation between MELD score and postoperative mortality, although specific adaptation for clinical practice has varied. One approach has been to define a MELD cutoff for poor outcomes. A retrospective review of 100 abdominal operations performed in patients with cirrhosis found a significantly higher risk of postoperative morbidity and mortality at MELD greater than or equal to 15.[10] Several studies have found a similar turning point in mortality risk at approximately MELD 15,[64–66] notable as the threshold above which most transplant centers consider the benefits of liver transplant to outweigh the risks of the transplant operation and long-term immunosuppression.[67]

Another approach, analyzing mortality by empirically chosen MELD score ranges, lends itself to comparison with CTP classes. Postoperative mortality of 3% to 9% has been reported for MELD less than 10, corresponding with CTP class A; whereas mortalities of 8% to 19% and 29% to 57% have been reported for MELD 10 to 15 and MELD greater than 15, consistent with CTP classes B and C, respectively (**Table 3**).[10,35,65] This approach trades the discriminatory potential of the continuous

Table 3
Perioperative mortality among cirrhotic patients undergoing nontransplant surgery, by preoperative Model for End-stage Liver Disease score and corresponding equivalent Child-Turcotte-Pugh class

MELD Score Range	Mortality (%)	Equivalent CTP Class
<10	3–9	A
10–15	8–19	B
>15	29–57	C

Data from Refs.[10,35,65]

MELD range for the ease of use of categories. An example of the former was shown in a 2015 National Surgical Quality Improvement Program (NSQIP) study of 17,812 patients who underwent herniorrhaphy (inguinal or umbilical) or colectomy. By procedure, postoperative complication rates showed a 7.8%, 13.8%, and 11.6% increase, respectively, per 1-point increase in MELD score more than the mean MELD, approximately 8.5.[68] A near-linear relationship between MELD score and postoperative morbidity enabled the investigators to define this point-wise rule of thumb, which could be applied to each patient's preoperative MELD to describe score-specific expected postoperative outcome.

Despite the apparent attraction of granular mortality predictions that could be derived from preoperative MELD score, but not CTP, empirical analyses have yielded a wide range of heuristics. Teh and colleagues[13] performed the largest single-center retrospective study, of 772 cirrhotic patients undergoing major surgeries (digestive, orthopedic, cardiovascular), comparing them with 2 control groups: cirrhotic patients who had minor surgeries or who did not have surgery and were seen in the ambulatory care setting. MELD score was the most important univariate predictor of postoperative mortality at 30 days, 90 days, 1 year, and beyond, and remained significant on multivariate analysis. Throughout the first year after surgery, for patients with preoperative MELD greater than or equal to 8, each additional MELD score point was associated with a 14% to 15% increase in mortality, with a 6% additional per-point mortality risk thereafter. By comparison, Northup and colleagues[69] retrospectively reviewed a comparable mix of 140 surgical procedures in patients with cirrhosis and similarly found that MELD independently predicted 30-day postoperative mortality. However, the investigators found a much lower mortality predictive heuristic: each 1-point increase in the MELD up to a score of 20 was associated with a 1% increase in mortality risk in their study, and an additional 2% mortality risk per MELD point beyond that.

The wide difference in mortality prediction generated by these 2 major studies highlights the practical challenges of applying the MELD score as a continuous prognosticator for cirrhotic patients undergoing surgery. MELD score does generally correlate with postoperative mortality, but the absolute size of that effect is strongly influenced by study-specific parameters and not easily generalizable to other patients or surgical practices. Furthermore, both studies identified a significant inflection point in the overall linear relationship between preoperative MELD and postoperative mortality, but at very different absolute MELD scores (8 vs 20). A clinical interpretation of this statistical turning point may be the long-recognized difference between compensated and decompensated cirrhosis. The MELD score is calculated independent of clinical decompensation, which may occur within a range of low to moderate scores. Patients with high laboratory MELD scores are likely to have decompensated liver disease, but the inverse does not necessarily hold true. Some patients with decompensated liver disease have inappropriately low MELD scores that underrepresent the severity of their illness and underestimate their true mortality risk.[70–72]

Introduced into wide clinical practice recently, the MELD-Na has yet to be fully studied in the context of outcomes after general surgical procedures. Causey and colleagues[55] compared CTP, MELD, and MELD-Na among a retrospective cohort of 64 cirrhotic patients undergoing unspecified nontransplant operations. Although CTP was the most sensitive scoring system to 30-day mortality, MELD-Na was the best independent predictor of morbidity and 1-year mortality. Again, a near-linear relationship between preoperative MELD-Na score and predicted postoperative mortality was found (**Fig. 2**).

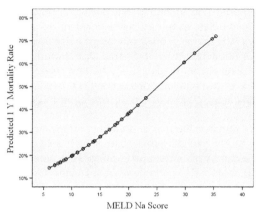

Fig. 2. Predicted probability curve for 1-year mortality after nontransplant surgery in cirrhotic patients shows a linear relationship with preoperative MELD-Na score. (*From* Causey MW, Steele SR, Farris Z, Lyle DS, Beitler AL. An assessment of different scoring systems in cirrhotic patients undergoing nontransplant surgery. *Am J Surg.* 2012;203(5):591; with permission.)

Portal Hypertension

Thrombocytopenia, which develops as portal hypertension progresses because of increasing platelet sequestration in the spleen, is widely viewed as a relative contraindication to hepatectomy in patients with hepatocellular carcinoma (HCC).[73] In one of the largest contemporary series, reported by Maithel and colleagues,[74] preoperative platelet count less than $150 \times 10^3/\mu L$ independently predicted major postoperative complications and 60-day mortality, and almost quadrupled the risk of postoperative hepatic insufficiency. The threshold count of less than $150 \times 10^3/\mu L$ was chosen by optimizing the receiver-operating characteristic model for postoperative liver insufficiency in the study cohort. Although CTP score, American Society of Anesthesiologists (ASA) physical status score of 4, and tumor burden beyond Milan criteria also showed prognostic value for certain outcomes, thrombocytopenia was the only factor predictive of all 3. Although nonhepatic surgery causes less direct insult to the liver, and therefore lower risk of postoperative liver insufficiency, similar platelet count thresholds, less than $150 \times 10^3/\mu L$ or less than $100 \times 10^3/\mu L$, were also associated with postoperative mortality in studies of general abdominal surgery in cirrhotic patients.[11,75]

Remarkably, successful hepatectomy with thrombocytopenia has been reported.[76–79] Cucchetti and colleagues[76] performed a propensity score matched analysis of patients with and without portal hypertension (defined as esophageal varices on endoscopy, or splenomegaly >12 cm with thrombocytopenia $<100 \times 10^3/\mu L$) undergoing hepatectomy for HCC. Overall, postoperative liver failure occurred more frequently in patients with portal hypertension, low serum albumin level, increased total bilirubin level, higher CTP and MELD scores, and in those who had more extensive hepatectomy or received intraoperative blood transfusion. However, when patients with and without portal hypertension were matched by all covariates for the outcome of postoperative liver failure, the investigators found that both groups had similar intraoperative course, postoperative complications, recovery from postoperative liver dysfunction, hospital length of stay, and mortality. Multivariate logistic regression in matched patients showed that only MELD and extent of hepatectomy, but not presence of portal hypertension, independently predicted postoperative liver failure. In this and several other studies, even clinically significant portal hypertension did not change postoperative liver failure or other outcomes when liver function was well preserved and extent of hepatectomy comparable. Although thrombocytopenia is still widely considered a relative contraindication to hepatic resection, these studies suggest that severity of liver dysfunction does not entirely overlap with degree of portal hypertension. In such cases, degree of hepatic reserve is more prognostic of postoperative outcome.

Few studies have examined the role of portal hypertension on nonhepatic surgical outcomes. A recent study by Kadry and colleagues[80] analyzed NSQIP data for all 1574 patients with esophageal varices who underwent general surgery operations over an 8-year period, matched to patients without varices. Overall, patients with varices had a higher risk of complications and death than those without varices. On multivariate analysis adjusting for patient characteristics, low-MELD patients (which they defined as MELD $\leq$ 15) with varices still had almost double the adjusted odds of death compared with patients without varices. The investigators concluded that portal hypertension is associated with significant additional risk of complications and death after surgery, even in apparently well-compensated low-MELD patients.

American Society of Anesthesiologists Physical Status Classification

Originally described in 1941 as a statistical tool for collecting data in anesthesiology, the ASA score has become synonymous with preoperative risk assessment (**Table 4**).[81,82] Inherently subjective and dependent on preoperatively available medical information,[83] the ASA score has shown variable inter-rater reliability[84–86] but has still proved to be a valuable predictor of general postoperative outcomes.[87] Among cirrhotic patients, several retrospective studies of nontransplant surgery have found ASA score greater than 3 or 4 to predict mortality.[8,10,13] In the largest study, by Teh and colleagues[13] described earlier, ASA score was the strongest predictor of 7-day postoperative mortality, and an ASA score of 4 conferred an additional mortality risk equivalent to a 5.5-point increase in the MELD score.

Malnutrition

Nutritional status, part of the original Child-Turcotte grading system, was recognized early on as an important determinant of mortality risk in cirrhotic patients undergoing surgery.[53,88] Orloff and colleagues[89] performed a prospective study of 138 consecutive patients with alcoholic cirrhosis undergoing emergency portacaval shunting for bleeding esophageal varices, and found approximately 50% higher mortality among patients with severe muscle wasting compared with those with mild or moderate muscle wasting. Another early study of 100 consecutive shunt surgeries defined

Table 4		
American Society of Anesthesiologists physical status classification		
ASA Class	**Description**	
1	Normal healthy patient	
2	Patient with mild systemic disease	
3	Patient with activity-limiting systemic disease	
4	Patient with severe systemic disease that is a constant threat to life	
5	Moribund patient who is not expected to survive 24 h without the operation	
6	Brain-dead patient whose organs are being procured for donation	

preoperative malnutrition by observed muscle wasting, cachexia, or greater than 10% weight loss over the prior 6 months.[90] In that cohort of patients, among whom 75% had alcohol-related liver disease and 75% underwent emergency surgery, malnutrition was found to be associated with 30-day and 1-year postoperative mortality. A preoperative diagnosis of malnutrition was also found to be significantly associated with postoperative complications and 30-day mortality in a study of nonshunt abdominal surgeries.[54]

The lack of a simple, widely available, accurate, and reproducible method of measuring nutritional status is a major challenge to using it in preoperative risk stratification. Widespread measures of nutrition in the general population are inaccurate in patients with liver disease: body mass index and percentage weight change over time may be affected by fluid retention and ascites; levels of biochemical markers such as serum albumin, prealbumin, and transferrin are decreased because of the liver's impaired synthetic function irrespective of nutritional status. The European Society for Clinical Nutrition and Metabolism (ESPEN) 2006 guideline in liver disease recommends using bedside methods such as subjective global assessment (SGA), anthropometric measurements such as midarm circumference or triceps skin thickness, or handgrip strength to evaluate for malnutrition.[91] SGA is a clinical assessment tool that reviews dietary intake, gastrointestinal symptoms, weight change, and physical examination findings of sarcopenia and ascites. It is simple to administer and does not require specialized equipment. A prospective study of 541 outpatients with cirrhosis or chronic hepatitis found that handgrip dynamometry was more accurate than anthropometric measurements at diagnosing malnutrition, compared with SGA as the standard.[92] Handgrip strength has the benefit of being a functional test, unlike SGA, but does require specialized equipment, a trained operator to do the assessment, and a patient who can follow instructions. In studies of liver transplant outcomes, severe malnutrition assessed by SGA has been associated with postoperative infection, respiratory failure, and intensive care unit and hospital lengths of stay.[93–95] More studies are needed to determine whether these measures of malnutrition are prognostic in cirrhotic patients undergoing nontransplant operations.

Coagulopathy

Cirrhotic patients have an abnormal coagulation profile caused by decreased hepatic synthesis of both procoagulant and anticoagulant factors. Consumptive coagulopathy is also relevant perioperatively when there is a risk of blood loss. It is worth noting that the CTP and MELD scores, which originally included PT and INR, respectively, were described in the setting of invasive procedures (shunt surgery, esophageal transection, TIPS placement) for recent or active esophageal variceal hemorrhage.[49,53,59] Prolonged PT, INR, and intraoperative transfusion of fresh frozen plasma have all been associated with increased postoperative mortality in patients with cirrhosis.[5,8,9,35,54,75] However, meaningful prognostication based on abnormal coagulation parameters is limited because studies have used varied cutoffs for PT and INR, or focused on CTP or MELD instead of their individual components. As a therapeutic target, abnormal coagulation parameters do not necessarily portend autoanticoagulation in patients with cirrhosis, and the decision to correct them by transfusion is best informed by the clinical context.[96] In cirrhotic patients with active surgical bleeding, our transfusion practice is guided by viscoelastic point-of-care testing available in the operating room, in conjunction with conventional coagulation tests. Depending on the severity of ongoing bleeding, transfusion may be initiated for a platelet count less than $50 \times 10^3/\mu L$, INR greater than 2, and fibrinogen level less than 100 mg/dL. Hypothermia and acidosis also exacerbate coagulopathy and must be assiduously corrected.

Related to coagulopathy, blood loss and the need for intraoperative blood transfusion have also been associated with inferior outcomes in several studies of general surgery in patients with cirrhosis.[10,35,54] del Olmo and colleagues[9] compared 135 cirrhotic patients undergoing nonhepatic surgery with 86 matched surgical patients without liver disease, and were the first to show that patients with cirrhosis need intraoperative blood transfusion more frequently than those without, about twice as often in their study. That study also showed that intraoperative blood transfusion was an independent risk factor for developing cirrhosis-related complications. In a study of 138 abdominal surgeries in patients with cirrhosis, Neeff and colleagues[35] found that patients who needed any intraoperative blood transfusion had higher postoperative mortality (43%, vs 5% if no transfusion) and that intraoperative transfusion was a multivariate predictor of mortality. The exact mechanism of how intraoperative transfusion increases postoperative risk is unclear, but may reflect greater surgical stress caused by the technical difficulty of the operation; immune sequelae of transfusion in patients who are already immunocompromised because of their liver disease[97]; or cirrhosis-related factors that may increase the expected blood loss during a given operation, such as coagulopathy, friable portosystemic collateral vessels that are not a part of normal surgical anatomy, and increased portal pressure.

Renal Dysfunction

Renal dysfunction is a frequent complication of chronic liver disease, and multiple studies of surgery in patients with cirrhosis have found increased serum creatinine level to be predictive of postoperative mortality.[8,11] However, as with coagulopathy (discussed earlier), a range of cutoff values from greater than or equal to 1.1 to 1.5 mg/dL have been tested, and many studies have favored testing MELD rather than its individual components. In addition, patients with chronic liver disease may have renal dysfunction despite a serum creatinine level within the normal laboratory range because of malnutrition and sarcopenia.

Emergency Surgery

Emergency surgery has higher morbidity and mortality compared with elective. In cirrhotic patients, mortalities after emergency operations range from 19% to 57% compared with 6% to 18% if not emergent (**Table 5**).[7,35,54,65] Cirrhotic patients undergoing emergency operations have higher CTP and MELD scores.[13,35] Several studies have found that emergent operation remained predictive of perioperative mortality on multivariate analysis when patient factors such as severity of liver disease have been controlled for.[10,35,55,80] Emergent nonshunt abdominal operations in early studies were most commonly for perforated viscus caused by peptic ulcer disease or ischemic bowel, whereas recent series have reported fewer of these relative to incarcerated hernias.[7,10,35,54] These retrospective studies likely reflect a selection bias because patients with decompensated liver disease may not be offered emergency surgery depending on how moribund they are on presentation. Cirrhotic patients undergoing electively planned operations likely represent a different risk profile that extends beyond the operation chosen for them and the elective, rather than emergent, circumstances.

STRATEGIES FOR MITIGATING PERIOPERATIVE RISK
Specialist Teams

Posing a unique pathophysiologic challenge and the potential to decompensate quickly, patients with portal hypertension and cirrhosis may benefit from care by

Table 5
Indications and mortality after emergent surgery in patients with cirrhosis

Study	Indications for Emergent Operation	Emergent Operations in Study (%)	Mortality After Emergent vs Elective Operations (%)
Garrison et al,[54] 1984	PUD, diverticulitis, trauma, strangulated hernia, exploration for infection	42	57 vs 10
Mansour et al,[7] 1997	GIB, perforated viscus (PUD, colonic), ischemic bowel, trauma	26	50 vs 18
Farnsworth et al,[65] 2004	NA	40	19 vs 17
Telem et al,[10] 2010	Incarcerated umbilical hernia, colonic perforation, GIB	32	25 vs 6
Neeff et al,[35] 2011	Perforated viscus, GIB, incarcerated hernia	49	47 vs 9
Causey et al,[55] 2012	NA	16	20 vs 9

Abbreviations: GIB, gastrointestinal bleeding; NA, not available; PUD, peptic ulcer disease.

specialists, particularly those who may facilitate their access to lifesaving liver transplant. Telem and colleagues[10] reviewed 100 general surgery operations in patients with cirrhosis. They reported similar postoperative complications rates compared with the literature, but remarkably low mortalities overall and by CTP class, despite half of the patients being CTP class B or C, one-third of operations being emergent, and a case mix including major operations such as colectomy and pancreaticoduodenectomy. The investigators cite their institutional volume, experience with intraoperative and postoperative management of cirrhotic patients, and their model of multidisciplinary care as important factors in their good outcomes. The ability to anticipate potential risk preoperatively and minimize it or delay surgery, and the ability to recognize morbidity early and take immediate steps to rescue and prevent mortality, are keys to minimizing perioperative complications and death. These benefits have been found in specialization for other operations, disease processes, and surgical patient groups, and more research is needed for patients with cirrhosis.[98–101]

Nutritional Optimization

Nutritional supplementation may improve outcomes in patients with cirrhosis, and studies of hepatectomy patients suggest perioperative benefit as well. A meta-analysis found evidence that tube feeding may decrease overall mortality in patients with chronic liver disease, formulas featuring branched-chain amino acids may improve hepatic encephalopathy, and oral supplemental nutrition may decrease the development of ascites and reduce overall disease complications.[102] ESPEN consensus guidelines recommend oral nutritional supplements and tube feeding for patients with chronic liver disease based on studies showing improved nutritional status and survival.[91] Evidence is of a lower grade regarding parenteral nutrition, which ESPEN recommends is safe, may improve mental status in patients with chronic liver disease, and may reduce perioperative complications.[103] Although studies of nutritional support in cirrhotic patients undergoing nonhepatic general surgery are scarce, research in patients undergoing hepatectomy suggest benefit. A randomized controlled trial of perioperative parenteral supplementation including branched-chain amino acids and medium chain triglycerides showed decreased postoperative complications in 124 patients undergoing hepatectomy for HCC.[104] Although only 58% of patients had cirrhosis and presence of portal hypertension was not mentioned, benefits were seen predominantly in the cirrhotic patients and included decreased septic complications and postoperative ascites, and better preservation of postoperative liver function and weight. Other trials comparing different formulas of parenteral nutrition for 7 days after hepatectomy for HCC found no difference between branched-chain and regular amino acids, but did show some benefit associated with high-glucose recipes, such as improved nitrogen balance, serum transaminase levels, and postoperative complications.[105–108]

Laparoscopy

Select patients with cirrhosis can safely undergo laparoscopic surgery. Procedures such as laparoscopic appendectomy and cholecystectomy are the most commonly reported in the literature, although laparoscopic colectomy and distal gastrectomy in cirrhotic patients have also been reviewed with favorable results.[109] With the caveat that studies have been primarily retrospective, nonrandomized, and focused on CTP class A patients, laparoscopy in cirrhotic patients has been associated with less postoperative pain, shorter postoperative hospital stay, and fewer wound infections and bleeding complications compared with open surgery.[10,64,110–112] Compared with noncirrhotic patients, a retrospective Nationwide Inpatient Survey (NIS) cohort of patients with cirrhosis undergoing laparoscopic appendectomy found similar length of stay, inpatient mortality, and postoperative complications.[113]

In laparoscopy, the decision to convert to an open surgical approach signals increased technical difficulty and the potential for greater perioperative complications. A study of NIS data for cirrhotic patients undergoing cholecystectomy compared laparoscopic versus open approaches and found a 14% rate of conversion, higher than previously reported in single-center reports.[112] Cholecystectomies that were laparoscopic converted to open were similar to open cases in having higher rates of blood transfusion, postoperative bleeding and infection, and reoperation compared with laparoscopic procedures. Despite this, postoperative liver failure and mortalities were similar between laparoscopic and laparoscopic conversion cases, compared with rates that were 5 to 6 times higher for open operations. The investigators concluded that laparoscopy should be the preferred initial approach in cirrhotic patients. Even when conversion is necessary, patients can be effectively rescued to maintain low perioperative mortality.

Management of Ascites and Neoadjuvant Transjugular Intrahepatic Portosystemic Shunt

The presence of preoperative ascites is an independent predictor of postoperative complications and death.[8,10,55] Although this is likely a reflection of the increased risk of portal hypertension, the mechanical pressure of ascites does increase the risk of abdominal wound dehiscence, leakage of ascites fluid, and secondary infection. Ascites may also develop newly or worsen postoperatively in patients who have a degree of hepatic decompensation as a result of surgery.

Various methods of managing ascites perioperatively have been described. Peritoneovenous shunting is seldom used anymore. Temporary placement of an abdominal drain or catheter allows frequent drainage of postoperative ascites. The indwelling foreign body increases the risk of introducing infection into the peritoneal cavity and seeding the ascites. Alternatively, repeated large-volume paracentesis (LVP) can be performed, at the risk of bleeding, visceral injury, or introducing infection with each

Table 6
Prophylactic transjugular intrahepatic portosystemic shunt placement in cirrhotic patients before undergoing nonhepatic surgery

Study	Planned Operation	N	CTP Class, N (A/B/C)	Mean MELD (Range)	Median Interval from TIPS to Surgery (d) (Range)	Complications (N)	1-y Mortality (%)
Azoulay, et al,[116] 2001	AAA repair, CA resections (renal, colonic, esophageal), Hartmann reversal	7	6/0/1	NA	90 (30–150)	Transfusion (3), liver failure (1)	14.3
Gil et al,[127] 2004	CA resections (gastric, colonic pancreatic)	3	2/1/0	NA	30 (14–45)	Right heart failure (1), HE (1)	0
Vinet et al,[128] 2006	Colectomy, antrectomy, pancreaticoduodenectomy	18	NA	NA	72[a]	Transfusion (6), HE (4), liver failure (3), ascites leak (2), ARDS (2)	44.4
Schlenker et al,[129] 2009	CA resections (renal, gastric, colonic, ovarian)	7	3/4/0	11 (7–16)	13 (1–32)	Infection (3), new ascites (1)	0
Kim et al,[4] 2009	AVR, colectomy, herniorrhaphy	6	2/3/1	11.7 (7–15)	22 (6–36)	HE (3), infection (2)	0
Menahem et al,[130] 2015	Colectomy, proctectomy with TME	8	3/2/3	10.4 (7–15)	39 (7–63)	Anastomotic leak (2), ascites (3), liver failure (1)	25

Abbreviations: AAA, abdominal aortic aneurysm; ARDS, acute respiratory distress syndrome; AVR, aortic valve replacement; CA, cancer; HE, hepatic encephalopathy; TME, total mesorectal excision.
[a] Mean reported, no range given.

tap. TIPS placement is the preferred approach in patients who can tolerate the procedure and have the opportunity to defer surgery. A randomized study comparing large-volume paracentesis with TIPS placement for cirrhotic patients with recurrent or refractory ascites showed a significantly higher rate of resolution of ascites at 3 months, with consequent improvement in CTP score, and higher survival with TIPS compared with LVP.[114] Laboratory measures of liver function and the incidence of hepatic encephalopathy did not differ between baseline and follow-up for either group. TIPS placement independently predicted transplant-free survival.

Beyond the management of ascites, TIPS placement has been studied as a means to decompress portal hypertension preoperatively. This approach (optimizing patients by decompressing their portal hypertension, effectively downgrading CTP class B patients to CTP class A) was originally described in the context of portacaval shunt surgery being combined with revision of biliodigestive anastomosis and other abdominal surgery.[115] The goal was to make surgical treatment options available to patients who would otherwise be considered too high risk for the operation they needed. Although TIPS is routinely used as secondary prophylaxis for recurrent variceal bleed or treatment of refractory ascites or hepatic hydrothorax after diuretics have failed, its use as primary prophylaxis to optimize patients specifically for major surgery is not yet widely accepted. The first prospective report of neoadjuvant TIPS placement in 2001 described 7 patients who underwent TIPS ahead of planned major surgery, including colectomy for cancer and repair of abdominal aortic aneurysm.[116] Mean HVPG decreased from 18 to 9 mm Hg, and there were no TIPS-related complications. Six patients had their planned operations at a median of 3 months after TIPS placement, whereas the seventh was found to have unresectable gastric adenocarcinoma of the cardia and was treated palliatively. Only 2 patients needed blood transfusion intraoperatively, and there was 1 perioperative mortality. This uncontrolled study and others have reported safe TIPS placement and low perioperative mortality (**Table 6**). However, there is no consensus on the optimal timing of surgery after TIPS placement, and more prospective studies will be needed to determine whether TIPS itself changes perioperative outcomes.

Alternatives to Surgery

Patient selection remains a critical means of risk reduction, and alternatives to surgery should be considered in patients with high risk of poor outcome. In small single-institution cohorts, endoscopic stenting of the cystic duct for symptomatic cholelithiasis is safe and effective in patients with decompensated cirrhosis awaiting liver transplant.[117,118] Percutaneous cholecystostomy has also been used successfully in patients with decompensated cirrhosis.[119,120]

SUMMARY

Patients with portal hypertension will increasingly present for nontransplant surgery because of the increasing incidence of, and improvements in, long-term survival for chronic liver disease. Because of the systemic pathophysiology of liver disease, these patients have increased perioperative morbidity and mortality. Preoperative assessment should focus on understanding the causes and severity of liver disease. Modifiable causes of liver injury may be addressed, and drawing the key distinction between compensated and decompensated cirrhosis may help health care providers anticipate potential perioperative concerns. Risk stratification, which is crucial to preparing patients and their families for surgery, relies on scores such as CTP and MELD to translate liver disease severity into quantified outcomes predictions. Other enduring risk factors for postoperative complications include portal hypertension, malnutrition, coagulopathy and bleeding, renal dysfunction, and emergency surgery. Strategies to mitigate perioperative risk include care by specialists in liver disease, nutritional optimization, a plan for ascites management and decompression of portal hypertension such as by TIPS placement, and careful patient selection.

REFERENCES

1. Xu J, Murphy S, Kochanek K, et al. Deaths: final data for 2016. In: Hurlburt J, editor. National vital statistics reports, vol. 67. Hyattsville (MD): Division of Vital Statistics, National Center for Health Statistics; 2018. p. 1–76.
2. Guirguis J, Chhatwal J, Dasarathy J, et al. Clinical impact of alcohol-related cirrhosis in the next decade: estimates based on current epidemiological trends in the United States. Alcohol Clin Exp Res 2015;39(11):2085–94.
3. Scaglione S, Kliethermes S, Cao G, et al. The epidemiology of cirrhosis in the United States: a population-based study. J Clin Gastroenterol 2015;49(8):690–6.
4. Kim JJ, Dasika NL, Yu E, et al. Cirrhotic patients with a transjugular intrahepatic portosystemic shunt undergoing major extrahepatic surgery. J Clin Gastroenterol 2009;43(6):574–9.
5. Aranha GV, Sontag SJ, Greenlee HB. Cholecystectomy in cirrhotic patients: a formidable operation. Am J Surg 1982;143(1):55–60.
6. Leonetti JP, Aranha GV, Wilkinson WA, et al. Umbilical herniorrhaphy in cirrhotic patients. Arch Surg 1984;119(4):442–5.
7. Mansour A, Watson W, Shayani V, et al. Abdominal operations in patients with cirrhosis: still a major surgical challenge. Surgery 1997;122(4):730–6.
8. Ziser A, Plevak DJ, Wiesner RH, et al. Morbidity and mortality in cirrhotic patients undergoing anesthesia and surgery. Anesthesiology 1999;90(1):42–53.
9. del Olmo JA, Flor-Lorente B, Flor-Civera B, et al. Risk factors for nonhepatic surgery in patients with cirrhosis. World J Surg 2003;27(6):647–52.
10. Telem DA, Schiano T, Goldstone R, et al. Factors that predict outcome of abdominal operations in patients with advanced cirrhosis. Clin Gastroenterol Hepatol 2010;8(5):451–7.
11. Neeff HP, Streule GC, Drognitz O, et al. Early mortality and long-term survival after abdominal surgery in patients with liver cirrhosis. Surgery 2014;155(4):623–32.
12. Modi A, Vohra HA, Barlow CW. Do patients with liver cirrhosis undergoing cardiac surgery have acceptable outcomes? Interact Cardiovasc Thorac Surg 2010;11(5):630–4.
13. Teh SH, Nagorney DM, Stevens SR, et al. Risk factors for mortality after surgery in patients with cirrhosis. Gastroenterology 2007;132(4):1261–9.
14. Meunier K, Mucci S, Quentin V, et al. Colorectal surgery in cirrhotic patients: assessment of operative morbidity and mortality. Dis Colon Rectum 2008;51(8):1225–31.
15. Nguyen GC, Correia AJ, Thuluvath PJ. The impact of cirrhosis and portal hypertension on mortality following colorectal surgery: a nationwide, population-based study. Dis Colon Rectum 2009;52(8):1367–74.
16. Csikesz NG, Nguyen LN, Tseng JF, et al. Nationwide volume and mortality after elective surgery in cirrhotic patients. J Am Coll Surg 2009;208(1):96–103.
17. Nathan H, Cameron JL, Choti MA, et al. The volume-outcomes effect in hepato-pancreato-biliary surgery: hospital versus surgeon contributions and specificity of the relationship. J Am Coll Surg 2009;208(4):528–38.

18. de Cleva R, Herman P, D'albuquerque LA, et al. Pre-and postoperative systemic hemodynamic evaluation in patients subjected to esophagogastric devascularization plus splenectomy and distal splenorenal shunt: a comparative study in schistomomal portal hypertension. World J Gastroenterol 2007;13(41):5471–5.

19. Brand M, Prodehl L, Ede CJ. Surgical portosystemic shunts versus transjugular intrahepatic portosystemic shunt for variceal haemorrhage in people with cirrhosis. Cochrane Database Syst Rev 2018;(10):CD001023.

20. Ede CJ, Nikolova D, Brand M. Surgical portosystemic shunts versus devascularisation procedures for prevention of variceal rebleeding in people with hepatosplenic schistosomiasis. Cochrane Database Syst Rev 2018;(8):CD011717.

21. Ferreira FG, Ribeiro MA, de Fátima Santos M, et al. Doppler ultrasound could predict varices progression and rebleeding after portal hypertension surgery: lessons from 146 EGDS and 10 years of follow-up. World J Surg 2009;33(10): 2136–43.

22. Silva Neto WBD, Tredicci TM, Coelho FF, et al. Portal pressure decrease after esophagogastric devascularization and splenectomy in schistosomiasis: long-term varices behavior, rebleeding rate, and role of endoscopic treatment. Arq Gastroenterol 2018;55(2):170–4.

23. Møller S, Henriksen JH, Bendtsen F. Extrahepatic complications to cirrhosis and portal hypertension: haemodynamic and homeostatic aspects. World J Gastroenterol 2014;20(42):15499–517.

24. Verbeeck RK. Pharmacokinetics and dosage adjustment in patients with hepatic dysfunction. Eur J Clin Pharmacol 2008;64(12):1147–61.

25. Starczewska MH, Mon W, Shirley P. Anaesthesia in patients with liver disease. Curr Opin Anaesthesiol 2017;30(3):392–8.

26. Dwyer JP, Jayasekera C, Nicoll A. Analgesia for the cirrhotic patient: a literature review and recommendations. J Gastroenterol Hepatol 2014;29(7):1356–60.

27. Northup PG, McMahon MM, Ruhl AP, et al. Coagulopathy does not fully protect hospitalized cirrhosis patients from peripheral venous thromboembolism. Am J Gastroenterol 2006;101(7):1524–8.

28. Barclay SM, Jeffres MN, Nguyen K, et al. Evaluation of pharmacologic prophylaxis for venous thromboembolism in patients with chronic liver disease. Pharmacotherapy 2013;33(4):375–82.

29. Bonnel AR, Bunchorntavakul C, Reddy KR. Immune dysfunction and infections in patients with cirrhosis. Clin Gastroenterol Hepatol 2011;9(9):727–38.

30. Edwards AF, Forest DJ. Preoperative laboratory testing. Anesthesiol Clin 2018; 36(4):493–507.

31. Ioannou GN, Boyko EJ, Lee SP. The prevalence and predictors of elevated serum aminotransferase activity in the United States in 1999–2002. Am J Gastroenterol 2006;101(1):76–82.

32. de Lédinghen V, Combes M, Trouette H, et al. Should a liver biopsy be done in patients with subclinical chronically elevated transaminases? Eur J Gastroenterol Hepatol 2004;16(9):879–83.

33. Benarroch-Gampel J, Sheffield KM, Duncan CB, et al. Preoperative laboratory testing in patients undergoing elective, low-risk ambulatory surgery. Ann Surg 2012;256(3):518–28.

34. Jan A, Narwaria M, Mahawar KK. A systematic review of bariatric surgery in patients with liver cirrhosis. Obes Surg 2015;25(8):1518–26.

35. Neeff H, Mariaskin D, Spangenberg HC, et al. Perioperative mortality after non-hepatic general surgery in patients with liver cirrhosis: an analysis of 138

operations in the 2000s using Child and MELD scores. J Gastrointest Surg 2011; 15(1):1–11.

36. Kwo PY, Cohen SM, Lim JK. ACG clinical guideline: evaluation of abnormal liver chemistries. Am J Gastroenterol 2017;112(1):18–35.

37. D'Amico G, Garcia-Tsao G, Pagliaro L. Natural history and prognostic indicators of survival in cirrhosis: a systematic review of 118 studies. J Hepatol 2006;44(1): 217–31.

38. Ripoll C, Groszmann R, Garcia–Tsao G, et al. Hepatic venous pressure gradient predicts clinical decompensation in patients with compensated cirrhosis. Gastroenterology 2007;133(2):481–8.

39. Fleming KM, Aithal GP, Card TR, et al. The rate of decompensation and clinical progression of disease in people with cirrhosis: a cohort study. Aliment Pharmacol Ther 2010;32(11–12):1343–50.

40. Fleming KM, Aithal GP, Card TR, et al. All-cause mortality in people with cirrhosis compared with the general population: a population-based cohort study. Liver Int 2012;32(1):79–84.

41. Jepsen P, Ott P, Andersen PK, et al. Clinical course of alcoholic liver cirrhosis: a Danish population-based cohort study. Hepatology 2010;51(5):1675–82.

42. Ginés P, Quintero E, Arroyo V, et al. Compensated cirrhosis: natural history and prognostic factors. Hepatology 1987;7(1):122–8.

43. D'Amico G, Pasta L, Morabito A, et al. Competing risks and prognostic stages of cirrhosis: a 25-year inception cohort study of 494 patients. Aliment Pharmacol Ther 2014;39(10):1180–93.

44. Greenwood SM, Leffler CT, Minkowitz S. The increased mortality rate of open liver biopsy in alcoholic hepatitis. Surg Gynecol Obstet 1972;134(4):600–4.

45. Strauss AA, Strauss SF, Schwartz AH, et al. Liver decompression by drainage of the common bile duct in subacute and chronic jaundice: report of seventy-three cases with hepatitis or concomitant biliary duct infection as cause. Am J Surg 1959;97(2):137–40.

46. Harville DD, Summerskill WH. Surgery in acute hepatitis: causes and effects. JAMA 1963;184(4):257–61.

47. Eslam M, Ampuero J, Jover M, et al. Predicting portal hypertension and variceal bleeding using non-invasive measurements of metabolic variables. Ann Hepatol 2013;12(4):588–98.

48. Jiménez JV, Carrillo-Pérez DL, Rosado-Canto R, et al. Electrolyte and acid-base disturbances in end-stage liver disease: a physiopathological approach. Dig Dis Sci 2017;62(8):1855–71.

49. Pugh RN, Murray-Lyon IM, Dawson JL, et al. Transection of the oesophagus for bleeding oesophageal varices. Br J Surg 1973;60(8):646–9.

50. Sugiura M, Futagawa S. A new technique for treating esophageal varices. J Thorac Cardiovasc Surg 1973;66(5):677–85.

51. Busuttil RW. Selective and nonselective shunts for variceal bleeding: a prospective study of 103 patients. Am J Surg 1984;148(1):27–35.

52. Orozco H, Mercado MA. The evolution of portal hypertension surgery: lessons from 1000 operations and 50 years' experience. Arch Surg 2000;135(12): 1389–93.

53. Child CG, Turcotte JG. Surgery and portal hypertension. Major Probl Clin Surg 1964;1:1–85.

54. Garrison RN, Cryer HM, Howard DA, et al. Clarification of risk factors for abdominal operations in patients with hepatic cirrhosis. Ann Surg 1984;199(6):648–55.

55. Causey MW, Steele SR, Farris Z, et al. An assessment of different scoring systems in cirrhotic patients undergoing nontransplant surgery. Am J Surg 2012; 203(5):589–93.
56. Christensen E, Schlichting P, Fauerholdt L, et al. Prognostic value of Child-Turcotte criteria in medically treated cirrhosis. Hepatology 1984;4(3):430–5.
57. Infante-Rivard C, Esnaola S, Villeneuve JP. Clinical and statistical validity of conventional prognostic factors in predicting short-term survival among cirrhotics. Hepatology 1987;7(4):660–4.
58. Kamath PS, Wiesner RH, Malinchoc M, et al. A model to predict survival in patients with end-stage liver disease. Hepatology 2001;33(2):464–70.
59. Malinchoc M, Kamath PS, Gordon FD, et al. A model to predict poor survival in patients undergoing transjugular intrahepatic portosystemic shunts. Hepatology 2000;31(4):864–71.
60. Kim WR, Biggins SW, Kremers WK, et al. Hyponatremia and mortality among patients on the liver-transplant waiting list. N Engl J Med 2008;359(10):1018–26.
61. Biggins SW, Kim WR, Terrault NA, et al. Evidence-based incorporation of serum sodium concentration into MELD. Gastroenterology 2006;130(6):1652–60.
62. Wiesner R, Edwards E, Freeman R, et al. Model for end-stage liver disease (MELD) and allocation of donor livers. Gastroenterology 2003;124(1):91–6.
63. Said A, Williams J, Holden J, et al. Model for end stage liver disease score predicts mortality across a broad spectrum of liver disease. J Hepatol 2004;40(6): 897–903.
64. Befeler AS, Palmer DE, Hoffman M, et al. The safety of intra-abdominal surgery in patients with cirrhosis: model for end-stage liver disease score is superior to Child-Turcotte-Pugh classification in predicting outcome. Arch Surg 2005; 140(7):650–4.
65. Farnsworth N, Fagan SP, Berger DH, et al. Child-Turcotte-Pugh versus MELD score as a predictor of outcome after elective and emergent surgery in cirrhotic patients. Am J Surg 2004;188(5):580–3.
66. Costa BP, Sousa FC, Serôdio M, et al. Value of MELD and MELD-based indices in surgical risk evaluation of cirrhotic patients: retrospective analysis of 190 cases. World J Surg 2009;33(8):1711–9.
67. Merion RM, Schaubel DE, Dykstra DM, et al. The survival benefit of liver transplantation. Am J Transplant 2005;5(2):307–13.
68. Zielsdorf SM, Kubasiak JC, Janssen I, et al. A NSQIP analysis of MELD and perioperative outcomes in general surgery. Am Surg 2015;81(8):755–9.
69. Northup PG, Wanamaker RC, Lee VD, et al. Model for End-Stage Liver Disease (MELD) predicts nontransplant surgical mortality in patients with cirrhosis. Ann Surg 2005;242(2):244–51.
70. Yoo HY, Edwin D, Thuluvath PJ. Relationship of the model for end-stage liver disease (MELD) scale to hepatic encephalopathy, as defined by electroencephalography and neuropsychometric testing, and ascites. Am J Gastroenterol 2003;98(6):1395–9.
71. Heuman DM, Abou-Assi SG, Habib A, et al. Persistent ascites and low serum sodium identify patients with cirrhosis and low MELD scores who are at high risk for early death. Hepatology 2004;40(4):802–10.
72. Atiemo K, Skaro A, Maddur H, et al. Mortality risk factors among patients with cirrhosis and a low model for end-stage liver disease sodium score ($\leq$15): an analysis of liver transplant allocation policy using aggregated electronic health record data. Am J Transplant 2017;17(9):2410–9.

73. Bruix J, Castells A, Bosch J, et al. Surgical resection of hepatocellular carcinoma in cirrhotic patients: prognostic value of preoperative portal pressure. Gastroenterology 1996;111(4):1018–22.
74. Maithel SK, Kneuertz PJ, Kooby DA, et al. Importance of low preoperative platelet count in selecting patients for resection of hepatocellular carcinoma: a multi-institutional analysis. J Am Coll Surg 2011;212(4):638–48.
75. Perkins L, Jeffries M, Patel T. Utility of preoperative scores for predicting morbidity after cholecystectomy in patients with cirrhosis. Clin Gastroenterol Hepatol 2004;2(12):1123–8.
76. Cucchetti A, Ercolani G, Vivarelli M, et al. Is portal hypertension a contraindication to hepatic resection? Ann Surg 2009;250(6):922–8.
77. Sugimachi K, Ikeda Y, Tomikawa M, et al. Appraisal of hepatic resection in the treatment of hepatocellular carcinoma with severe thrombocytopenia. World J Surg 2008;32(6):1077–81.
78. Capussotti L, Ferrero A, Viganò L, et al. Portal hypertension: contraindication to liver surgery? World J Surg 2006;30(6):992–9.
79. Santambrogio R, Kluger MD, Costa M, et al. Hepatic resection for hepatocellular carcinoma in patients with Child–Pugh's A cirrhosis: is clinical evidence of portal hypertension a contraindication? HPB (Oxford) 2013;15(1):78–84.
80. Kadry Z, Schaefer EW, Shah RA, et al. Portal hypertension: an underestimated entity? Ann Surg 2016;263(5):986–91.
81. Saklad M. Grading of patients for surgical procedures. Anesthesiology 1941; 2(3):281–4.
82. Dripps RD, Lamont A, Eckenhoff JE. The role of anesthesia in surgical mortality. JAMA 1961;178(3):261–6.
83. Marian AA, Bayman EO, Gillett A, et al. The influence of the type and design of the anesthesia record on ASA physical status scores in surgical patients: paper records vs. electronic anesthesia records. BMC Med Inform Decis Mak 2016; 16(1):29.
84. Ranta S, Hynynen M, Tammisto T. A survey of the ASA physical status classification: significant variation in allocation among Finnish anaesthesiologists. Acta Anaesthesiol Scand 1997;41(5):629–32.
85. Sankar A, Johnson SR, Beattie WS, et al. Reliability of the American Society of Anesthesiologists physical status scale in clinical practice. Br J Anaesth 2014; 113(3):424–32.
86. Shichino T, Hirao M, Haga Y. Inter-rater reliability of the American Society of Anesthesiologists physical status rating for emergency gastrointestinal surgery. Acute Med Surg 2017;4(2):161–5.
87. Hackett NJ, De Oliveira GS, Jain UK, et al. ASA class is a reliable independent predictor of medical complications and mortality following surgery. Int J Surg 2015;18:184–90.
88. Merli M, Nicolini G, Angeloni S, et al. Malnutrition is a risk factor in cirrhotic patients undergoing surgery. Nutrition 2002;18(11–12):978–86.
89. Orloff MJ, Charters AC 3rd, Chandler JG, et al. Portacaval shunt as emergency procedure in unselected patients with alcoholic cirrhosis. Surg Gynecol Obstet 1975;141(1):59–68.
90. Cello JP, Deveney KE, Trunkey DD, et al. Factors influencing survival after therapeutic shunts: results of a discriminant function and linear logistic regressions analysis. Am J Surg 1981;141(2):257–65.
91. Plauth M, Cabré E, Riggio O, et al. ESPEN guidelines on enteral nutrition: liver disease. Clin Nutr 2006;25(2):285–94.

92. Sharma P, Rauf A, Matin A, et al. Handgrip strength as an important bed side tool to assess malnutrition in patient with liver disease. J Clin Exp Hepatol 2017;7(1):16–22.
93. Merli M, Giusto M, Gentili F, et al. Nutritional status: its influence on the outcome of patients undergoing liver transplantation. Liver Int 2010;30(2):208–14.
94. Pikul J, Sharpe MD, Lowndes R, et al. Degree of preoperative malnutrition is predictive of postoperative morbidity and mortality in liver transplant recipients. Transplantation 1994;57(3):469–72.
95. Stephenson GR, Moretti EW, El-Moalem H, et al. Malnutrition in liver transplant patients: preoperative subjective global assessment is predictive of outcome after liver transplantation. Transplantation 2001;72(4):666–70.
96. Kozek-Langenecker SA, Ahmed AB, Afshari A, et al. Management of severe perioperative bleeding: guidelines from the European Society of Anaesthesiology: first update 2016. Eur J Anaesthesiol 2017;34(6):332–95.
97. Fragkou PC, Torrance HD, Pearse RM, et al. Perioperative blood transfusion is associated with a gene transcription profile characteristic of immunosuppression: a prospective cohort study. Crit Care 2014;18(5):541.
98. Hevesi ZG, Lopukhin SY, Mezrich JD, et al. Designated liver transplant anesthesia team reduces blood transfusion, need for mechanical ventilation, and duration of intensive care. Liver Transpl 2009;15(5):460–5.
99. Wong SL, Revels SL, Yin H, et al. Variation in hospital mortality rates with inpatient cancer surgery. Ann Surg 2015;261(4):632–6.
100. Callahan MA, Christos PJ, Gold HT, et al. Influence of surgical subspecialty training on in-hospital mortality for gastrectomy and colectomy patients. Ann Surg 2003;238(4):322–32.
101. Azagury D, Morton JM. Bariatric surgery outcomes in US accredited vs non-accredited centers: a systematic review. J Am Coll Surg 2016;223(3):469–77.
102. Koretz RL, Avenell A, Lipman TO, et al. Does enteral nutrition affect clinical outcome? A systematic review of the randomized trials. Am J Gastroenterol 2007;102(2):412–29.
103. Plauth M, Cabré E, Campillo B, et al. ESPEN guidelines on parenteral nutrition: hepatology. Clin Nutr 2009;28(4):436–44.
104. Fan ST, Lo CM, Lai EC, et al. Perioperative nutritional support in patients undergoing hepatectomy for hepatocellular carcinoma. N Engl J Med 1994;331(23): 1547–52.
105. Nakai T, Tanimura H, Mori K, et al. Total parenteral nutrition in posthepatectomy patients. Nutrition 1993;9(4):323–8.
106. Nishizaki T, Takenaka K, Yanaga K, et al. Nutritional support after hepatic resection: a randomized prospective study. Hepatogastroenterology 1996;43(9): 608–13.
107. Kanematsu T, Koyanagi N, Matsumata T, et al. Lack of preventive effect of branched-chain amino acid solution on postoperative hepatic encephalopathy in patients with cirrhosis: a randomized, prospective trial. Surgery 1988; 104(3):482–8.
108. Okuno M, Nagayama M, Takai T, et al. Postoperative total parenteral nutrition in patients with liver disorders. J Surg Res 1985;39(2):93–102.
109. Alshahrani AS, Gong GS, Yoo MW. Comparison of long-term survival and immediate postoperative liver function after laparoscopic and open distal gastrectomy for early gastric cancer patients with liver cirrhosis. Gastric Cancer 2017;20(4):744–51.

110. Puggioni A, Wong LL. A metaanalysis of laparoscopic cholecystectomy in patients with cirrhosis. J Am Coll Surg 2003;197(6):921–6.

111. Tsugawa K, Koyanagi N, Hashizume M, et al. A comparison of an open and laparoscopic appendectomy for patients with liver cirrhosis. Surg Laparosc Endosc Percutan Tech 2001;11(3):189–94.

112. Chmielecki DK, Hagopian EJ, Kuo YH, et al. Laparoscopic cholecystectomy is the preferred approach in cirrhosis: a nationwide, population-based study. HPB (Oxford) 2012;14(12):848–53.

113. Al-Azzawi Y, Al-Abboodi Y, Fasullo M, et al. The morbidity and mortality of laparoscopic appendectomy in patients with cirrhosis. Clin Med Insights Gastroenterol 2018;11. 1179552217746645.

114. Rössle M, Ochs A, Gülberg V, et al. A comparison of paracentesis and transjugular intrahepatic portosystemic shunting in patients with ascites. N Engl J Med 2000;342(23):1701–7.

115. Schwartz SI. Biliary tract surgery and cirrhosis: a critical combination. Surgery 1981;90(4):577–83.

116. Azoulay D, Buabse F, Damiano I, et al. Neoadjuvant transjugular intrahepatic portosystemic shunt: a solution for extrahepatic abdominal operation in cirrhotic patients with severe portal hypertension. J Am Coll Surg 2001;193(1):46–51.

117. Tujios SR, Rahnama-Moghadam S, Elmunzer JB, et al. Transpapillary gallbladder stents can stabilize or improve decompensated cirrhosis in patients awaiting liver transplantation. J Clin Gastroenterol 2015;49(9):771–7.

118. Schlenker C, Trotter JF, Shah RJ, et al. Endoscopic gallbladder stent placement for treatment of symptomatic cholelithiasis in patients with end-stage liver disease. Am J Gastroenterol 2006;101(2):278–83.

119. Jayadevan R, Garg M, Schiano T, et al. Is cholecystostomy a safe procedure in patients with cirrhosis? Am Surg 2014;80(11):1169–71.

120. Yao Z, Hu K, Huang P, et al. Delayed laparoscopic cholecystectomy is safe and effective for acute severe calculous cholecystitis in patients with advanced cirrhosis: a single center experience. Gastroenterol Res Pract 2014;2014: 178908.

121. Carbonell AM, Wolfe LG, DeMaria EJ. Poor outcomes in cirrhosis-associated hernia repair: a nationwide cohort study of 32,033 patients. Hernia 2005;9(4): 353–7.

122. Gray SH, Vick CC, Graham LA, et al. Umbilical herniorrhapy in cirrhosis: improved outcomes with elective repair. J Gastrointest Surg 2008;12(4):675–81.

123. Oh H-K, Kim H, Ryoo S, et al. Inguinal hernia repair in patients with cirrhosis is not associated with increased risk of complications and recurrence. World J Surg 2011;35(6):1229–33.

124. Fernandes NF, Schwesinger WH, Hilsenbeck SG, et al. Laparoscopic cholecystectomy and cirrhosis: a case-control study of outcomes. Liver Transpl 2000; 6(3):340–4.

125. Yeh CN, Chen MF, Jan YY. Laparoscopic cholecystectomy in 226 cirrhotic patients. Experience of a single center in Taiwan. Surg Endosc 2002;16(11): 1583–7.

126. Warnick P, Mai I, Klein F, et al. Safety of pancreatic surgery in patients with simultaneous liver cirrhosis: a single center experience. Pancreatology 2011; 11(1):24–9.

127. Gil A, Martınez-Regueira F, Hernández-Lizoain JL, et al. The role of transjugular intrahepatic portosystemic shunt prior to abdominal tumoral surgery in cirrhotic patients with portal hypertension. Eur J Surg Oncol 2004;30(1):46–52.

128. Vinet E, Perreault P, Bouchard L, et al. Transjugular intrahepatic portosystemic shunt before abdominal surgery in cirrhotic patients: a retrospective, comparative study. Can J Gastroenterol 2006;20(6):401–4.

129. Schlenker C, Johnson S, Trotter JF. Preoperative transjugular intrahepatic portosystemic shunt (TIPS) for cirrhotic patients undergoing abdominal and pelvic surgeries. Surg Endosc 2009;23(7):1594–8.

130. Menahem B, Lubrano J, Desjouis A, et al. Transjugular intrahepatic portosystemic shunt placement increases feasibility of colorectal surgery in cirrhotic patients with severe portal hypertension. Dig Liver Dis 2015;47(1):81–4.

Noncirrhotic Portal Hypertension

Current and Emerging Perspectives

Rajeev Khanna, MD, PDCC[a], Shiv Kumar Sarin, MD, DM, DSc, FNASc[b],*

KEYWORDS

- Idiopathic portal hypertension • Extrahepatic portal venous obstruction
- Animal models • Biliopathy • Rex shunt • Parenchymal extinction

KEY POINTS

- Non-cirrhotic portal hypertension refers to portal hypertension (PHT) in absence of cirrhosis and normal HVPG.
- Idiopathic portal hypertension (IPH) and extrahepatic portal venous obstruction (EHPVO) are two prototype disorders with different ages of presentation.
- Infections, toxins, and immunological, prothrombotic and genetic disorders are possible causes of IPH, while prothrombotic and local factors around the portal vein lead to EHPVO.
- Parenchymal extinction in the long term can lead to decompensation necessitating liver transplantation.
- Endoscopic and radiological interventions and surgical techniques have evolved to alter the natural history of these disorders.

INTRODUCTION

Portal hypertension (PHT) is defined as a portal venous pressure gradient between the portal vein (PV) and inferior vena cava (IVC) of more than 5 mm Hg. It is classified as prehepatic, hepatic, or posthepatic, which depends on the level of resistance in the portal venous system. Hepatic PHT is further classified as presinusoidal, sinusoidal, and postsinusoidal from involvement before, at, and after the level of sinusoids. Sinusoidal PHT secondary to cirrhosis is the commonest cause of PHT in adults and is characterized by increased hepatic venous pressure

Conflicts of Interest: None to declare.
Funding Sources: None to declare.
[a] Department of Pediatric Hepatology, Institute of Liver & Biliary Sciences (ILBS), D-1, Vasant Kunj, New Delhi 110 070, India; [b] Department of Hepatology, Institute of Liver & Biliary Sciences (ILBS), D-1, Vasant Kunj, New Delhi 110 070, India
* Corresponding author.
E-mail addresses: shivsarin@gmail.com; sksarin@ilbs.in

Clin Liver Dis 23 (2019) 781–807
https://doi.org/10.1016/j.cld.2019.07.006
1089-3261/19/© 2019 Elsevier Inc. All rights reserved.

gradient (HVPG); that is, the difference between wedge hepatic venous pressure (WHVP) and free hepatic venous pressure (FHVP).[1,2] The same is not true with presinusoidal and postsinusoidal causes of PHT (**Table 1**).[1,3,4] It is important to understand the differences between cirrhotic and noncirrhotic causes of PHT, in that the former is associated with increased transaminases and parenchymal dysfunction (coagulopathy, hypoalbuminemia), whereas the latter presents mostly with complications related to PHT (splenomegaly, variceal bleed, thrombocytopenia).[3,4] Based on the competent risk estimates in cirrhotics, variceal bleed represents stage 3 disease with a 5-year risk of further decompensation and mortality before further decompensation in 65% and 20%.[5] In contrast, well-tolerated variceal bleed is one of the major manifestations in noncirrhotic PHT without accompanying decompensation. This article discusses in detail the 2 common causes of noncirrhotic portal hypertension: idiopathic PHT (IPH) and extrahepatic portal venous obstruction (EHPVO).[1–4]

IDIOPATHIC PORTAL HYPERTENSION

IPH, known by various names such as noncirrhotic portal fibrosis (NCPF), hepatoportal sclerosis, obliterative portovenopathy, and idiopathic noncirrhotic PHT, is a presinusoidal cause of PHT in which the HVPG is normal or near normal but the intrasplenic and intravariceal pressures are markedly increased, with patent PV and hepatic veins. Clinically the disorder is characterized by features of PHT; moderate to massive splenomegaly, with or without hypersplenism and preserved liver functions.[6–17]

Geographical Variation and Epidemiology

IPH is a disease predominantly reported from the Indian subcontinent and Japan.[6–10] The disease is commonly seen in men in their third or fourth decades (Indian subcontinent) or women in their fifth decades (Japan and the West).[6–14] A decreasing trend in the prevalence of the disease in the high-prevalence populations was recorded in the 2007 consensus, and it was hypothesized that this was possibly related to the improvement in the sanitation, hygiene, and socioeconomic status of the people and to the decrease in prevalence of umbilical sepsis and diarrheal diseases.[18] Over the last decade there has been increase in the number of reports of IPH cases secondary to human immunodeficiency virus (HIV) infection.[15–17] IPH has also been described in children.[19,20] Around 10% to 30% of variceal bleeds worldwide are caused by IPH.[3,8,18,21] From the explants and liver histology data, it has been shown that about 41% to 81% of IPH cases may be misdiagnosed as cryptogenic cirrhosis in adults.[21,22]

Etiopathogenesis

Because the etiopathogenesis of IPH is not well understood, various theories have been proposed. Infections, prothrombotic states, immunologic disorders, toxins, and genetic factors are possible causal factors (**Table 2**) (Tripathi DM, Sarin SK. Role of heme-oxygenase and nitric oxide synthase in modulating the vascular tone in endotoxin induced portal hypertensive rabbits, unpublished data, 2013).[23–37] Various animal models and pathogenetic theories of IPH have been developed suggesting immunologic, infective, and vascular bases of disease (**Figs. 1 and 2**).[3,38–40]

Pathology

The histologic hallmark of IPH/NCPF is said to be obliterative portal venopathy; the main PV trunk is dilated with thick sclerosed walls, along with thrombosis in medium and small PV branches. Other features include approximation and atrophy of portal tracts, aberrant vessels in the portal tract (portal angiomatosis) and herniation of PV

Table 1
Causes of noncirrhotic portal hypertension from pressure studies

		Cause of Noncirrhotic Portal Hypertension			
		Hepatic			
	Prehepatic	Presinusoidal	Sinusoidal	Postsinusoidal	Posthepatic
FHVP	Normal	Normal	Normal	High	Normal or high
WHVP	Normal	Normal or near normal	High	High	High
RAP	Normal	Normal	Normal	Normal	Normal or high
HVPG	Normal	Normal or near normal	High	Normal to high	Normal or near normal
	EHPVO[b] PV thrombosis Splenic vein thrombosis Splanchnic arteriovenous fistula Massive splenomegaly Infiltrative diseases Storage disorders (Gaucher disease)	Congenital: polycystic disease, congenital hepatic fibrosis[b] Vascular: HHT, peliosis hepatis Biliary: PBC, PSC Granulomatous: Schistosomiasis/sarcoidosis[b] Idiopathic: IPH[b]	Alcoholic hepatitis[b] Drugs and toxins: Methotrexate,[b] amiodarone, vinyl chloride, copper Metabolic: NASH Infiltrative: Mastocytosis, myeloid metaplasia, amyloidosis Sinusoidal compression: Gaucher disease,[b] visceral leishmaniasis, alcoholic hepatitis, AFLP	Veno-occlusive disease (irradiation, drugs/toxins) Neoplastic: epithelioid hemangioendothelioma, angiosarcoma Granulomatous: sarcoidosis,[b] mycobacterial infections[b]	HVOTO[a,b] IVC obstruction[a,b] Constrictive pericarditis[b] Tricuspid regurgitation Severe right-sided heart failure[b] Restrictive cardiomyopathy

Abbreviations: AFLP, acute fatty liver of pregnancy; EHPVO, extrahepatic portal venous obstruction; HHT, hereditary hemorrhagic telangiectasia; HVOTO, hepatic venous outflow tract obstruction; IPH, idiopathic portal hypertension; NASH, nonalcoholic steatohepatitis; PBC, primary biliary cirrhosis; PSC, primary sclerosing cholangitis; RAP, right atrial pressure.

[a] HVPG may not be recordable in patients with HVOTO or IVC obstruction.

[b] Important causes.

Data from Refs.[1–3]

Table 2
Etiopathogenetic factors and animal models of idiopathic portal hypertension

Postulated Factors	Evidence from Literature		Comments
	Clinical Studies	Animal Models	
Infections	Decreasing prevalence in endemic regions associated with a concomitant decrease in rates of umbilical sepsis and diarrheal diseases[18]	Rabbit model: repeated intraportal injections of killed *Escherichia coli* antigen[23] Endotoxemia rabbit model: *E coli* antigen administered intramuscularly as well as via gastrosplenic vein[24]	Weak evidence (hypothesis) Animal models not well reproduced and accepted Role of endothelial dysfunction as suggested by endotoxemia model (Tripathi DM, Sarin SK. Role of heme-oxygenase and nitric oxide synthase in modulating the vascular tone in endotoxin induced portal hypertensive rabbits, unpublished data, 2013)[24]
HIV	Prevalence around 0.45%–1% Male homosexuals, prolonged infection (median 11.5 y) with immune reconstitution Usage of didanosine (± stavudine) PVT in 25%–75%[15–17]	None	Exact prevalence not known Multiple factors: direct effect of HIV, HAART (didanosine), opportunistic pathogens, hypercoagulability[15–17]
Prothrombotic states	Prothrombotic states in 8%–11%: FVL, prothrombin, and MTHFRase[11–13,26]	None	Association in a limited subgroup of patients
ADAMTS13	Lower levels of ADAMTS13 in IPH livers[27]	None	Deficiency of ADAMTS13 leads to ultralarge uncleaved von-Willebrand factor within IPH livers with a tendency to remain anchored and interact with platelet glycoprotein 1b, thereby activating formation of platelet thrombi[27]

PVT	Prevalence of PVT in IPH variable: 2.2% (Japan),[28] 13%–46% (West)[11–13]	Rat model of repetitive PV embolization: injection of colored microspheres into the PV at weekly intervals[29]	Low incidence of PVT (on biopsy, autopsy, and on transhepatic portography), insidious onset, increased (rather than decreased) splenic blood flow are points that refute PVT as a causal factor; it may be an effect of the disease itself[3,6,28,30]
Immunologic	SLE, scleroderma, POEMS syndrome[31] Celiac disease (present in 16%–20% of IPH)[31,32]	Rabbit model: intraportal injections or indwelling catheter infusion of albumin or splenic extract into gastrosplenic vein[24]	Female preponderance favors immunologic basis.[11–14] 37% of IPH have at least 1 serum antibody: ANA, ASMA, ACLA, antiactin, anti–gastric parietal cell, or anti–thyroid peroxidise[31]
Immune deficiency	Association with CVID and XLA Splenomegaly, dilated PV, varices/collaterals, and evidence of IPH on histology in 60.7%, 25.6%, 4.2%, and 4.2% patients, respectively[33]	None	IPH related to more aggressive phenotype with a higher prevalence of bronchiectasis, gastroenteritis, lymphoid nodular hyperplasia, and autoimmune manifestations, with low switched memory B-cell levels[33]
Medications and toxins	Arsenic, vinyl chloride, $CuSO_4$, Mtx, 6-Mercaptopurine azathioprine, oxaliplatin, didanosine, irradiation, vitamin A, herbs[3,34]	Rat model: chronic arsenic exposure leads to changes similar to IPH[35]	High arsenic levels in IPH livers in contrast with cirrhosis and controls[34]
Genetic factors	Syndromes (Turner, Noonan, and Adams-Oliver)[3,19] HLA-DR3[36] KCNN3 mutation[37]	None	Weak association KCNN3 channel regulates arterial and venous vascular tone by causing smooth muscle activation or relaxation, suggesting vascular mechanism[37]

Abbreviations: ACLA, anticardiolipin antibody; ADAMTS13, disintegrin and metalloprotease with thrombospondin type 1 motif, member 13; ANA, antinuclear antibody; ASMA, anti–smooth muscle antibody; CVID, common variable immunodeficiency; FVL, factor-V Leiden; HAART, highly active antiretroviral therapy; HLA, human leukocyte antigen; KCNN3, gene encoding small conductance calcium-activated potassium channel 3; MTHFRase, methylene tetrahydrofolate reductase; Mtx, methotrexate; POEMS, polyneuropathy, organomegaly, endocrinopathy or edema, M-protein, skin changes; PVT, PV thrombosis; SLE, systemic lupus erythematosus; XLA, X-linked agammaglobulinemia.

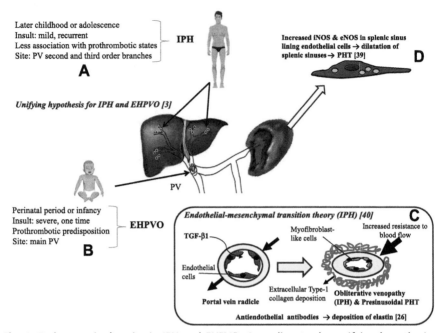

Fig. 1. Pathogenetic theories in IPH and EHPVO. According to the unifying hypothesis, a major thrombotic event occurring at a young age involving main PV results in EHPVO, whereas repeated microthrombotic events later in life that involve small or medium branches of PV lead to IPH[3] (A, B). Endothelial-mesenchymal transition theory says that vascular endothelial cells of portal venules acquire myofibroblastic features leading to collagen synthesis and subsequent occlusion of small PV branches.[39] There is also development of antiendothelial antibodies[25] (C). Development of IPH is also explained secondary to increased splenic blood flow caused by high inducible nitric oxide synthase (iNOS) level leading to portal hypertension[38] (D). eNOS, endothelial nitric oxide synthase; TGF-β1, transforming growth factor beta 1).

radicles, portal and perisinusoidal fibrosis, and nodular regenerative hyperplasia.[3,8,18,39] For grading severity of IPH, a staging system has been proposed by Nakanuma: stage I, absence of peripheral parenchymal atrophy; stage II, presence of peripheral parenchymal atrophy in a nonatrophic liver; stage III, presence of peripheral parenchymal atrophy in an atrophic liver; and stage IV, presence of obstructive thrombosis in intrahepatic large branches or trunk of PV.[41] In order to better define the portal and periportal vascular changes of IPH, a consensus of expert pathologists recently suggested usage of terms PV stenosis, herniated PV, hypervascularized portal tract, and periportal abnormal vessels, and avoidance of terms like sclerosis, venopathy, aberrant or shunt vessels, or angiomatosis.[42] A positive correlation between portal inflammation and antinuclear antibody titer, and between sinusoidal fibrosis and transaminases, has been shown. In the same study, platelets were shown to correlate inversely with portal angiomatosis, sinusoidal dilatation, increased central veins, and diffuse sinusoidal capillarization.[26]

Clinical Features

As per most literature available on the topic, the commonest presentation of IPH/NCPF includes episodes of variceal bleed, long-standing splenomegaly, and anemia. Although earlier series mentioned splenomegaly and variceal bleed in 60% to 97%

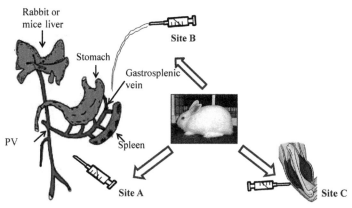

Fig. 2. Animal models of IPH. Various rabbit models of IPH with various interventions at different sites: site A (into PV via ileocecal vein), site B (gastrosplenic vein), and site C (intramuscularly), or site B and C. Studies using splenic extract[24] favor an immunologic basis, those using *Escherichia coli* antigen favor an infective or endotoxin basis (Tripathi DM, Sarin SK. Role of heme-oxygenase and nitric oxide synthase in modulating the vascular tone in endotoxin induced portal hypertensive rabbits, unpublished data, 2013),[23] and those using colored microspheres favor a prothrombotic basis of IPH.[29] Interventions for creation of animal models of IPH: (1) sensitization with *E coli* antigen with Freud adjuvant (site C) on days 0, 1, 2, 7, 14 followed by cannulation of gastrosplenic vein on day 15 and injection of heat-killed *E coli* antigen (lipopolysaccharide) on days 15, 16, 17, 22, 29, 43 (site B) (Tripathi DM, Sarin SK. Role of heme-oxygenase and nitric oxide synthase in modulating the vascular tone in endotoxin induced portal hypertensive rabbits, unpublished data, 2013)[23]; (2) rabbit splenic extract (site C) every 2 weeks for 3 months[24]; (3) weekly injections of 150,000 colored microspheres (week 1, *violet*; week 2, *blue*; week 3, *yellow*) (site A).[29]

and 65% to 84% patients respectively,[3,6–10] the recent data from the West reported that a sizable proportion (20%–58%) of patients with IPH may be asymptomatic.[11–14,26] An Italian study has shown that around 19.5% of noncirrhotic cryptogenic chronic liver disorders without clinical PHT have almost all histologic features similar to diagnosed IPH cases, with comparable liver function tests, prothrombotic predisposition, and extrahepatic autoimmune conditions. Liver histology of some of these patients showed nodular regenerative hyperplasia and incomplete fibrous septa, thus indicating a less severe disease and hence less clinical PHT. Thus, a sizable number of IPH cases may not have PHT and are often missed in the absence of clinical features such as splenomegaly. Such individuals have been shown to develop PHT and PV thrombosis (PVT) during follow-up at similar rates as typical IPH cases.[26] It is possible that with increase in understanding of the disease, early referrals, and multidisciplinary approach, more IPH cases may be found in the preclinical stage in future. Duration of symptoms at presentation varies from 15 days to 18 years. Frequency of variceal bleeding increases with age with a median of 1 (range, 1–20) bleeding episode before presentation. Bleeding from nongastrointestinal sites is reported in about 20%.[7–9] Ascites is seen in 10% to 34% of cases.[11–14,26] Pain over the left upper quadrant may occur because of perisplenitis or splenic infarction.[8] Clinically, there is moderate to massive splenomegaly.[3,8] Liver is either normal sized, enlarged, or shrunken, with absence of peripheral stigmata of chronic liver disease. Jaundice and hepatic encephalopathy are rare (~2%) and are usually seen after either a major bleed or shunt surgery.[8,9]

Laboratory Evaluation

Hypersplenism is present in 27% to 87% of patients, the commonest being anemia followed by thrombocytopenia and leukopenia.[3,7–10] However, this depends on the stage of the disease and degree of PHT and may be absent in patients diagnosed early.[12,26] Anemia is related to multiple variceal bleeds, hypersplenism, and iron deficiency. Liver function tests are mostly normal, but a proportion have derangements in liver enzymes, prothrombin time, and albumin.[3,11–14] Autonomic dysfunction, and coagulation and platelet function abnormalities, may also be seen.[43,44] Patients with IPH have low vitamin B_{12} levels ($\leq$250 pg/mL), which may be helpful in distinguishing them from cirrhotics; higher levels in cirrhotics are possibly caused by excessive release or reduced clearance.[45]

Hemodynamics

Intrasplenic pressure (ISP) and intravariceal pressure (IVP) are significantly increased in NCPF compared with WHVP and intrahepatic pressures (IHPs), suggesting a presinusoidal level of block. There are 2 independent pressure gradients: one between ISP and IHP, and another between IHP and WHVP.[3,46] Mean HVPG is 7.1 ± 3.1 mm Hg, significantly lower than the values in cirrhosis. Value of HVPG is normal ($\leq$5 mm Hg) in 16%, increased mildly (6–10 mm Hg) in 44%, and increased significantly ($\geq$11 mm Hg) in 40%. Hepatic venovenous communications are present in almost half of these patients, which impairs proper hepatic vein occlusion and precludes proper HVPG measurement.[47]

Endoscopic Findings

Earlier series have reported presence of esophageal varices in about 80% to 90% of patients.[7–10] Compared with cirrhotics, esophageal varices are more often large (90% vs 70%), gastric (gastroesophageal varices [GOV] 1 and GOV2) varices (31%–44% vs 22%) and anorectal varices (89% vs 56%) are more prevalent, whereas portal hypertensive gastropathy is less prevalent (5.4% vs 10.9%).[7–10,48–51] From the recent data from the West, patients without varices develop them at rates of 10%, 20%, and 69%, and those with small ones show progression at rates of 13%, 35%, and 44% at 1, 2, and 5 years, respectively. Moreover, in patients with large esophageal varices, the age at diagnosis and presence of red wale marks are factors significantly associated with first bleed, with respective odds of 1.10 and 9.22.[14]

Radiological Features

Doppler ultrasonography (USG) is the first radiological investigation in evaluation of IPH. Liver is mostly normal in size and echotexture. Spleen is enlarged with presence of Gandy-Gamna bodies; splenoportal axis is dilated and patent. Thickened PV (>3 mm) with echogenic walls is characteristic. There is sudden narrowing or cutoff of intrahepatic second-degree and third-degree PV branches: so-called withered-tree appearance along with approximation of vascular channels.[3,8] A layered appearance of PV has been described.[52] Splenic index and PV inflow are high. Spontaneous shunts (paraumbilical and gastroadrenorenal) are seen in 16%.[8] There is delayed periportal enhancement on contrast-enhanced USG using perflubutane microbubbles, which is caused by distribution of contrast into abnormal intrahepatic vascular branches and may be of help in differentiating IPH from cryptogenic cirrhosis.[53] MRI and computed tomography (CT) show a nonnodular liver with enlarged caudate lobe, atrophic right lobe, and preserved liver volume amid features of portal hypertension. Other features include intrahepatic PV abnormalities (nonvisualization, reduced caliber, occlusive thrombosis), focal nodular hyperplasia–like nodules, and perfusion defects.[54] Radionuclide scintigraphy using 99mTc-Sn colloid shows absence of increased bone marrow uptake.[55] A ratio of spleen/liver stiffness greater than 1.71 on acoustic radiation force impulse may be helpful in differentiating IPH from cirrhosis and chronic hepatitis.[56] Transient elastography value of IPH livers (8.4 $\pm$ 3.3 kPa) is higher than those with EHPVO (6.4 $\pm$ 2.2 kPa) but significantly lower than in cirrhotics (40.9 $\pm$ 20.5 kPa).[47]

Liver Biopsy

Liver biopsy is indicated in all patients with PHT with a suspicion of IPH in order to exclude cirrhosis and other causes. The diagnosis should be made in a liver biopsy specimen longer than 1 cm with at least 5 complete portal tracts regularly alternating with central veins along with absence of cirrhosis and features of IPH in at least two-thirds of them.[12]

Metabolomics and Gene Signatures in Idiopathic Portal Hypertension

Two studies from Spain have studied the role of metabolomics in differentiating IPH from cirrhosis. Of the total 582 metabolites analyzed, 5 lipid metabolites were found to be associated with IPH on logistic regression analysis; levels of 4 of them, belonging to the fatty acid, acyl carnitine, lysophosphatidylethanolamine, and sphingomyelin families, were decreased, whereas 1, related to the bile acid family, was increased. A decision tree constructed using these metabolite signatures helped in diagnosing 88% of patients with IPH.[57,58] From Japan, comprehensive analysis of gene expression using microarray analysis showed involvement of genes related to the immune system in IPH. There was compromised function of immunocompetent cells with a range of abnormalities in the metabolism of nucleic acids and inflammatory cytokines.[59] Such data need external validation in larger cohorts and have limitations of cost and expertise.

Idiopathic Portal Hypertension in Children

Two recent series have described 67 children less than 18 years of age with histologically proven IPH.[19,20] The French series presented younger children with most being familial, or with syndromic features, or secondary to malignancy and chemotherapy.[19] The Indian study described older children without any predisposition, with median ages at presentation and diagnosis of 10 and 14 years.[20] Overall in pediatric IPH, PHT was present in 81% to 100%, hypersplenism in 62% to 90%, esophageal varices in 81%, variceal bleed in 16% to 40%, and growth failure in 74%. Liver transplant was required in 10% because of hepatopulmonary syndrome or portopulmonary hypertension. The pediatric counterpart of IPH represents a more aggressive phenotype, and around 44% have some genetic component.[19,20]

Diagnosis

The diagnosis of IPH is mainly clinical (moderate to massive splenomegaly, evidence of PHT [varices and/or collaterals]); patent splenoportal axis and hepatic veins, without any evidence of liver dysfunction; liver histology showing absence of cirrhosis or parenchymal injury; and absence of any known cause of liver disease.[3] As per Baveno VI, liver biopsy is mandatory and a normal or near-normal HVPG is recommended for diagnosis.[60] Presence of PVT, which can be present in IPH cases, either at presentation or at follow-up, does not exclude IPH. An algorithm with major and minor criteria taking into account clinical, histologic, and imaging criteria has been proposed.[40]

Natural History

The natural course of IPH is dominated by repeated attacks of uncontrolled bleeding and development of PVT, and in a minority occurrence of hepatopulmonary syndrome (HPS) (**Fig. 3**). Long-term survival following eradication of esophagogastric varices and after a properly timed shunt surgery is nearly 100% and 80%, respectively.[3,7–10] Liver functions usually remain well preserved, but, in time, 20% to 33% patients develop parenchymal atrophy with subsequent decompensation, HPS, and need for liver transplant (LT) (**Fig. 4**).[13,22] Development of ascites, seen in about a quarter over time, is not necessarily a terminal event.[9,11,14] The commonest causes of death are bacterial infection (31%), followed by progressive liver failure (25%), uncontrolled variceal bleeding (17%), and intestinal infarction (8%).[61]

Development of portal venous thrombosis

The development of PVT in an IPH liver has been variably reported from 2.2% to 46%.[3,11–14] In a prospective study by Siramolpiwat and colleagues,[14] PVT developed in 36% over a mean follow-up period of 6.7 years, the actuarial probability of this event being 9%, 16%, 33%, and 42% at 1, 2, 5, and 10 years, respectively, and was related to presence of HIV infection, variceal bleeding at diagnosis, and high bilirubin level. Usage of anticoagulant therapy recanalized the PV in almost half the patients. From a French cohort, it has been shown that ascites and PVT develop in almost half of cases, and liver failure in 21% over a mean follow-up period of 7.6 years.[11] A worsening of preexisting PHT in half and development of new PVT in almost one-third of cases, occasionally requiring LT, has been reported.[12] Hence, development of PVT is a serious event in the natural history of IPH leading to progressive PHT, liver dysfunction, and increased mortality.

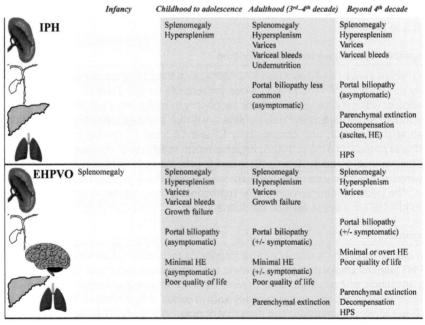

Fig. 3. Time line of events in the natural history of IPH and EHPVO from infancy to adulthood. Although EHPVO is a childhood disease and presents during early years of life, IPH is an adult disease. HE, hepatic encephalopathy.

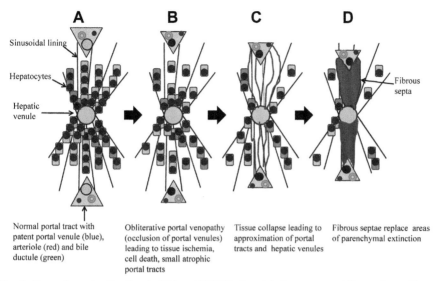

Normal portal tract with patent portal venule (blue), arteriole (red) and bile ductule (green)

Obliterative portal venopathy (occlusion of portal venules) leading to tissue ischemia, cell death, small atrophic portal tracts

Tissue collapse leading to approximation of portal tracts and hepatic venules

Fibrous septae replace areas of parenchymal extinction

Fig. 4. Parenchymal extinction in IPH and EHPVO. Panel A shows normal liver acinus. Chronically obliterated (thrombosed) PV leads to tissue ischemia, cell death, and atrophy of portal tracts (*Panel B*) followed by tissue collapse resulting in approximation of portal and hepatic venules (*Panel C*), culminating in parenchymal extinction (*Panel D*).

Hepatocellular carcinoma (HCC) in the setting of IPH liver has been reported. Presence of hyperplastic nodules (1.5–7 cm) were evaluated in 7 patients with IPH; 4 patients had 3 or more nodules; Ki-67 labeling index was increased in 2 patients (1 was HCC). It was hypothesized that marked narrowing of peripheral PVs induces atrophy of hepatocytes leading to compensatory increase in blood flow of patent PVs and aberrant vessels. This condition causes hyperplasia of hepatic lobules adjacent to atrophic ones, and some progress to form nodules.[62]

Pregnancy outcomes have recently been reported from 24 pregnancies of 16 women from a multinational cohort. There were 4 miscarriages, 1 ectopic pregnancy, 1 medical termination of pregnancy, and 9 preterm deliveries with 2 newborn deaths. Six PHT-related complications were observed: 3 worsening ascites, 2 variceal bleeds, and 1 portopulmonary hypertension, requiring transjugular intrahepatic portosystemic shunt (TIPSS) in patient. Three patients had vaginal bleeds; 1 required uterine artery embolization.[63]

Ten-year survival in patients with IPH from the Asia-Pacific region has been reported to be around 86% to 95%.[18] Contrastingly, the report from Schouten and colleagues[13] mentioned 5-year and 10-year survival of 78% and 56%, respectively; the difference may be related to preponderance of hematological and immunologic conditions in their cohort. Further differences in survival may have been affected by genetics, ethnicity, and prevalence of HIV infection. Indications of LT in IPH, although not very clear, may include presence of PVT, decompensation, HPS, and refractory variceal bleed. HVPG and Model for End-stage Liver Disease (MELD) score are not associated with poor outcome or need of LT.[11–14,22]

EXTRAHEPATIC PORTAL VENOUS OBSTRUCTION

EHPVO is another prehepatic cause of PHT and is considered the pediatric counterpart of adult IPH. The two disorders are similar in the mode of presentation, normal liver functions, and a small but significant risk of parenchymal extinction. However, they differ with regard to the age of presentation, prothrombotic predisposition, and natural history. It is a major cause of PHT (54%) and upper gastrointestinal bleeding in children (68%–84%) from the developing world.[64,65] In the West, noncirrhotic, nontumoral PVT is the second most frequent cause of PHT in adults after cirrhosis,[4] whereas in children it constitutes a small proportion (11%–12%).[66] The largest cohort on pediatric PHT from France has described EHPVO to comprise 12% of overall causes, and is the second common single cause of PHT after biliary atresia.[67] As per the Asian Pacific Association for the Study of the Liver (APASL) consensus (2006), EHPVO is defined as "a vascular disorder of liver, characterized by obstruction of the extra-hepatic PV with or without involvement of intra-hepatic PV radicles or splenic or superior mesenteric veins."[65] The Baveno VI consensus definition includes recent thrombus in the PV along with presence of cavernoma; however, excludes cirrhosis and other liver diseases such as IPH, as well as HCC from the definition, and emphasizes that EHPVO in these settings is a different entity. Isolated occlusion of the splenic vein or superior mesenteric vein has a different causal spectrum and clinical presentation, and is hence removed from the defining criteria of EHPVO. Hence, EHPVO is a distinct disease rather an event in the natural history or an extension or association of a primary liver disease.[60]

Etiopathogenesis

Causal factors

The causal profile of EHPVO in adults has been extrapolated mostly from studies on acute PVT. The predisposing factors, as in other venous thrombosis states, have been divided into within the vessel lumen, within the vessel wall, and outside the vessel. Predisposing risk factors are present in 72% to 87% of adults with EHPVO; local factors in the form of trauma, tumor, or inflammation are present in 19% to 64%. Corresponding figures in children are 38% to 74% and 18% to 68%, respectively.[3,68–80] A combination of local and systemic factors is seen in 19% to 64% of adult patients.[68,70] In a study with 73 adult patients with EHPVO, JAK2 mutation was detected in 36%, whereas the bone marrow biopsy and clonality assay were able to identify myeloproliferative states in 94% and 87%, respectively.[71] As per 1 meta-analysis, estimated prevalences of myeloproliferative disorders and JAK2 mutations in the setting of EHPVO in adults are 31.5% and 27.7%, respectively.[80] Overall, at least 1 prothrombotic state is seen in 28% to 62% of cases; however, a detailed evaluation was absent in most of them.[68–73] In children, data are limited; however, data from nonsplanchnic thromboses indicate that the risk of recurrent thromboses in the presence of single and multiple genetic prothrombotic factors is 2.7 (95% confidence interval [CI], 1.8–4.1) and 10.6 (95% CI, 3.2–31.6), respectively.[81] Common local causes leading to EHPVO are pancreatitis, liver abscess, omphalitis, PV phlebitis, umbilical vein catheterization (UVC), surgery around PV (splenectomy, cholecystectomy, Billroth-II procedure), and malignancies (pancreatic, hepatic, or duodenal).[3,4,68,73] Congenital anomalies have been reported in 30% of children with EHPVO (most often in those without history of omphalitis), the commonest ones were cardiovascular and urinary tract abnormalities, but there were also Turner syndrome, cleft lip and palate, coloboma, and external ear and limb deformities.[76,82] Perinatal insults are known to predispose to EHPVO in 30% to 66% of children: UVC, omphalitis, necrotizing enterocolitis, or neonatal sepsis.[74–79] Of these, UVC has ever been a matter of debate as a cause of EHPVO. A prospective series of neonates who had undergone UVC showed that, despite development of PVT in 45%, there is spontaneous recanalization of PV within 3 months. The study inferred that prolonged or traumatic cannulation or presence of omphalitis or sepsis are risk factors and need careful surveillance for PVT.[83] Additional local factors culminating in EHPVO in children are diarrheal illnesses, abdominal sepsis, and nephrotic syndrome.[3] Despite elaborate history taking and extensive work-up, around 13% to 28% of adults and 26% to 62% of children with EHPVO do not have a defined cause.

Pathogenesis

In most of the children and adults with EHPVO, the acute inciting event leading to EHPVO goes unrecognized and thrombus gradually becomes organized with formation of multiple tortuous hepatopetal collaterals around and inside the PV. This group of collaterals, termed cavernoma, appear within a span of 6 to 20 days following PV flow interruption. These collaterals tend to overcome the prehepatic obstruction and terminate in middle-sized intrahepatic PV branches but remain insufficient to decompress high pressure in the splanchnic bed and to compensate the reduction of total hepatic blood flow. Hence, hepatofugal vessels develop at the sites of porto-systemic communications and transform into varices, hemorrhoids, collaterals, and spontaneous shunts.[3,4]

Stringer and colleagues[84] gave the first description of various patterns of occlusion of PV: first, involvement of small intrahepatic PV branches, termed hepatoportal sclerosis, a synonym of IPH; second, involvement of main PV, which is commonest and is mostly congenital; third, involvement of main PV and superior mesenteric vein, which happens secondary to intra-abdominal sepsis; and, last, widespread thrombosis of portal venous system, which happens secondary to a hypercoagulable state. The relative proportions of these patterns in a group of 53 children were 6%, 47%, 19%, and 28%, respectively.[84] Recently, an anatomic-functional classification of PVT in the setting of cirrhosis has been proposed and it is suggested that it can be applied in the noncirrhotic setting as well and may be helpful for management decisions such as type of shunt surgery or TIPSS, and will also be helpful to define the natural history.[85]

Animal models

Partial PV ligation is the most widely used animal model to study the hemodynamic changes in EHPVO, which can be extrapolated to UVC or acute PVT-related EHPVO. However, it is not helpful to understand the natural history of congenital anomalies and prothrombotic and inflammatory states leading to EHPVO.[3,4]

Pathology

On histology, there is cavernomatous transformation of the PV, which includes a cluster of varying-sized vessels replacing PV arranged haphazardly within connective tissue support at the liver hilum. This group of collaterals may extend for a variable length inside and outside the liver. Liver architecture is well preserved. Mild periportal fibrosis may be seen.[3,4]

Clinical Features

Depending on the predisposing event causing PVT, a bimodal presentation of EHPVO has been described. In the setting of UVC, omphalitis, or perinatal events causing EHPVO, children often present early (~3 years). In contrast, those secondary to intra-abdominal infections or unknown cause manifest in late childhood (~8 years) or adolescence or early adulthood.[3,4] Variceal bleed (49%–85%) and splenomegaly (63%–88%) are the commonest presentations in children. Mean age of first bleeding episode is around 3.8 to 5.2 years.[64–66] From the developed world, children with perinatal risk factors are frequently diagnosed early, at a mean age of 3 years before the development of variceal bleed with an incidental finding of splenomegaly, thrombocytopenia, or PHT.[76,77] In contrast, in the developing world, the diagnosis is mostly delayed up to a mean age of 6.3 to 9.3 years until the children have a mean number of 1.8 to 3.1 bleeding episodes before presentation.[64,75] From a recent series of noncirrhotic nontumoral chronic PVT in 178 adults, variceal bleeding was seen in 32%; 15% at presentation and 17% at a median follow-up of 4 years. The source of bleeding was esophageal varices in 84%, gastric varices in 7%, portal hypertensive gastropathy (PHG) in 7%, and ectopic varices in 2%.[86] Variceal bleeding episodes are often recurrent and relate to febrile illnesses and usage of nonsteroidal antiinflammatory drugs, and they increase in frequency and severity with age until adolescence. In contrast with cirrhosis, such bleeding episodes do not cause decompensation in view of preserved liver synthetic functions. Moderate splenomegaly is characteristically present, which increases with the age of the child, but without any correlation with frequency and severity of bleeds.[3,4] Ascites is present in 4% of children and in up to 21% of adults and is often transient, related to the bleeding episode, growth failure, and hypoalbuminemia.[64,87] Persistent ascites is usually seen late in the course of disease as part of prolonged duration of PHT with subsequent progressive deterioration of liver functions.[87]

Laboratory Evaluation

Liver functions are well preserved in most individuals; a proportion (4%–9%) have abnormal transaminase levels. Increases of alkaline phosphatase and gamma-glutamyl transpeptidase levels are seen with development of portal biliopathy. Hypoalbuminemia is seen in the setting of malnutrition or transiently during variceal bleed episodes.[3,4]

Thrombocytopenia is commonly seen, up to 85%, but is mostly asymptomatic.

Hemodynamics

Similar to IPH, there is increase of ISP and IVP in EHPVO, whereas HVPG is normal. IVP reliably predicts severity of PHT in this setting.[2,3] Hepatic blood flow is normal or decreased, depending on collateral flow and hepatic arterial buffer response. Hyperdynamic circulatory state, similar to cirrhosis, is also described, possibly related to increased nitric oxide levels.[3,88]

Endoscopic Findings

In contrast with cirrhosis, esophageal, gastric, and anorectal varices are more common (90% vs 70%, 31%–44% vs 22%, and 89% vs 56%), whereas PHG is less frequent (5% vs 11%) in adults with EHPVO.[1,48,49,65] Esophageal varices are most often large. Isolated gastric varices (IGV1) are present in up to 6% of patients with EHPVO. Bleeding from gastric varices, particularly IGV1, is less frequent but torrential.[48] Comparable data in pediatric population also reveal that children with EHPVO have a greater proportion of high-risk varices than the cirrhotic causes (70% vs 32%): esophageal varices are seen in 85% to 94%, two-thirds have large varices with red color signs.[67] The prevalences of gastric varices, PHG, and duodenal and anorectal varices in children are 30% to 64%, 12% to 40%, 11%, and 41% to 76%, respectively.[89,90] PHG usually develops after variceal eradication and is often transient, nonprogressive, and asymptomatic.[49,89] Small or absent esophageal varices should alert to a possibility of gastric varix or spontaneous shunt.[48,89] Rectal endoscopic USG has been shown to be superior to sigmoidoscopy for detecting rectal varices.[90]

Radiological Features

Doppler USG of splenoportal axis reveals cavernoma and is the diagnostic investigation of choice, with a sensitivity and specificity of more than 95%.[3,4] Splenoportography and arterial portography, used in earlier days, have now become obsolete and have been replaced by noninvasive methods: CT and magnetic resonance (MR) portovenography. These two techniques also provide an anatomic road map before shunt surgery and sometimes need supplementation by retrograde or wedge hepatic venous portography.[91] Transient elastography of spleen is high in patients with EHPVO and a value more than 42.8 kPa has been shown to predict variceal bleed with a sensitivity and specificity of 88% and 94%, respectively.[92]

Liver Biopsy

Liver biopsy is not required in children with EHPVO unless and until there is a strong clinical suspicion of underlying liver disease. In adults with EHPVO, it may be required to exclude cirrhosis.[60]

Diagnosis

Diagnosis of EHPVO is based on Baveno VI consensus; that is, demonstration of portal cavernoma on USG Doppler in the absence of features of cirrhosis or chronic liver disease. Liver biopsy and HVPG are recommended only if the liver is dysmorphic on imaging or with abnormal liver function tests.[49]

Natural History

The long-term survival of children and adults with EHPVO is usually more than 95%. From a large series of 178 adults, the 1-year, 3-year, and 5-year survival is 99%, 98%, and 96%.The 1-year, 3-year, and 5-year actuarial probability of variceal development is 2%, 22%, and 22%, whereas that of variceal growth (from small to large)is 13%, 40%, and 54%, respectively.[86] Following eradication of esophageal varices with endoscopic sclerotherapy (EST) or endoscopic variceal ligation (EVL), gastroesophageal varices (GOV1, toward the lesser curve) also decrease, whereas GOV2 (toward greater curve), isolated (fundal) gastric varix (IGV1), and PHG increase.[48,49,89,93,94] Mortality related to variceal bleed and intestinal infarction is less than 5%.[86] However, various factors affect the quality of life (QoL) of these children and young adults. Growth failure, problems related to big spleen, portal biliopathy, minimal hepatic encephalopathy, parenchymal extinction, and complications related to myeloproliferative state are some of the factors that affect the natural history of these groups of patients.[3,4] **Fig. 3** shows the age-wise natural history of EHPVO from infancy to adulthood in contrast with IPH.

Growth retardation

Almost one-third to one-half of these children have wasting and stunting.[95,96] The severity of growth failure is related to duration of PHT and is independent of appropriate energy intake.[95] Growth failure in EHPVO is multifactorial and is caused by chronic reduction of hepatic blood flow with concomitant decrease in hepatotropic factors, malabsorptive state caused by portal hypertensive enteropathy, early satiety caused by massive splenomegaly, a state of growth hormone (GH) resistance shown by high levels of GH and low levels of insulinlike growth factor (IGF)-1 and IGF-binding protein-3, and lastly caused by anemia and thrombocytopenia.[3,95,96]

Impaired quality of life

Children with EHPVO have poor health-related QoL with lower median scores in physical, social, emotional, and school functioning health domains in contrast with healthy children. Poor scores are affected by spleen size and growth failure, but are unrelated to variceal eradication. A nonsignificant trend toward improving QoL has been shown following shunt surgery.[97]

Portal biliopathy

The term portal biliopathy (PB) was coined to describe biliary ductal (extrahepatic and intrahepatic) and gall-bladder wall abnormalities in patients with cirrhotic or noncirrhotic PHT, which take the form of intrahepatic biliary radicle dilatation, indentations, caliber irregularities, displacements, angulations, ectasias, strictures, stones, filling defects, compressions, gall bladder and pericholedochal varices, or a mass (pseudocholangiocarcinoma sign). The definition needs exclusion of other biliary diseases.[98] Pathogenesis is related to 2 mechanisms: compression of the pliable common bile duct by dilated collaterals and neovascularization secondary to long-standing PVT, and bile duct ischemia caused by prolonged compression by collaterals, thrombosis of smaller veins draining the duct, or excessive deposition of connective tissue forming a tumorlike cavernoma.[3,98] Compression of paracholedochal venous plexus leads to a varicoid type of PB involving the entire biliary system, giving a wavy or undulating contour, and may show favorable response following shunt surgery. Contrastingly, chronic inflammation and ischemia lead to scarring of the bile duct wall, causing a fibrotic type of PB producing single or multiple segmental strictures with upstream dilatation, changes that may be nonreversible.[99] Frequency of PB is highest in patients with EHPVO (80%–100%) in contrast with cirrhosis (0%–33%) and IPH (9%–40%). Most (62%–95%) patients are without any symptoms. Left hepatic duct is involved most commonly (38%–100%) and severely. Symptomatic patients present with jaundice, biliary colic, abdominal pain, and recurrent cholangitis, most often with increasing age, long-standing disease, choledocholithiasis, and abnormal liver function tests.[98–102] In EHPVO, it has been shown that those symptoms caused by PB usually start a decade later than variceal bleed and are common when PVT extends into mesenteric veins or when the bile duct is more acutely angulated.[100–103] ERCP is the diagnostic gold standard but is now being replaced by noninvasive magnetic resonance cholangiopancreatography, which, when combined with portovenography, helps in detection of choledochal and epicholedochal varices.[101] Endoscopic USG is also useful for detection of perforators and intracholedochal varices.[102] Natural history of biliopathy is poorly defined but a slow progression is well known with development of symptoms over a decade. Overall 4% to 10% of patients develop complications like choledocholithiasis, cholangitis, and secondary biliary cirrhosis.[98,100,103]

Minimal hepatic encephalopathy

Minimal hepatic encephalopathy (MHE) in the setting of EHPVO can develop with or without shunt surgery.[104–107] Following shunt surgery, toxic substances directly enter from portal blood into systemic circulation, and hence MHE is more prevalent with nonselective compared with selective shunts. However, MHE is also seen in 32% to 35% of cases in the absence of shunt and this has been shown from abnormalities in critical flicker frequency, psychometric tests, and P300 auditory event–related potential.[104,105] The reason for these abnormalities is possibly chronic deprivation of hepatic blood flow leading to parenchymal extinction, and is shown by increased brain glutamine and glutamine/creatine ratio on ^{1}H-MR spectroscopy, high blood ammonia and proinflammatory cytokine levels (tumor necrosis factor-alpha and interleukin-6), and increased mean diffusivity on diffusion tensor imaging in several areas of brain, suggesting a mechanism similar to that seen in chronic liver disease.[105,106] MHE is shown to persist in 75%, whereas a new episode of MHE develops in 5% over 1 year.[107]

Pregnancy outcomes have been reported from a European cohort of 45 pregnancies. There were 9 miscarriages, 64% had favorable outcome with delivery of a term healthy infant in 58%, whereas preterm births occurred in 38%. Three had variceal bleeding, whereas 4 had genital or parietal bleeding. Unfavorable outcome was related to increased platelet count at diagnosis.[108]

Parenchymal extinction and liver dysfunction
Progressive deterioration of liver functions, ascites, and encephalopathy may develop with increasing age and prolonged duration of disease, and is associated with more severe PB changes[87] (see **Fig. 4**).

MANAGEMENT OF IDIOPATHIC PORTAL HYPERTENSION AND EXTRAHEPATIC PORTAL VENOUS OBSTRUCTION

The key management issues in both IPH and EHPVO are centered on PHT and its complications: varices and splenomegaly. In addition, children and adults with EHPVO have concerns of growth failure, PB, MHE, and poor QoL. Later in life, both of these disorders run a risk of parenchymal extinction with subsequent decompensation.

Control and Prophylaxis of Variceal Bleed

As per the Baveno VI consensus, the same principles related to vasoconstrictor drugs, endotherapy, and propanolol applicable to cirrhotic PHT should be applied to patients with IPH and patients with EHPVO with variceal bleed. Vasoconstrictors should be started early. Endoscopic management includes sclerotherapy (EST) and variceal band ligation (EVL), which are equally efficacious for variceal eradication.[60] As per 2 randomized controlled trials (RCTs) and several cohort studies from India, EVL eradicates varices in fewer sessions (4 vs 5–6), with less risk of stricture formation (0%–4% vs 10%–25%) and rebleeding (4%–6% vs 21%–25%) but with a higher rate of variceal recurrence (17%–29% vs 8%–20%). After esophageal variceal eradication, GOV1 decreases, whereas IGV1, PHG, and ectopic varices increase.[89,93,109–111] For GOV2-related or IGV1-related bleed, glue injection with N-butyl-cyanoacrylate is considered helpful, but depends on its availability and endoscopic expertise.[3] Band ligation followed by sclerotherapy may be a better alternative than sclerotherapy alone in children.[111] For secondary prophylaxis of variceal bleed, usage of nonselective β-blockers in a single RCT in adults with IPH and EHPVO has been shown to have comparable efficacy to EVL, although 18% had minor adverse events.[112] In children, there are concerns regarding usage of β-blockers with regard to hemodynamic instability and hyper-reactive airway. Hence, usage of β-blockers is apparently prevalent at most of the pediatric hepatology centers worldwide, but their usage is not yet recommended because of lack of sufficient evidence on their safety and efficacy.[91]

Role of Surgery

Most IPH is easily manageable with successive endotherapies, hence there are very few indications for surgery: uncontrolled or recurrent variceal bleed, or bleeding from ectopic sites. Moreover, there are long-term risks of MHE, glomerulonephritis, pulmonary arteriovenous fistula, and ascites following shunt procedures in IPH.[113]

In contrast, in EHPVO, with advancement in technical expertise and risk of later complications such as PB and MHE, surgery is gradually becoming the first-line treatment.[91,114] Meso-Rex shunt or mesenterico-left PV bypass (MLPVB) decompresses the superior mesenteric vein into the left PV (LPV) via an autologous graft and is the surgical shunt of choice in EHPVO. This shunt restores hepatic portal blood flow in the closest possible physiologic manner, and in a long run protects liver from parenchymal extinction.[114–116] In the absence of a patent Rex vein (LPV), the indications for shunt should be carefully looked for. Nonphysiologic portosystemic shunts are still the commonest surgeries performed worldwide for EHPVO. From the south-east Asian region, there is vast literature on feasibility, patency, and long-term outcomes of these shunt surgeries.[117–119] However, in a recent report, the long-term patency has been questioned.[120] Although nonselective shunts, such as the proximal splenorenal shunt, decompress the whole system, taking care of PB as well, the distal splenorenal shunt takes care of the left-sided (sinistral) PHT. In young children, there are issues related to technical feasibility and shunt thrombosis, but these have largely been overcome with improvement in surgical expertise.[91] From clinically significant varices, variceal eradication on endotherapy, degree of thrombocytopenia, and patency of Rex vein, a stepwise approach for these children has been suggested.[121] With Rex shunt, the patency rates are lower than with traditional shunts. However, in addition to causing improvements in spleen size, hypersplenism, varices, growth, and PB, Rex shunt, in contrast with nonphysiologic shunts, also leads to improvement in liver volume, MHE, and neurocognitive outcome in the long term, and hence is now the surgery of choice in applicable settings[91,114–116] (**Fig. 5**).

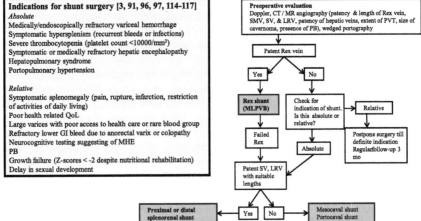

Fig. 5. Surgical management of EHPVO. Indications for shunt and prerequisites. GI, gastrointestinal; IJV, internal jugular vein; LRV, left renal vein; SMV, superior mesenteric vein; SV, splenic vein.

Head-to-head comparison of surgical shunt with EST was done in a single small RCT from India with comparable mortality and treatment failure but with a high rebleeding rate and transfusion requirement in the EST group.[122]

Surgical ablative procedures, such as esophageal devascularization and transection or splenectomy, have become obsolete because of the advancement in endoscopic and radiological techniques.[3,4]

Liver Transplantation

Around 6% of patients with IPH may need LT, although the decompensation secondary to parenchymal extinction is around 20% over 20 years.[13] Two series on IPH mentioned that indications of LT in this setting are ascites (62%), hepatic encephalopathy (31%), SBP (19%), and hepatopulmonary syndrome (12%). Even with onset of decompensation in IPH, MELD scores at the time of transplant are low (median 13; range 9–22).[22,123]

Role of Interventional Radiology Techniques

TIPSS is a feasible option in noncirrhotic PVT, the indications being PHT complications (recurrent bleed, refractory ascites) that are getting difficult to manage medically, or need of anticoagulation in the presence of large varices. Literature review suggests feasibility of the procedure in 83%, although the decision should be individualized in view of the risks of encephalopathy (34%), variceal rebleed (28%), hemoperitoneum (10%), liver failure (5%), and death (12%).[124,125] TIPSS has been done in children with EHPVO, but the rate of successful placement is low (61%). Of the 17 children in whom it was successfully placed, in 3 of them insertion was done into a major collateral because of complete occlusion of the PV. Shunt dysfunction was present in 35%, which was managed with reinsertion and/or balloon dilatation.[126] Partial splenic artery embolization is sometimes offered as a safer alternative to splenectomy for hypersplenism. However, the effect on improvement in cell lines is only transient, and postembolization syndrome is almost universal.[127] Percutaneous transhepatic/transsplenic variceal embolization using sclerosants, glue, or coils is sometimes done in patients with life-threatening variceal hemorrhage, especially when the bleeding is from isolated gastric varix. Percutaneous transhepatic biliary drainage is done in settings of cholangitis or choledocholithiasis secondary to PB when endoscopic techniques have failed. In addition, shunt reduction or closure can be done using coils or balloon-occluded transvenous obliteration in the setting of postshunt encephalopathy.[125]

Role of Anticoagulation

In IPH with PVT, anticoagulation usage has been shown to recanalize thrombus in half of the patients.[11] Recent data from the Vascular Liver Disease Interest Group (VALDIG) on 58 noncirrhotic adults with PVT treated with direct-acting oral anticoagulants have shown that their usage is safe with episodes of bleeding in 18%.[128] Although there is a lack of controlled trials and consensus, the authors propose that, in the presence of underlying prothrombotic state in IPH or EHPVO, anticoagulation can be started, taking into consideration the risk of bleeding from the varices.

Management of Portal Biliopathy

Treatment is indicated only for symptomatic PB: jaundice, cholangitis, choledocholithiasis, or biliary stricture. Endoscopic decompression is favored. However, in the long run, most of these patients require a shunt surgery. Biliary diversion procedures are rarely needed if symptoms of biliary obstruction persist after shunt surgery.[1,91,129,130]

Surveillance

Regular 6-monthly follow-up of all patients with IPH and EHPVO is mandatory to look for spleen size, growth, QoL, school performance, development of jaundice, decompensation, PB, and HPS, and to assess their laboratory values and imaging for PVT and PB.[3]

SUMMARY

IPH and EHPVO are noncirrhotic vascular causes of PHT in adults and children. Proposed pathogenetic mechanisms for IPH include infection, prothrombotic status, immunologic injuries, toxins, and genetic predisposition. In contrast, the cause of EHPVO is related to local or prothrombotic risk factors. The diagnosis is easy in presence of splenomegaly and variceal bleed. It is often a diagnosis of exclusion of cirrhosis with near-normal HVPG and synthetic functions of the liver. The management of noncirrhotic portal hypertension is mostly management of variceal bleeding by endoscopic interventions with a good long-term outcome. Rex shunt for EHPVO is the surgical modality of choice but needs technical expertise. MHE and parenchymal extinction are poorly understood scenarios and need further research.

REFERENCES

1. Bosch J, Iwakiri Y. The portal hypertension syndrome: etiology, classification, relevance, and animal models. Hepatol Int 2018;12(Suppl 1):1–10.
2. Abraldes JG, Sarlieve P, Tandon P. Measurement of portal pressure. Clin Liver Dis 2014;18(4):779–92.
3. Khanna R, Sarin SK. Non-cirrhotic portal hypertension. J Hepatol 2014;60: 421–41.
4. Garcia-Pagan JC, Hernandez-Guerra M, Bosch J. Extrahepatic portal vein thrombosis. Semin Liver Dis 2008;28(3):282–92.
5. D'Amico G, Pasta L, Morabito A, et al. Competing risks and prognostic stages of cirrhosis: a 25-year inception cohort study of 494 patients. Aliment Pharmacol Ther 2014;39(10):1180–93.
6. Aoki H, Hasumi A, Yoshida K. A questionnaire study on treatment of idiopathic portal hypertension and extrahepatic portal obstruction. In: Kameda H, editor. Annual report on portal hemodynamics abnormalities (in Japanese). Tokyo: Japan Ministry of Health and Welfare; 1988. p. 179–89.
7. Vakili C, Farahvash MJ, Bynum TE. 'Endemic' idiopathic portal hypertension. Report on 32 patients with noncirrhotic portal fibrosis. World J Surg 1992;16: 118–25.
8. Dhiman RK, Chawla Y, Vasishta RK, et al. Non-cirrhotic portal fibrosis (idiopathic portal hypertension): experience with 151 patients and a review of the literature. J Gastroenterol Hepatol 2002;17:6–16.
9. Pande C, Kumar A, Sarin SK. Non-Cirrhotic Portal Fibrosis: a clinical profile of 366 patients. Am J Gastroenterol 2006;101(S2):191 (abstract: 439).
10. Madhu K, Avinash B, Ramakrishna B, et al. Idiopathic non-cirrhotic intrahepatic portal hypertension: common cause of cryptogenic intrahepatic portal hypertension in a Southern Indian tertiary hospital. Indian J Gastroenterol 2009; 28(3):83–7.
11. Hillaire S, Bonte E, Denninger MH, et al. Idiopathic non-cirrhotic intrahepatic portal hypertension in the West: a re-evaluation in 28 patients. Gut 2002; 51(2):275–80.

12. Cazals-Hatem D, Hillaire S, Rudler M, et al. Obliterative portal venopathy: portal hypertension is not always present at diagnosis. J Hepatol 2011;54(3):455–61.

13. Schouten JNL, Nevens F, Hansen B, et al. Idiopathic noncirrhotic portal hypertension is associated with poor survival: results of a long-term cohort study. Aliment Pharmacol Ther 2012;35(12):1424–33.

14. Siramolpiwat S, Seijo S, Miquel R, et al. Idiopathic portal hypertension: natural history and long-term outcome. Hepatology 2014;59:2276–85.

15. Vispo E, Moreno A, Maida I, et al. Noncirrhotic portal hypertension in HIV-infected patients: unique clinical and pathological findings. AIDS 2010;24: 1171–6.

16. Schouten JN, Van der Ende ME, Koëter T, et al. Risk factors and outcome of HIV-associated idiopathic noncirrhotic portal hypertension. Aliment Pharmacol Ther 2012;36(9):875–85.

17. Chang PE, Miquel R, Blanco JL, et al. Idiopathic portal hypertension in patients with HIV infection treated with highly active antiretroviral therapy. Am J Gastroenterol 2009;104:1707–14.

18. Sarin SK, Kumar A, Chawla YK, et al. Noncirrhotic portal fibrosis/idiopathic portal hypertension: APASL recommendations for diagnosis and treatment. Hepatol Int 2007;1:398–413.

19. Franchi-Abella S, Fabre M, Mselati E, et al. Obliterative portal venopathy: a study of 48 children. J Pediatr 2014;165(1):190–3.e2.

20. Sood V, Lal BB, Khanna R, et al. Noncirrhotic portal fibrosis in pediatric population. J Pediatr Gastroenterol Nutr 2017;64(5):748–53.

21. Goel A, Madhu K, Zachariah U, et al. A study of aetiology of portal hypertension in adults (including the elderly) at a tertiary centre in southern India. Indian J Med Res 2013;137(5):922–7.

22. Krasinskas AM, Eghtesad B, Kamath PS, et al. Liver transplantation for severe intrahepatic noncirrhotic portal hypertension. Liver Transpl 2005;11(6):627–34.

23. Omanwar S, Rizvi MR, Kathayat R, et al. A rabbit model of non-cirrhotic portal hypertension by repeated injections of E. coli through indwelling cannulation of the gastrosplenic vein. Hepatobiliary Pancreat Dis Int 2004;3:417–22.

24. Kathayat R, Pandey GK, Malhotra V, et al. Rabbit model of non-cirrhotic portal fibrosis with repeated immunosensitization by rabbit splenic extract. J Gastroenterol Hepatol 2002;17:1312–6.

25. Sato Y, Ren XS, Harada K, et al. Induction of elastin expression in vascular endothelial cells relates to hepatoportal sclerosis in idiopathic portal hypertension: possible link to serum anti-endothelial cell antibodies. Clin Exp Immunol 2012;167(3):532–42.

26. Guido M, Sarcognato S, Sonzogni A, et al. Obliterative portal venopathy without portal hypertension: an underestimated condition. Liver Int 2016;36(3):454–60.

27. Eapen CE, Nightingale P, Hubscher SG, et al. Non-cirrhotic intrahepatic portal hypertension: associated gut diseases and prognostic factors. Dig Dis Sci 2011;56(1):227–35.

28. Sawada S, Sato Y, Aoyama H, et al. Pathological study of idiopathic portal hypertension with an emphasis on cause of death based on records of Annuals of Pathological Autopsy Cases in Japan. J Gastroenterol Hepatol 2007;22(2): 204–9.

29. Klein S, Hinüber C, Hittatiya K, et al. Novel rat model of repetitive portal venous embolization mimicking human non-cirrhotic idiopathic portal hypertension. PLoS One 2016 2;11(9):e0162144.

30. Okudaria M, Ohbu M, Okuda K. Idiopathic portal hypertension and its pathology. Semin Liver Dis 2002;22:59–71.

31. Saito K, Nakanuma Y, Takegoshi K, et al. Nonspecific immunological abnormalities and association of autoimmune diseases in idiopathic portal hypertension. A study by questionnaire. Hepatogastroenterology 1993;40:163–6.

32. Maiwall R, Goel A, Pulimood AB, et al. Investigation into celiac disease in Indian patients with portal hypertension. Indian J Gastroenterol 2014;33(6):517–23.

33. Pulvirenti F, Pentassuglio I, Milito C, et al. Idiopathic non cirrhotic portal hypertension and spleno-portal axis abnormalities in patients with severe primary antibody deficiencies. J Immunol Res 2014;2014:672458.

34. Santra A, Das Gupta J, De BK, et al. Hepatic manifestations in chronic arsenic toxicity. Indian J Gastroenterol 1999;18(4):152–5.

35. Sarin SK, Sharma G, Banerjee S, et al. Hepatic fibrogenesis using chronic arsenic ingestion: studies in a murine model. Indian J Exp Biol 1999;37:147–51.

36. Sarin SK, Mehra NK, Agarwal A, et al. Familial aggregation in noncirrhotic portal fibrosis: a report of four families. Am J Gastroenterol 1987;82:1130–3.

37. Koot BG, Alders M, Verheij J, et al. A de novo mutation in KCNN3 associated with autosomal dominant idiopathic non-cirrhotic portal hypertension. J Hepatol 2016;64(4):974–7.

38. Sato Y, Sawada S, Kozaka K, et al. Significance of enhanced expression of nitric oxide synthases in splenic sinus lining cells in altered portal hemodynamics of idiopathic portal hypertension. Dig Dis Sci 2007;52:1987–94.

39. Sato Y, Nakanuma Y. Role of endothelial-mesenchymal transition in idiopathic portal hypertension. Histol Histopathol 2013;28(2):145–54.

40. Hernández-Gea V, Baiges A, Turon F, et al. Idiopathic portal hypertension. Hepatology 2018;68(6):2413–23.

41. Nakanuma Y, Tsuneyama K, Ohbu M, et al. Pathology and pathogenesis of idiopathic portal hypertension with an emphasis on the liver. Pathol Res Pract 2001; 197(2):65–76.

42. Guido M, Alves VAF, Balabaud C, et al, International Liver Pathology Study Group. Histology of portal vascular changes associated with idiopathic non-cirrhotic portal hypertension: nomenclature and definition. Histopathology 2019;74(2):219–26.

43. Rangari M, Sinha S, Kapoor D, et al. Prevalence of autonomic dysfunction in cirrhotic and non-cirrhotic portal hypertension. Am J Gastroenterol 2002;97(3): 707–13.

44. Bajaj JS, Bhattacharjee J, Sarin SK. Coagulation profile and platelet function in patients with extrahepatic portal vein obstruction and non-cirrhotic portal fibrosis. J Gastroenterol Hepatol 2001;16:641–6.

45. Goel A, Ramakrishna B, Muliyil J, et al. Use of serum vitamin B12 level as a marker to differentiate idiopathic noncirrhotic intrahepatic portal hypertension from cryptogenic cirrhosis. Dig Dis Sci 2013;58(1):179–87.

46. Sarin SK, Sethi KK, Nanda R. Measurement and correlation of wedged hepatic, intrahepatic, intrasplenic and intravariceal pressure in patients with cirrhosis of liver and non-cirrhotic portal fibrosis. Gut 1987;28:260–6.

47. Seijo S, Reverter E, Miquel R, et al. Role of hepatic vein catheterisation and transient elastography in the diagnosis of idiopathic portal hypertension. Dig Liver Dis 2012;44(10):855–60.

48. Sarin SK, Lahoti D, Saxena SP, et al. Prevalence, classification and natural history of gastric varices: a long-term follow up study in 568 portal hypertension patients. Hepatology 1992;16:1343–9.

49. Sarin SK, Shahi HM, Jain M, et al. The natural history of portal hypertensive gastropathy: influence of variceal eradication. Am J Gastroenterol 2000;95: 2888–93.
50. Chawla Y, Dilawari JB. Anorectal varices—their frequency in cirrhotic and non-cirrhotic portal hypertension. Gut 1991;32:309–11.
51. Ganguly S, Sarin SK, Bhatia V, et al. The prevalence and spectrum of colonic lesions in patients with cirrhosis and noncirrhotic portal hypertension. Hepatology 1995;21:1226–31.
52. Arora A, Sarin SK. Multimodality imaging of obliterative portal venopathy: what every radiologist should know. Br J Radiol 2015;88:20140653.
53. Maruyama H, Shimada T, Ishibashi H, et al. Delayed periportal enhancement: a characteristic finding on contrast ultrasound in idiopathic portal hypertension. Hepatol Int 2012;6(2):511–9.
54. Glatard AS, Hillaire S, d'Assignies G, et al. Obliterative portal venopathy: findings at CT imaging. Radiology 2012;263(3):741–50.
55. Qureshi H, Kamal S, Khan RA, et al. Differentiation of cirrhotic vs idiopathic portal hypertension using 99mTc-Sn colloid dynamic and static scintigraphy. J Pak Med Assoc 1991;41:126–9.
56. Furuichi Y, Moriyasu F, Taira J, et al. Noninvasive diagnostic method for idiopathic portal hypertension based on measurements of liver and spleen stiffness by ARFI elastography. J Gastroenterol 2013;48(9):1061–8.
57. Seijo S, Lozano JJ, Alonso C, et al. Metabolomics discloses potential biomarkers for the noninvasive diagnosis of idiopathic portal hypertension. Am J Gastroenterol 2013;108(6):926–32.
58. Seijo S, Lozano JJ, Alonso C, et al. Metabolomics as a diagnostic tool for idiopathic non-cirrhotic portal hypertension. Liver Int 2016;36(7):1051–8.
59. Kotani K, Kawabe J, Morikawa H, et al. Comprehensive screening of gene function and networks by DNA microarray analysis in Japanese patients with idiopathic portal hypertension. Mediators Inflamm 2015;2015:349215.
60. de Franchis R, Baveno VI Faculty. Expanding consensus in portal hypertension Report of the Baveno VI Consensus Workshop: stratifying risk and individualizing care for portal hypertension. J Hepatol 2015;63:743–52.
61. Murai Y, Ohfuji S, Fukushima W, et al. Prognostic factors in patients with idiopathic portal hypertension: two Japanese nationwide epidemiological surveys in 1999 and 2005. Hepatol Res 2012;42(12):1211–20.
62. Hidaka H, Ohbu M, Kokubu S, et al. Hepatocellular carcinoma associated with idiopathic portal hypertension: review of large nodules in seven non-cirrhotic portal hypertensive livers. J Gastroenterol Hepatol 2005;20(3):493–4.
63. Andrade F, Shukla A, Bureau C, et al. VALDIG investigators. Pregnancy in idiopathic non-cirrhotic portal hypertension: a multicentric study on maternal and fetal management and outcome. J Hepatol 2018;69(6):1242–9.
64. Poddar U, Thapa BR, Rao KL, et al. Etiological spectrum of esophageal varices due to portal hypertension in Indian children: is it different from the West? J Gastroenterol Hepatol 2008;23:1354–7.
65. Sarin SK, Sollano JD, Chawla YK, et al. Members of the APASL working party on portal hypertension. Consensus on extra-hepatic portal vein obstruction. Liver Int 2006;26(5):512–9.
66. Fagundes ED, Ferreira AR, Roquete ML, et al. Clinical and laboratory predictors of esophageal varices in children and adolescents with portal hypertension syndrome. J Pediatr Gastroenterol Nutr 2008;46(2):178–83.

67. Duché M, Ducot B, Ackermann O, et al. Portal hypertension in children: high-risk varices, primary prophylaxis and consequences of bleeding. J Hepatol 2017; 66(2):320–7.
68. Denninger MH, Chaït Y, Casadevall N, et al. Cause of portal or hepatic venous thrombosis in adults: the role of multiple concurrent factors. Hepatology 2000; 31(3):587–91.
69. Janssen HL, Wijnhoud A, Haagsma EB, et al. Extrahepatic portal vein thrombosis: aetiology and determinants of survival. Gut 2001;49(5):720–4.
70. Bhattacharyya M, Makharia G, Kannan M, et al. Inherited prothrombotic defects in Budd-Chiari syndrome and portal vein thrombosis: a study from North India. Am J Clin Pathol 2004;121(6):844–7.
71. Primignani M, Barosi G, Bergamaschi G, et al. Role of the JAK2 mutation in the diagnosis of chronic myeloproliferative disorders in splanchnic vein thrombosis. Hepatology 2006;44(6):1528–34.
72. Amitrano L, Guardascione MA, Scaglione M, et al. Prognostic factors in noncirrhotic patients with splanchnic vein thromboses. Am J Gastroenterol 2007; 102(11):2464–70.
73. Sogaard KK, Astrup LB, Vilstrup H, et al. Portal vein thrombosis; risk factors, clinical presentation and treatment. BMC Gastroenterol 2007;7:34.
74. El-Karaksy H, El-Koofy N, El-Hawary M, et al. Prevalence of factor V Leiden mutation and other hereditary thrombophilic factors in Egyptian children with portal vein thrombosis: results of a single-center case-control study. Ann Hematol 2004;83:712–5.
75. El-Karaksy HM, El-Koofy N, Mohsen N, et al. Extrahepatic portal vein obstruction in Egyptian children. J Pediatr Gastroenterol Nutr 2015;60(1):105–9.
76. Abd El-Hamid N, Taylor RM, Marinello D, et al. Aetiology and management of extrahepatic portal vein obstruction in children: King's College Hospital experience. J Pediatr Gastroenterol Nutr 2008;47:630–4.
77. Pietrobattista A, Luciani M, Abraldes JG, et al. Extrahepatic portal vein thrombosis in children and adolescents: influence of genetic thrombophilic disorders. World J Gastroenterol 2010;16(48):6123–7.
78. Weiss B, Shteyer E, Vivante A, et al. Etiology and long-term outcome of extrahepatic portal vein obstruction in children. World J Gastroenterol 2010;16: 4968–72.
79. Ferri PM, Rodrigues Ferreira A, Fagundes ED, et al. Evaluation of the presence of hereditary and acquired thrombophilias in brazilian children and adolescents with diagnoses of portal vein thrombosis. J Pediatr Gastroenterol Nutr 2012; 55(5):599–604.
80. Smalberg JH, Arends LR, Valla DC, et al. Myeloproliferative neoplasms in Budd-Chiari syndrome and portal vein thrombosis: a meta-analysis. Blood 2012; 120(25):4921–8.
81. Nowak-Göttl U, Junker R, Kreuz W, et al, Childhood Thrombophilia Study Group. Risk of recurrent venous thrombosis in children with combined prothrombotic risk factors. Blood 2001;97(4):858–62.
82. Odièvre M, Pigé G, Alagille D. Congenital abnormalities associated with extrahepatic portal hypertension. Arch Dis Child 1977;52(5):383–5.
83. Yadav S, Dutta AK, Sarin SK. Do umbilical vein catheterization and sepsis lead to portal vein thrombosis? A prospective, clinical and sonographic evaluation. J Pediatr Gastroenterol Nutr 1993;17:392–6.
84. Stringer MD, Heaton ND, Karani J, et al. Patterns of portal vein occlusion and their aetiological significance. Br J Surg 1994;81:1328–31.

85. Sarin SK, Philips CA, Kamath PS, et al. Toward a comprehensive new classification of portal vein thrombosis in patients with cirrhosis. Gastroenterology 2016 Oct;151(4):574–7.e3.
86. Noronha Ferreira C, Seijo S, Plessier A, et al. Natural history and management of esophagogastric varices in chronic noncirrhotic, nontumoral portal vein thrombosis. Hepatology 2016;63(5):1640–50.
87. Rangari M, Gupta R, Jain M, et al. Hepatic dysfunction in patients with extrahepatic portal venous obstruction. Liver Int 2003;23(6):434–9.
88. Jha SK, Kumar A, Sharma BC, et al. Systemic and pulmonary hemodynamics in patients with extrahepatic portal vein obstruction is similar to compensated cirrhotic patients. Hepatol Int 2009;3:384–91.
89. Itha S, Yachha SK. Endoscopic outcome beyond esophageal variceal eradication in children with extrahepatic portal venous obstruction. J Pediatr Gastroenterol Nutr 2006;42(2):196–200.
90. Yachha SK, Dhiman RK, Gupta R, et al. Endosonographic evaluation of the rectum in children with extrahepatic portal venous obstruction. J Pediatrgastroenterol Nutr 1996;23(4):438–41.
91. Shneider BL, de Ville de Goyet J, Leung DH, et al. Primary prophylaxis of variceal bleeding in children and the role of meso-rex bypass: summary of the Baveno VI pediatric satellite symposium. Hepatology 2016;63(4):1368–80.
92. Sharma P, Mishra SR, Kumar M, et al. Liver and spleen stiffness in patients with extrahepatic portal vein obstruction. Radiology 2012;263(3):893–9.
93. Zargar SA, Yattoo GN, Javid G, et al. Fifteen-year follow up of endoscopic injection sclerotherapy in children with extrahepatic portal venous obstruction. J Gastroenterol Hepatol 2004;19:139–45.
94. Thomas V, Jose T, Kumar S. Natural history of bleeding after esophageal variceal eradication in patients with extrahepatic portal venous obstruction: a 20-year follow-up. Indian J Gastroenterol 2009;28:206–11.
95. Sarin SK, Bansal A, Sasan S, et al. Portal-vein obstruction in children leads to growth retardation. Hepatology 1992;15:229–33.
96. Mehrotra RN, Bhatia V, Dabadghao P, et al. Extrahepatic portal vein obstruction in children: anthropometry, growth hormone and insulin-like growth factor I. J Pediatr Gastroenterol Nutr 1997;25:520–3.
97. Krishna YR, Yachha SK, Srivastava A, et al. Quality of life in children managed for extrahepatic portal venous obstruction. J Pediatr Gastroenterol Nutr 2010; 50(5):531–6.
98. Chandra R, Kapoor D, Tharakan A, et al. Portal biliopathy. J Gastroenterol Hepatol 2001;16:1086–92.
99. Shin SM, Kim S, Lee JW, et al. Biliary abnormalities associated with portal biliopathy: evaluation on MR cholangiography. AJR Am J Roentgenol 2007;188(4): W341–7.
100. Khuroo MS, Yattoo GN, Zargar SA, et al. Biliary abnormalities associated with extrahepatic portal venous obstruction. Hepatology 1993;17:807–13.
101. Jabeen S, Robbani I, Choh NA, et al. Spectrum of biliary abnormalities in portal cavernoma cholangiopathy (PCC) secondary to idiopathic extrahepatic portal vein obstruction (EHPVO)-a prospective magnetic resonance cholangiopancreaticography (MRCP) based study. Br J Radiol 2016;89(1068):20160636.
102. Rai GP, Nijhawan S, Madhu MP, et al. Comparative evaluation of magnetic resonance cholangiopancreatography/magnetic resonance splenoportovenography and endoscopic ultrasound in the diagnosis of portal cavernoma cholangiopathy. Indian J Gastroenterol 2015;34(6):442–7.

103. Chattopadhyay S, Govindasamy M, Singla P, et al. Portal biliopathy in patients with non-cirrhotic portal hypertension: does the type of surgery affect outcome? HPB (Oxford) 2012;14(7):441–7.

104. Sharma P, Sharma BC, Puri V, et al. Minimal hepatic encephalopathy in patients with extrahepatic portal vein obstruction. Am J Gastroenterol 2008;103(6): 1406–12.

105. Yadav SK, Srivastava A, Srivastava A, et al. Encephalopathy assessment in children with extra-hepatic portal vein obstruction with MR, psychometry and critical flicker frequency. J Hepatol 2010;52:348–54.

106. Srivastava A, Yadav SK, Yachha SK, et al. Pro-inflammatory cytokines are raised in extrahepatic portal venous obstruction with minimal hepatic encephalopathy. J Gastroenterol Hepatol 2011;26(6):979–86.

107. Sharma P, Sharma BC, Puri V, et al. Natural history of minimal hepatic encephalopathy in patients with extrahepatic portal vein obstruction. Am J Gastroenterol 2009;104(4):885–90.

108. Hoekstra J, Seijo S, Rautou PE, et al. Pregnancy in women with portal vein thrombosis: results of a multicentric European study on maternal and fetal management and outcome. J Hepatol 2012;57(6):1214–9.

109. Sarin SK, Govil A, Jain AK, et al. Prospective randomized trial of endoscopic sclerotherapy versus variceal band ligation for esophageal varices: influence on gastropathy, gastric varices and variceal recurrence. J Hepatol 1997;26(4): 826–32.

110. Zargar SA, Javid G, Khan BA, et al. Endoscopic ligation compared with sclerotherapy for bleeding esophageal varices in children with extrahepatic portal venous obstruction. Hepatology 2002;36:666–72.

111. Poddar U, Bhatnagar S, Yachha SK. Endoscopic band ligation followed by sclerotherapy: is it superior to sclerotherapy in children with extrahepatic portal venous obstruction? J Gastroenterol Hepatol 2011;26:255–9.

112. Sarin SK, Gupta N, Jha SK, et al. Equal efficacy of endoscopic variceal ligation and propranolol in preventing variceal bleeding in patients with noncirrhotic portal hypertension. Gastroenterology 2010;139(4):1238–45.

113. Pal S, Radhakrishna P, Sahni P, et al. Prophylactic surgery in non-cirrhotic portal fibrosis: is it worthwhile? Indian J Gastroenterol 2005;24(6):239–42.

114. Superina R, Bambini DA, Lokar J, et al. Correction of extrahepatic portal vein thrombosis by the mesenteric to left portal vein bypass. Ann Surg 2006;243: 515–21.

115. Lautz TB, Keys LA, Melvin JC, et al. Advantages of the meso-Rex bypass compared with portosystemic shunts in the management of extrahepatic portal vein obstruction in children. J Am Coll Surg 2013;216(1):83–9.

116. Mack CL, Zelko FA, Lokar J, et al. Surgically restoring portal blood flow to the liver in children with primary extrahepatic portal vein thrombosis improves fluid neurocognitive ability. Pediatrics 2006;117(3):e405–12.

117. Prasad AS, Gupta S, Kohli V, et al. Proximal splenorenal shunts for extrahepatic portal venous obstruction in children. Ann Surg 1994;219:193–6.

118. Sharma BC, Singh RP, Chawla YK, et al. Effect of shunt surgery on spleen size, portal pressure and oesophageal varices in patients with non-cirrhotic portal hypertension. J Gastroenterol Hepatol 1997;12(8):582–4.

119. Sharma N, Bajpai M, Kumar A, et al. Portal hypertension: a critical appraisal of shunt procedures with emphasis on distal splenorenal shunt in children. J Indian Assoc Pediatr Surg 2014;19(2):80–4.

120. Mishra PK, Patil NS, Saluja S, et al. High patency of proximal splenorenal shunt: a myth or reality ? - a prospective cohort study. Int J Surg 2016;27:82–7.

121. Alberti D, Colusso M, Cheli M, et al. Results of a stepwise approach to extrahepatic portal vein obstruction in children. J Pediatr Gastroenterol Nutr 2013;57(5): 619–26.

122. Wani AH, Shah OJ, Zargar SA. Management of variceal hemorrhage in children with extrahepatic portal venous obstruction – shunt surgery versus endoscopic sclerotherapy. Indian J Surg 2011;73(6):409–13.

123. Saigal S, Nayak NC, Jain D, et al. Non-cirrhotic portal fibrosis related end stage liver disease in adults: evaluation from a study on living donor liver transplant recipients. Hepatol Int 2011;5(4):882–9.

124. Bissonnette J, Garcia-Pagán JC, Albillos A, et al. Role of the transjugular intrahepatic portosystemic shunt in the management of severe complications of portal hypertension in idiopathic noncirrhotic portal hypertension. Hepatology 2016; 64(1):224–31.

125. Pargewar SS, Desai SN, Rajesh S, et al. Imaging and radiological interventions in extra-hepatic portal vein obstruction. World J Radiol 2016;8(6):556–70.

126. Lv Y, He C, Guo W, et al. Transjugular intrahepatic portosystemic shunt for extrahepatic portal venous obstruction in children. J Pediatr Gastroenterol Nutr 2016; 62(2):233–41.

127. Ozturk O, Eldem G, Peynircioglu B, et al. Outcomes of partial splenic embolization in patients with massive splenomegaly due to idiopathic portal hypertension. World J Gastroenterol 2016;22(43):9623–30.

128. De Gottardi A, Trebicka J, Klinger C, et al. VALDIG Investigators. Antithrombotic treatment with direct-acting oral anticoagulants in patients with splanchnic vein thrombosis and cirrhosis. Liver Int 2017;37(5):694–9.

129. Chaudhary A, Dhar P, Sarin SK, et al. Bile duct obstruction due to portal biliopathy in extrahepatic portal hypertension: surgical management. Br J Surg 1998; 85:326–9.

130. Agarwal AK, Sharma S, Singh S, et al. Portal biliopathy: a study of 39 surgically treated patients. HPB (Oxford) 2011;13:33–9.

1. Publication Title	2. Publication Number		3. Filing Date
CLINICS IN LIVER DISEASE	016 – 754		9/18/2019

4. Issue Frequency	5. Number of Issues Published Annually	6. Annual Subscription Price
FEB, MAY, AUG, NOV	4	$304.00

7. Complete Mailing Address of Known Office of Publication (Not printer) (Street, city, county, state, and ZIP+4®)

ELSEVIER INC.
230 Park Avenue, Suite 800
New York, NY 10169

Contact Person
STEPHEN R. BUSHING

Telephone (Include area code)
215-239-3688

8. Complete Mailing Address of Headquarters or General Business Office of Publisher (Not printer)

ELSEVIER INC.
230 Park Avenue, Suite 800
New York, NY 10169

9. Full Names and Complete Mailing Addresses of Publisher, Editor, and Managing Editor (Do not leave blank)

Publisher (Name and complete mailing address)

TAYLOR BALL, ELSEVIER INC.
1600 JOHN F KENNEDY BLVD. SUITE 1800
PHILADELPHIA, PA 19103-2899

Editor (Name and complete mailing address)

KERRY HOLLAND, ELSEVIER INC.
1600 JOHN F KENNEDY BLVD. SUITE 1800
PHILADELPHIA, PA 19103-2899

Managing Editor (Name and complete mailing address)

PATRICK MANLEY, ELSEVIER INC.
1600 JOHN F KENNEDY BLVD. SUITE 1800
PHILADELPHIA, PA 19103-2899

10. Owner (Do not leave blank. If the publication is owned by a corporation, give the name and address of the corporation immediately followed by the names and addresses of all stockholders owning or holding 1 percent or more of the total amount of stock. If not owned by a corporation, give the names and addresses of the individual owners. If owned by a partnership or other unincorporated firm, give its name and address as well as those of each individual owner. If the publication is published by a nonprofit organization, give its name and address.)

Full Name	Complete Mailing Address
WHOLLY OWNED SUBSIDIARY OF REED/ELSEVIER, US HOLDINGS	1600 JOHN F KENNEDY BLVD. SUITE 1800 PHILADELPHIA, PA 19103-2899

11. Known Bondholders, Mortgagees, and Other Security Holders Owning or Holding 1 Percent or More of Total Amount of Bonds, Mortgages, or Other Securities. If none, check box ▶ ☐ None

Full Name	Complete Mailing Address
N/A	

12. Tax Status (For completion by nonprofit organizations authorized to mail at nonprofit rates) (Check one)
The purpose, function, and nonprofit status of this organization and the exempt status for federal income tax purposes:

☒ Has Not Changed During Preceding 12 Months
☐ Has Changed During Preceding 12 Months (Publisher must submit explanation of change with this statement)

PS Form 3526, July 2014 (Page 1 of 4 (see instructions page 4)) PSN: 7530-01-000-9931   PRIVACY NOTICE: See our privacy policy on www.usps.com.

13. Publication Title	14. Issue Date for Circulation Data Below
CLINICS IN LIVER DISEASE	AUGUST 2019

15. Extent and Nature of Circulation		Average No. Copies Each Issue During Preceding 12 Months	No. Copies of Single Issue Published Nearest to Filing Date
a. Total Number of Copies (Net press run)		130	114
b. Paid Circulation (By Mail and Outside the Mail)	(1) Mailed Outside-County Paid Subscriptions Stated on PS Form 3541 (Include paid distribution above nominal rate, advertiser's proof copies, and exchange copies)	40	41
	(2) Mailed In-County Paid Subscriptions Stated on PS Form 3541 (Include paid distribution above nominal rate, advertiser's proof copies, and exchange copies)	0	0
	(3) Paid Distribution Outside the Mails Including Sales Through Dealers and Carriers, Street Vendors, Counter Sales, and Other Paid Distribution Outside USPS®	30	42
	(4) Paid Distribution by Other Classes of Mail Through the USPS (e.g. First-Class Mail®)	0	0
c. Total Paid Distribution (Sum of 15b (1), (2), (3) and (4))		70	83
d. Free or Nominal Rate Distribution (By Mail and Outside the Mail)	(1) Free or Nominal Rate Outside-County Copies included on PS Form 3541	45	16
	(2) Free or Nominal Rate In-County Copies Included on PS Form 3541	0	0
	(3) Free or Nominal Rate Copies Mailed at Other Classes Through the USPS (e.g. First-Class Mail)	0	0
	(4) Free or Nominal Rate Distribution Outside the Mail (Carriers or other means)	0	0
e. Total Free or Nominal Rate Distribution (Sum of 15d (1), (2), (3) and (4))		45	16
f. Total Distribution (Sum of 15c and 15e)		115	99
g. Copies not Distributed (See Instructions to Publishers #4 (page #3))		15	15
h. Total (Sum of 15f and g)		130	114
i. Percent Paid (15c divided by 15f times 100)		60.87%	83.84%

* If you are claiming electronic copies, go to line 16 on page 3. If you are not claiming electronic copies, skip to line 17 on page 3.

16. Electronic Copy Circulation		Average No. Copies Each Issue During Preceding 12 Months	No. Copies of Single Issue Published Nearest to Filing Date
a. Paid Electronic Copies	▶		
b. Total Paid Print Copies (Line 15c) + Paid Electronic Copies (Line 16a)	▶		
c. Total Print Distribution (Line 15f) + Paid Electronic Copies (Line 16a)	▶		
d. Percent Paid (Both Print & Electronic Copies) (16b divided by 16c × 100)	▶		

☒ I certify that 50% of all my distributed copies (electronic and print) are paid above a nominal price.

17. Publication of Statement of Ownership

☒ If the publication is a general publication, publication of this statement is required. Will be printed in the NOVEMBER 2019 issue of this publication.   ☐ Publication not required.

18. Signature and Title of Editor, Publisher, Business Manager, or Owner

STEPHEN R. BUSHING – INVENTORY DISTRIBUTION CONTROL MANAGER

Date 9/18/2019

I certify that all information furnished on this form is true and complete. I understand that anyone who furnishes false or misleading information on this form or who omits material or information requested on the form may be subject to criminal sanctions (including fines and imprisonment) and/or civil sanctions (including civil penalties).

PS Form 3526, July 2014 (Page 3 of 4)   PRIVACY NOTICE: See our privacy policy on www.usps.com

Moving?

Make sure your subscription moves with you!

To notify us of your new address, find your **Clinics Account Number** (located on your mailing label above your name), and contact customer service at:

Email: journalscustomerservice-usa@elsevier.com

800-654-2452 (subscribers in the U.S. & Canada)
314-447-8871 (subscribers outside of the U.S. & Canada)

Fax number: 314-447-8029

Elsevier Health Sciences Division
Subscription Customer Service
3251 Riverport Lane
Maryland Heights, MO 63043

*To ensure uninterrupted delivery of your subscription, please notify us at least 4 weeks in advance of move.

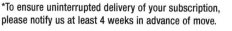
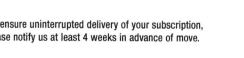

Printed and bound by CPI Group (UK) Ltd, Croydon, CR0 4YY

03/10/2024

01040407-0007